The Consumer's Guide to

HOMEOPATHY

ALSO BY DANA ULLMAN

Homeopathic Medicine for Children and Infants

Everybody's Guide to Homeopathic Medicines
(with Stephen Cummings, M.D.)

The One-Minute (or So) Healer

Discovering Homeopathy

The Consumer's Guide to

HOMEOPATHY

*The Definitive Resource for
Understanding Homeopathic Medicine
and Making It Work for You*

Dana Ullman, M.P.H.

A JEREMY P. TARCHER/PUTNAM BOOK
published by
G. P. PUTNAM'S SONS *New York*

Notice: *The Consumer's Guide to Homeopathy* will inform readers of the most recent developments in homeopathic medicine, the research and experience using these natural medicines, and the homeopathic approach to understanding and treating a wide variety of health problems. This book, however, is not meant to replace the need for medical care. Readers are encouraged to seek out the best medical resources available so that well-informed decisions can be made.

A Jeremy P. Tarcher / Putnam Book
Published by G. P. Putnam's Sons
Publishers Since 1838
200 Madison Avenue
New York, NY 10016

Most Tarcher/Putnam books are available at special quantity discounts for bulk purchases for sales promotions, premiums, fund-raising, and educational needs. Special books or book excerpts also can be created to fit specific needs.

For details, write or telephone Special Markets, The Putnam Publishing Group, 200 Madison Avenue, New York, NY 10016: (212) 951-8891.

Library of Congress Cataloging-in-Publication Data

Ullman, Dana.
The consumer's guide to homeopathy : the definitive resource for understanding homeopathic medicine and making it work for you / Dana Ullman.
p.   cm.
"A Jeremy P. Tarcher / Putnam book."
Includes bibliographical references and index.
ISBN 0-87477-813-1 (acid-free paper)
1. Homeopathy—Popular works.   2. Homeopathy—Materia medica and therapeutics.
RX76.U45   1996   95-18442 CIP
615.5'32—dc20

Design by Mauna Eichner
Cover design by Susan Shankin
Cover illustration © by Don Weller

Printed in the United States of America

3   5   7   9   10   8   6   4   2

This book is printed on acid-free/recycled paper. ∞

CONTENTS

P A R T   I I I   *Can Homeopathy Help Me?*
Specific Conditions

PART IV   *Homeopathic Resources*

ACKNOWLEDGMENTS

This book stands on the shoulders and back of all homeopaths, past and present. I give special thanks to those homeopaths who performed research, who systematically observed their clinical results, and who recorded their experiences with these powerfully healing natural medicines. This book is, in part, a result of and a tribute to their efforts.

This book is also the result of the strong spirit of homeopaths before me who withstood the dramas of practicing an unconventional type of healing at a time when there was no tolerance of medical diversity.

I want to give specific thanks to my colleagues who reviewed large portions of this manuscript, including Jay Borneman, Dennis Chernin, M.D., M.P.H., Mitchell Fleisher, M.D., George Guess, M.D., Nicholas Nossaman, M.D., and Julian Winston. I also wish to thank colleagues who reviewed various parts of this book, including Franne Berez, M.D., Michael Carlston, M.D., Cindy Dykes, Jean Hoaglund, Randall Neustaedter, C.A., O.M.D., and Mahlon Wagner, Ph.D.

People who provided me with information that I included in this book include Gina Casey, Ted Chapman, M.D., Bill Gray, M.D., Asa Hershoff, D.C., N.D., Ifeoma Ikenze, M.D., Alan Levine, M.D., Thierry Montfort, David Riley, M.D., Patty Smith, Vincent Speck-hardt, M.D., and Janet Zand, L.Ac., O.M.D.

An extra special thanks goes to my editor, Donna Zerner. More than cleaning up my grammar, she helped me be precise in describing what I was trying to say. She helped me write so that the book would be clear to readers new to homeopathy, as well as to serious students and practitioners of homeopathy. She was so convincing and so friendly when she insisted on editorial surgery of various chapters, I couldn't help but heartily support her recommendations. Most of all, she knew that she was the midwife and I was the mother of the book, so when we disagreed, she usually let my preferences prevail.

I also wish to thank my wife, Clare, who is the editor of my life. She helps me punctuate my life appropriately, encouraging me to use commas to take a breath, to use periods to stop and rest, and to use exclamation points to express the excitement that I often feel about life. She reminds me to dot my *i*'s, cross my *t*'s, and keep food off my face and lap. She also makes certain that I don't socially or professionally stick my foot in my mouth, or at least not both feet. Her generous soul and spirit are continually teaching me how to be a good parent to our new son, Jacob.

I thank my son Jacob (born July 7, 1994) for being my spiritual teacher, for he has already taught me the importance of selflessness and compassion, two vital characteristics of being a good parent.

Finally, I thank my father, Dr. Sanford Ullman. As a pediatrician, he was my first doctor. It is ironic that he is also an allergist, because this medical specialty utilizes small doses of substances that actually cause the condition in order to treat it. It seems that the homeopathic principle of similars is in my genes.

INTRODUCTION

"First, do no harm," is the best-known passage from the writings of Hippocrates, the father of medicine, which he wrote as advice to practicing physicians. This statement implores physicians to consider safe healing methods before resorting to potentially more dangerous therapeutics for the treatment of acute and chronic ailments. This book will teach physicians *and* consumers what to do *first*.

Homeopathic medicines can and should be considered as the *first* method of treatment for healing ailments because they are often effective and are considerably safer than conventional drugs. Needless to say, it makes sense to use safer therapeutic methods before resorting to more invasive ones. Sadly, health care seekers usually try conventional drugs first and consider homeopathy and other alternatives only when the drugs don't work. By this time, however, these people may have considerably more symptoms and a more deeply developed disease, in part because of the side effects of the drugs and in part because the disease has continued to worsen.

Still, because homeopathic medicines strengthen the body's own immune and defense system, they have the capacity to heal a wide assortment of ailments, even those that are complicated by previous drug use. Homeopathy's two-hundred-year history of clinical successes is gaining worldwide recognition (see Chapter 3), and a growing body of research is confirming its efficacy (see Chapter 4).

Our society and, specifically, our medical and scientific community, has focused its attention on treating symptoms and diseases. Although this approach to creating health certainly seems to be rational and logical, it is not the only valid approach to healing.

In fact, since Hippocratic times there have been two distinct schools of thought in medicine. One school of medical thought sought to understand the physiochemical workings of the human body and created ever-changing and seemingly rational theories about disease causation. It defined health as the absence of symptoms and defined disease as an entity and as a localized condition. People with similar symptoms were considered to have a specific disease, and unusual or idiosyncratic symptoms that didn't fit the specific pathology were generally ignored. Practitioners sought to extract the disease or intervene between the presumed physiochemical cause and its effect. The practitioners of this school of thought called themselves Rationalists, and this approach developed into the modern biomedical model.

The other school of thought, whose practitioners called themselves Empiricists, was less interested in *explaining* why a specific treatment worked and, more important, sought to observe *what actually worked* to heal people. According to Empiricists, health was not simply the absence of symptoms but a high level of physical and psychological vitality. Diseases were not simply entities that were localized to a unhealthy body part, but rather, represented a response to an imbalance of the entire body and mind. It was not enough to treat a diseased part without treating the whole individual. Rather than focusing on getting rid of symptoms and diseases, Empiricists applied natural methods to augment the body's own defenses so that it could heal itself. Distinct from the Rationalist approach that sought to give everyone who had the same illness the same treatment, the Empiricists sought to treat the entire bodymind *syndrome* and provided more individualized care according to a person's idiosyncratic characteristics. This school of thought developed into the modern natural medicine model in which homeopathy plays an integral part.

Although both schools of thought in medicine have their own rationale and body of experience, the Rationalist school today has dominated and even oppressed the Empiricists and any other potential competitors. Despite the Rationalists' dominance in Western civilization, more people in the world today actually utilize empirical methods, which include various folk-healing practices, than modern conventional medical therapies (the World Health Organization estimates that 80 percent of the world's population uses "traditional healing methods" as their primary form of health care).

In addition to the popularity of traditional healing practices in developing countries, there is, as Chapter 3 of this book highlights, significant and growing interest in homeopathy in virtually every developed country. This book will explain why further growth in the field of homeopathic medicine is not only desirable but inevitable.

WHAT THIS BOOK WILL DO FOR YOU

This book will introduce you to homeopathic medicine, its principles and methodology, its formal research and body of clinical experience, its applications in self-care and professional care, its potential and limitations, and its organizations and assorted resources. This consumer's guide will not advocate for homeopathy or any system of healing as much as it will advocate for you, the consumer who is looking for safe, effective health care. Readers will learn what research exists and what clinical experiences homeopaths have had in the treatment of common acute and chronic ailments. Information on what results to expect (and how soon to expect them from homeopathic care) is provided in the descriptions of most conditions. This information will help readers learn if self-care is appropriate, when they should seek professional homeopathic care, when they should seek a second opinion, and when they should try some other therapies.

As a graduate of the School of Public Health at the University of California at Berkeley and as a professional public health educator, I am trained to help individuals and populations of people take care of themselves so that disease can be prevented and health can be promoted. While most public health educators focus on improving nutrition and other lifestyle influences on health, and on reducing environmental stresses that tend to cause disease, I have added to these appropriate concerns knowledge of homeopathy and homeopathic medicines. Early in my professional career it became clear to me that conventional medicine, as valuable as it can be, has real limitations and serious side effects. People need alternatives, and after studying homeopathy and using the medicines, I soon learned that it offers much to consumers and to health professionals.

However, when I first got involved in homeopathy in 1972, almost all of the literature in the field consisted of books that were published prior to 1900. Although the information was good, the books weren't easily accessible, the writing wasn't easily understandable, and the medicines, which were listed by their Latin names, weren't easily comprehendible.

Instead of choosing to be a homeopathic practitioner, I decided to take a more difficult role: I chose to try to make homeopathy more user-friendly, both to consumers and health professionals. By writing articles and books (this is my fifth book on homeopathy) and publishing books of my colleagues (my company has published thirty so far), I am doing what health educators try to do—that is, I'm trying to make information more accessible so that people can make more informed decisions about their health.

This book is my most comprehensive effort to answer many of the common questions and concerns that people have about homeopathic medicine.

Chapter 1 of this book attempts to explain homeopathy in modern, user-friendly language. Sadly, most previous books on homeopathy tend to describe it in antiquated language, making homeopathy seem like an idiosyncratic nineteenth-century healing art. This book attempts to explain it as a contemporary, even futuristic medical science.

Chapter 2 describes basic underlying assumptions about homeopathy, including the homeopathic definition of health and disease. Clear definitions of health and disease are vital, for they help define what is meant by "cure," which is the ultimate goal of medical therapeutics. This chapter also discusses the difference between curing and suppressing disease. Because the possibility of suppressing disease isn't even considered by modern physicians or the general public, the information provided here will encourage greater caution in using certain treatments, especially many conventional medications. To understand the homeopaths' view of disease and its treatment, this chapter also gives insight into their perspective on genetic components of disease and into homeopathic "constitutional care," which is a highly individualized and profoundly effective means to augment healing of deeply ingrained disease.

While other parts of this book will help the reader understand why homeopathy is growing, Chapter 3 describes specifics about the significant growth that homeopathy has experienced in the past several years. Readers will be surprised at how popular homeopathy is in many countries. It is so popular in some parts of Europe and Asia that it is not appropriate to consider it an "alternative" medicine.

Advocates and skeptics alike tend to ask what research there is using homeopathic medicine, and in response, Chapter 4 provides a review of laboratory and clinical studies. Information about homeopathic research is also sprinkled throughout the clinical chapters in Part III.

Users of homeopathy are often faced with ridicule or doubt from skeptical doctors and family members. Following the research chapter, it is appropriate to answer the various questions and concerns that skeptics have. Although skeptics tend to be ill informed or uninformed about homeopathy, Chapter 5 (and this entire book) will help to "cure" this disease.

Part I of this book concludes with a chapter that discusses the interface between homeopathy and conventional medicine. While there are times when these two different approaches to healing can complement each other, at other times each person must sometimes decide which of the two to begin treatment with and at what point the other approach should be considered.

Part II will give readers the practical information they need to know when using homeopathic medicines for self-care and when seeking professional homeopathic care.

Chapter 7 teaches readers about the method for finding the correct homeopathic remedy, potency, and dosage. It will bring out the "inner homeopath" in anyone interested in learning. In contrast to most conventional physicians, homeopaths encourage self-care for common acute problems (except if a person has just taken a homeopathic constitutional remedy from a homeopath). Homeopaths believe that patients who are better informed about homeopathy are better patients (and are easier to treat!).

Because self-care has its limitations, it is important to know what professional homeopaths have to offer, and Chapter 8 answers many common questions that consumers have about professional homeopathic care. This chapter will help you make informed choices in finding a good homeopath.

A visit to a professional homeopath is quite different from a visit to a conventional family physician. Chapter 9 will help prepare you for the experience by describing the questions that homeopaths typically ask their patients, and suggesting ways you can help your homeopath to be most effective in finding the correct remedy for you.

More and more people are getting introduced to homeopathy through homeopathic combination medicines (also called homeopathic formulas). Chapter 10 discusses their applications and limitations as well as the controversy about their use.

Chapter 11 provides recommendations for home medicine kits

and various specialty kits, and Chapter 12 covers practical issues in using homeopathic medicines, including what can possibly antidote them and how to properly store and handle homeopathic medicines. Because a little bit of knowledge about homeopathy (and about virtually any subject) can create a lot of misunderstandings, there are inevitably myths and misconceptions about this healing system. Part of this chapter attempts to "treat" these problems to prevent them from infecting other people. The chapter also deals with thorny issues that include how to be careful in purchasing homeopathic medicines to ensure that you are getting a quality and legally made product. A discussion of the limitations of homeopathy ends this important chapter.

Part III is the clinical section of the book, which describes the recommended homeopathic treatment of many common ailments. Also included are conditions that are rarely covered in homeopathic texts, including AIDS, chronic fatigue syndrome, arthritis, cancer, heart disease, addictions, and pre- and postsurgical care.

Information on using homeopathic medicines for self-care is provided when appropriate, and when it isn't, on what to expect from professional homeopath care. References to controlled clinical and laboratory studies and to clinical experience are interspersed throughout these chapters to give insight into the potential and limitations of treating people with each condition.

This book is not a comprehensive self-care guide, and the purpose of Part III is to list key remedies and to describe only their primary indications, as well as to provide information about the potential and limitations of homeopathic self-care for each condition. Therefore, a list of recommended resources that provide additional information is included at the end of each chapter.

Part IV provides access to homeopathic resources. Because this book will hopefully be a seed for your further study of and involvement in homeopathic medicine, I've provided this section to help you access more information and products related to homeopathic medicine.

Ultimately, this book will not just introduce you to homeopathy, it will also help you to better understand conventional medicine. Just as travel to foreign countries helps us to understand the many things we take for granted in our own country, introduction to a different and unconventional model of health and medicine helps us to better understand our conventional model of medicine.

Whether you are a parent concerned about health care for your child, a senior citizen concerned about increasing health problems, or an average Joe or Jane Citizen who simply experiences painful or aggravating symptoms, it is both logical and prudent to consider using safer healing methods before using potentially dangerous ones.

It is my personal hope that this book will help inform you of additional health care choices available to you. Besides informing you of choices, it will provide you with tools for better understanding your own health as well as specific medicines for helping to improve it. It is also my hope that health professionals read this book so that they will be inspired to integrate homeopathic medicines into their practice. Health care will become truly comprehensive when it integrates the best of conventional medical technologies with the best of natural therapeutics. This book will hopefully educate and empower you so that you can help create the best possible health care for yourself and your family.

Introduction to Homeopathic Medicine

ONE

Homeopathy: A Modern View

THE WISDOM OF THE BODY

The human organism has survived several hundred thousand years because it is an amazing miracle worker at defending and healing itself. Although conventional medicine has created some of its own technological miracles, they don't compare to the depth and breadth of miracles that the body creates every moment of every day as it staves off innumerable infective agents and adapts to untold subtle and not so subtle stresses.

The inner doctor works continuously, and one does not have to tell the inner doctor what to do: it does its work automatically and with an evolved sophistication that is truly inspired.

Conventional physicians know about this innate wisdom, but tend to ignore it and intervene too often, thinking that they know more than the inner doctor. Inevitably, this arrogance creates its own problems, such as when doctors overprescribe drugs that lead to side effects and addiction.

A fundamental flaw in conventional medical thinking is that physicians tend to assume that symptoms represent the disease itself, that symptoms signify that something is wrong with the person's health, and that these symptoms need to be controlled, managed, or elimi-nated. In fact, the word "symptom" is derived from Greek and means "sign" or "signal." A symptom is *not* a disease itself but a sign or signal of it. Getting rid of the signal does not necessarily affect the original reason for its being there. Seeking to eliminate a symptom is akin to unplugging a car's low-oil-warning light when it comes on. Needless to say, although this "treatment" may "work," it doesn't change the fundamental cause of the signaling.

Although symptoms may indeed suggest that a person's health is disturbed, homeopaths and a growing number of modern physiolo-gists recognize that symptoms are adaptive responses of the organism to stress or infection. As such, symptoms are efforts of the body to de-fend and heal itself.

Because symptoms are inherent defenses of the body, eliminating them without affecting the original source of the problem tends to suppress the body's innate healing responses (a more detailed discus-sion on suppressing symptoms is provided in Chapter 2). This suppres-sion inhibits healing, and because the organism always seeks to defend and heal itself in the most effective way possible based on its present abilities, secondary treatments are not as effective or as efficient as ef-forts to affect the original source of the problem.

For instance, a nasal discharge is a response of the body to viruses that cause the common cold. This nasal discharge is composed of dead virus and dead white blood cells. If a person with a cold takes a med-ication that dries up mucous membranes, he or she will be unable to eliminate this dead matter through the nose, which inevitably leads to head and chest congestion. The body is not as efficient in spitting out mucus through the mouth as it is in discharging it from the nose, and the resulting chest congestion is more likely to lead to more serious health problems than those which occur from a common cold.

A profoundly different perspective on health and healing emerges when one realizes that a person's symptoms are actually defenses of the body. Instead of treating, controlling, inhibiting, managing, or sup-pressing symptoms, as is commonly the approach in conventional medicine, therapies that augment the body's own defenses and that support and even mimic them ultimately make more sense.

Such is the approach used in homeopathic medicine.

The Principle of Similars: The Basis
for Homeopathic Medicine

Homeopathic medicine is based on the principle of similars—that is, whatever symptoms and syndromes a substance causes in large or toxic doses, it can heal when given in specially prepared, exceedingly small doses. In fact, homeopathy derives its name from this similars principle. In Greek, *homoios* means "similar" and *pathos* means "disease" or "suffering."[1] Although homeopathy was formally developed into a systematic method of applying the similars principle in the early 1800s, the use of this healing approach is an ancient pharmacological strategy that was used by the ancient Egyptians, Chinese, Incas, Aztecs, and Native Americans.

At first, the principle of similars doesn't seem to make sense. One would think that giving a dose of something that creates symptoms similar to those that a person is experiencing would exacerbate symptoms, not heal them. And yet modern physiologists recognize that symptoms are inherent responses of the organism to adapt to and defend against infection or stress; therefore, using small doses of whatever causes symptoms similar to those that sick people are experiencing augments their defenses. Even conventional medicine applies the similars principle in its use of immunizations and allergy treatment. Giving small doses of bacteria or viruses has been found to stimulate a person's immune system to create antibodies to protect against infection, and giving small doses of an allergen helps the body's defenses to desensitize the person to larger amounts of a particular allergen. It is worth noting that immunizations and allergy treatment represent two of the few conventional medical procedures that do something to augment the body's own recuperative processes, and they are based on the homeopathic principle of similars.

An example of the body's wisdom in creating symptoms as defenses is the common symptom of fever. Fever is now recognized by physiologists and physicians alike to be an important defense of the body. Fever is the body's effort to create an internally heated state that makes it more difficult for bacteria and viruses to multiply and survive. Although prolonged high fever has been associated with serious health problems and even death, it is not the fever that kills the person; it is the infection. The fever is the body's best effort to defend itself against the infection.

Using exceedingly small doses of medicinal agents that have the capacity to cause the similar symptoms of fever that the sick person is experiencing actually helps the fever resolve more quickly. *Belladonna* (deadly nightshade) and *Aconitum* (monkshood) are two such substances that cause fever when given in large doses and help to heal it when given in small doses to people who exhibit symptoms that correspond to each substance's unique characteristics.

THE EXPERIMENTAL BASIS OF EVERY HOMEOPATHIC MEDICINE

Every homeopathic medicine is tested for its toxicology, for homeopaths have found that whatever a substance *causes* in overdose, it can *cure* when prescribed in small doses. For the past two hundred years homeopaths have performed experiments called provings (derived from the German word *pruefung,* which means "test"), in which healthy subjects are given repeated doses of a substance from the plant, mineral, or animal kingdom. These experiments are conducted only on human subjects because what a substance causes in an animal is not always applicable to humans. Also, human subjects are able to communicate the precise symptoms they are experiencing, and a high level of precision and detail is critical for knowing the specific symptoms and syndromes that a substance causes and cures. The substances are tested only on healthy subjects because if they were tested on ill people, it would be difficult to differentiate their own symptoms from those that the substance creates.

These careful experiments have been collected in volumes of books and now even sophisticated software programs which have helped establish homeopathy as containing the most detailed information on toxicology presently available. Although homeopathic literature does not provide information about the specific doses that cause a specific symptom, it describes the many common and unusual symptoms that various substances cause in greater detail than any other source.

The information from these experiments is written in homeopathic texts called *materia medica* and repertories. *Materia medica* (from the Latin, "materials of medicine") are books that have chapters on common homeopathic medicines, along with detailed descriptions of the symptoms associated with each substance. A repertory is a complementary book to a *materia medica*, and its many chapters list thousands of symptoms as well as the various substances that have been found to cause or cure each symptom.

Computer-minded people will be pleased to know that homeopathic texts have been computerized, and expert systems have been developed for several programs. The incredible detail that homeopaths have collected for the past two hundred years is perfect for the modern computer age.

It should be noted that homeopathic provings are conducted with substances either in crude form or in homeopathic potentized dose (the definition of homeopathic potentized dose is provided later in this chapter). For example, when conducting a proving of coffee, homeopaths will sometimes give continual doses of the crude form of coffee to subjects, but more often, they will give continual specially prepared, highly diluted ("potentized") doses of coffee to subjects. Homeopaths collect the experiences from these subjects. While most people will feel the stimulating effects of coffee, some will feel restless physically and/or mentally, some will feel anxious, some will develop a headache, some will experience irregular heart palpitations, and some will have idiosyncratic symptoms. The symptoms that are experienced by most people are written in boldface letters in homeopathic texts, symptoms that are experienced by large numbers of subjects are listed in italic, and symptoms that are experienced infrequently are listed in plain type.

Subjects who volunteer for provings are never given crude doses of poisonous substances. Instead, potentized doses of these substances are tested. Subjects of provings are informed to stop taking the potentized substance once any symptoms have developed, thus reducing the danger from these experiments. In fact, homeopaths have found that subjects of provings experience health benefits from provings because these tests challenge a person's immune and defense system and therefore strengthen it.

That homeopaths use potentized doses of substances to test what their remedies cause is one fact of which skeptics of homeopathy are commonly ignorant. Evidence that homeopathic microdoses have biological effect is apparent not only by the clinical results of homeopaths but also by homeopathic provings because they can cause symptoms if taken beyond their medicinal dose. Because so much of homeopathy is based on these experiments, it is unlikely that homeopathic texts could have developed with such consistent information if the microdoses of substances they were testing were simply placebos.

The other lesson that homeopathic provings have for consumers is that the basic rule of thumb in using homeopathic medicines is to stop taking them if symptoms have begun to improve. If no improvement is obvious within forty-eight hours in acute ailments, it is likely that the homeopathic medicine was not the correct one. Repeating doses is not beneficial and may, in fact, cause symptoms of a proving. The good news here is that if such symptoms develop, they rarely last very long, unless the person unwittingly continues to take the medicine.

The lesson that homeopaths teach consumers is that homeopathic remedies are medicines, not vitamins or supplements that need to be taken every day. Homeopathic medicines should be taken only when a person's symptoms match the symptoms that the substance causes.

INDIVIDUALIZATION OF CARE: DESIGNER MEDICINE

Imagine a medical system which individualizes medicines based on the totality of unique and idiosyncratic symptoms that a person experiences. This "designer medicine" is homeopathic medicine.

From a homeopathic perspective, there are no diseases, only diseased people. To diagnose a person as having a specific disease is too limiting, because we all experience disease syndromes in subtly and sometime overtly different ways. One person with a migraine will have pain on one side of the head, another will have it on the other, and yet another will have it on both sides. One person will feel relief by applying heat, while another's pain would be aggravated by that. One person will have nausea with the migraine, while another might have dizziness. In addition to the various unique physical symptoms, people have varying psychological symptoms. One person with a migraine will feel depressed, another anxious, and another irritable. And of course, there are different types of depression, anxiety, and irritability that each person experiences.

Ultimately, homeopaths believe that ailing people do not simply have a disease, they have a *syndrome*. This syndrome is a bodymind constellation of symptoms. This homeopathic perspective is considerably more modern, if not futuristic, than the limited medical model which tends to assume that disease is somehow localized. Conventional medicine, however, is finally changing, as witnessed by the growing acceptance of psychoneuroimmunology, the scientific field that investigates the effects of the mind on the body and the body on the mind. This field is also slowly developing a perspective that perceives an increasing number of diseases as syndromes, though it is still far from the homeopathic perspective that sees all disease in this light.

From this perspective, homeopathy is a system of finding a medicine that fits the *totality* of physical and psychological symptoms that each person experiences. This may at first sound like a difficult and extremely complex process, and sometimes it is, but often people fit common patterns of symptoms which match specific remedies. Also, as one learns about homeopathy, one is taught to place more weight on certain symptoms than on others (see page 88, "How to Find the Correct Homeopathic Medicine" in Chapter 7 for details).

Individualizing a medicine to a person and his or her unique pattern of symptoms makes sense, and at some time in the near future it will probably seem strange that physicians ever believed that they could effectively give the same medicine to everyone who shared only a small number of similar symptoms. The biological individuality that geneticists have long recognized is appreciated and integrated within the homeopathic method.

Despite the emphasis on individualizing a homeopathic medicine to a sick person, consumers today often see homeopathic remedies sold in natural food stores and pharmacies labeled to treat specific ailments, ranging from "allergy" and "arthritis" to "PMS" and "teething. " It is easy to see how some people can be confused by this and wonder if it is a legitimate form of homeopathy. Homeopathic formulas, also called combination remedies or complexes, are mixtures of two to eight medicines which may each be known to be effective for treating slightly different variations of a certain ailment. Homeopathic formulas are useful when one does not know how to find an individualized single remedy or if that single remedy is not readily available. (A more detailed discussion of homeopathic formulas is provided in Chapter 10.)

THE SMALL DOSES OF HOMEOPATHIC MEDICINES

Abraham Lincoln once said, "Homeopathy is a soup made from the shadow of the wing of a pigeon that starved to death."

This quote is probably more an example of his wry sense of humor than a true critique of homeopathy, as his most trusted political adviser, Secretary of State William Seward, was a strong advocate for homeopathy.

People who know very little about homeopathy tend to know only that extremely small doses of medicines are used. But homeopathic medicines are not simply small doses, for if they were, then the people of Los Angeles (or any major metropolitan area), who regularly inhale small doses of innumerable toxic substances, would probably be cured of everything.

Homeopathic medicines are specially prepared small doses which undergo a specific process of consecutive dilution and succussion (vigorous shaking). A substance is diluted one part to nine parts water (1:10) or one part to ninety-nine parts water (1:100), usually in distilled water, and shaken, then diluted again and shaken, and the process is repeated.[2]

When a substance is diluted 1:10 three times, the medicine is called "3x" (x is the Roman numeral that stands for 10). When a substance is diluted 1:100 three times, the medicine is called "3c" (c is the Roman numeral that stands for 100).

This pharmacological process is called potentization, and homeopaths have observed from two hundred years of clinical practice that the more a substance is potentized, the longer and more deeply the medicine acts and the fewer doses are necessary for treatment. Although it does not initially make sense that this potentization process would *increase* the clinical strength of a medicine, the results have been experienced by hundreds of thousands of homeopathic physicians and tens of millions of homeopathic patients. (Further discussion of this phenomenon is provided in the next section.)

One interesting note about homeopathy's use of small doses involves homeopathy's founder, Dr. Samuel Hahnemann. Dr. Hahnemann conducted his first experiments on the homeopathic principle of similars in 1790, but he did not write his first book about homeopathy until 1810, after conducting experiments for twenty years. For these first twenty years Hahnemann primarily used medicines that were not potentized very much, usually 1c to 6c.

Later in his life as his colleagues began experimenting in higher potencies such as the 1,000th, the 2,500th, and higher, he admonished them by saying, "I do not approve of your potentizing the medicines higher [than the 30th potency]; there must be a limit to the thing."[3] But then, after Hahnemann himself began experimenting with these highly potentized microdoses, he acknowledged that they were effective and, in fact, were more powerful than the less potentized doses. Hahnemann encouraged his colleagues to use these medicines sparingly and carefully because of their power.

Despite the initial skepticism that is common when people are first introduced to the concept that such extremely small doses can have any healing effect, there is actually a considerable body of literature from a wide variety of scientific fields investigating and proving microdose phenomena. Many of these studies are discussed in Chapter 4.

THE WISDOM AND WONDER OF SMALL DOSES

"Nature uses as little as possible of anything," wrote Johannes Kepler.

Scientists readily acknowledge that virtually all animals have one or more incredible senses which provide them with exquisite sensitivity to exceedingly small amounts of whatever substances they need for their survival. For instance, sharks are known to detect small concentrations of blood in the water at a great distance, despite the large volume of water that exists in oceans. Dogs have an incredible sense of smell and can follow a human trail despite the fact that a person leaves only approximately four billionths of a gram of odorous sweat per step.[4] This feat becomes even more impressive when you consider that people wear shoes which considerably cuts down on the amount of sweat that reaches the ground.

In addition to these amazing feats, biologists recognize that animals emit pheromones, which are sexually attracting hormones. Male night moths can find females on dark moonless nights, and if necessary, even against the wind. A male silkworm will fly many miles to find its female insects.[5] These are not exceptions, for many insects can smell as little as a single molecule of their species' pheromones. Perhaps these insects are not smelling molecules at all; perhaps they are sensing some type of magnetic or energetic field. Whatever it is, it is a real phenomenon of nature and is an amazing example of the hypersensitivity that living organisms have for what they need to survive.

It is hard to believe that human beings are not as sophisticated as most other living creatures, especially when one considers the incredible abilities of the human brain and its cerebral cortex. Scientists readily acknowledge that exceedingly small doses of certain neurotransmitters in the brain can dramatically affect one's emotional, mental, and behavioral states. Further, very slight changes in hormones can likewise have significant effects on the body. Some pituitary hormones can produce contraction of muscle tissue in doses as dilute as one part in 19 billion parts of water. Also, animal musk is so chemically close to testosterone that we can smell it in portions of as little as .000000000000032 (thirteen zeros!) ounces.[6]

If these facts and figures are difficult to grasp, simply witness a person who is allergic to cats. Even though the person may only have briefly passed through a room through which a single cat had simply walked earlier, this person may exhibit a powerful allergic response. What is particularly surprising is that the person is fully clothed, and it is likely that he did not physically touch anything in the room except the ground, and even then, his shoes protected him from direct contact with the floor. Allergists assume that the person breathed in trace amounts of cat hair in the air. Sensitivity to small amounts of substances is obvious.

However, it is not as if small amounts of anything have an effect on everyone. People and animals are sensitive to certain substances but not to others. Ants, for instance, can smell the trails created by ants of their own species, but they can't smell the trails created by other species. Likewise, animals can sense the pheromones from their own species, but not from others.

Ultimately, the hypersensitivity seems, in part, to be based on the principle of similars in nature. Homeopathy is simply the medicinal application of this natural law, and the law of similars is homeopathy's method of individualizing microdoses of a substance to a person who needs this substance and is thus hypersensitive to it. Homeopathy's similars principle may, in fact, be one of the important laws in nature that will explain many phenomena that are presently a part of nature's mysteries.

How Homeopathic Medicines Work

(This section of the book explores various scientific theories that may help explain how homeopathy works. Some of the information may seem a bit technical and hard to understand, particularly if you do not have a scientific background. If you are not especially interested in the theories about *how* homeopathy works, feel free to skip this section.)

Just as physicians do not understand how many of their drugs work, homeopaths do not understand the precise mechanism of action of homeopathic medicines. Still, by drawing from research from several scientific fields and by exploring known phenomena, we may get a better sense of how and why the microdoses that homeopaths use can have such profound clinical effects.

It is known that all matter consists of and radiates energy. Some substances, such as radium, radiate a great deal, while other substances, such as the chair you are sitting on, radiate much less. Some things can even store frequencies, whether it be a tape, a CD, or a computer disk. Homeopaths have found that water, the substance in which most homeopathic medicines are made, likewise stores frequencies.

All things produce their own frequencies, and like a snowflake, each substance is unique. Researchers have discovered that snow crystals, after melting, resume their previous form when they are frozen again. Not only does water store frequencies, it stores some form of memory. Some homeopathic researchers theorize that the double-distilled water used in the preparation of homeopathic medicines maintains the memory of the original substance that has been diluted in it, even when repeated dilutions of 1:10 or 1:100 have in all probability exceeded the point at which there should be no remaining molecules of the original substance.

Another way to understand that something remains in the water despite repeated dilutions comes from what is understood about holograms. Holograms are high-resolution, laser-created photographs that look three-dimensional. One astonishing feature of holograms is that if a hologram of, for example, a tree is broken into pieces, each small piece of the photographic plate maintains a picture of the whole tree, albeit a smaller and less clear picture of it. A similar situation of a pattern within a pattern within a pattern occurs in a phenomenon known as fractals, a frequently discussed topic in current science. A potentized homeopathic medicine may therefore be a holographic fractal.

The holographic effect may seem illogical or even impossible, but it is unquestionably true. Further, the human body's DNA is another example of a hologram. Each person's DNA is an integral part of every cell of an individual's body, and like a holograph, the DNA in each cell contains all of a person's genetic information.

While holograms bring to homeopathy evidence that some imprint or resonance of a substance will remain no matter how many times it is diluted and shaken, it still remains a mystery how or why the exceedingly small doses used in homeopathy have any effect, let alone increasingly larger effect the more times the medicine is potentized.

Evidence from the cutting edge of current science may provide some insight into the homeopathic microdose phenomenon.[7] Modern chaos theory, for instance, recognizes the power of infinitesimal changes. One of the basis assumptions of chaos theory is that minute changes can lead to huge differences. Another basic principle of chaos theory is that significant effects from minute changes tend to be most commonly observed in dynamic systems that are raised to high levels of energy or turbulence (what physicists call "far from equilibrium"). It can be theorized that the diluting and shaking process which is a vital part of making homeopathic medicines creates these high levels of energy.

Homeopathic medicines consist of extremely small doses of substances that may be able to sift through the blood-brain barrier which normally impedes large and potentially dangerous molecules from entering the brain; perhaps homeopathic medicines are able to affect brain chemistry and thereby disease in significant ways.

Some research in health physics has suggested that small doses of medicines may have a more significant effect than large doses because of a "therapeutic window." This effect from small doses is more likely when an organism is in a state of "metastable excitation," a hypersensitive state which is "cocked and ready to go" as soon as a specific stimulus triggers the cascade effect. For instance, it is widely acknowledged in science that large changes can occur in living organisms when specific key enzymes, hormones, or tissues are activated, even if only slightly activated. The homeopathic principle of similars may ultimately be the vital link to finding a substance in nature that when individually prescribed can trigger this avalanche effect.

It has previously been noted that all living and nonliving things have their own resonance. As science writer K. C. Cole wrote, "Planets and atoms and almost everything in between vibrate at one or more natural frequencies. When something else nudges them periodically at one of those frequencies, resonance results."[8] Cole goes on to say that "resonance" means to resound, to sound again, or to echo, and the power of resonance is in the pushing or pulling in the same direction that the force is already going. Synchronized small pushes can add up to create a significant change. A classic example of the force of resonance is witnessed in the phenomenon of soldiers walking in place over a bridge, causing it to collapse from the natural resonance created.

What is also interesting about resonance is that it is more powerful when there is a little friction—when the force is similar to though not exactly the same as the initial force. The resonance becomes broader, creating something similar to a chord rather than a single note. The relationship of this concept to healing is that homeopaths find that the most effective homeopathic medicine is one that in overdose creates symptoms that are the most similar to, not necessarily the same as, the symptoms the person is experiencing.

What is also interesting about resonance is that there is a hypersensitivity that the C note on a piano has to other C notes on the piano. Even if two pianos are several hundred feet away, hitting the C note on one piano will be felt by and will cause resonance in all the C notes on both pianos. The B note immediately next to the C will not resonate at all. The small doses that homeopaths use will likewise be felt only by people who have symptoms similar to those that a substance causes.

Using small doses of the wrong substance or of the right substance at the wrong time creates no effect, because there is no similar resonance between the substance and the person's symptoms. This is why incorrect homeopathic medicines don't do anything. It is like the lack of action when a magnet is placed near something that does not have iron in it. The magnet will not draw it closer.

Homeopaths have also noted that homeopathic medicines can become neutralized if subjected to high temperatures or certain magnetic fields, suggesting that some type of memory or information is encoded in the water which can be erased by certain physical influences.

Although the precise mechanism of action is not yet known, and although it may not be a single or knowable mechanism of action, researchers at the California Institute of Technology have made a discovery that may shed some light on the homeopathic phenomenon. The researchers discovered magnetic particles called magnetite throughout the human brain.[9] The purpose and function of magnetite remains unknown, though its discovery is significant because it establishes the existence of an electromagnetic component of the brain. Perhaps the increased number of times a homeopathic medicine is diluted and shaken creates a higher level of electromagnetic field to which the brain's magnetite is hypersensitive.

It is further intriguing to note that a piece of iron becomes magnetized when it is rubbed with another piece of iron. Also, a weakened magnet regains its previous magnetic field when the north and south poles of another magnet are aligned to the north and south poles of the weakened magnet. These widely known facts about magnets may help us understand something about the homeopathic process of potentizing medicines and the principle of similars. For instance, the homeopathic process of shaking a substance between each dilution may be, like the rubbing of pieces of iron together to create a magnet, a way for the substance to create its own magnetic or energetic field. And the regeneration of a weakened magnet by aligning the same poles of the magnet next to another's may be another example of the regenerative and "healing" effects of the principle of similars.

Although these explanations may be perfectly understandable to some people, half-baked to others, and totally ludicrous to still others, they cannot prove or disprove homeopathy. Explanations and theories only explain or theorize; they do not prove anything. Still, the human mind tends to try to understand both the fathomable and the unfathomable.

The mystery of homeopathic microdoses is a serious challenge to science. It is not, however, a phenomenon that one should simply dismiss because it does not fit within our presently limited understanding of the laws of nature. Rather, because the phenomenon is quite real, the attitude of the real scientist needs to be: How can we change or expand our present understanding of nature to incorporate the real but mysterious phenomenon of homeopathic medicine.

Resources

Trevor Cook, *Homeopathic Medicine Today*. New Canaan: Keats, 1989.

Stephen Cummings and Dana Ullman, *Everybody's Guide to Homeopathic Medicine*. Los Angeles: Tarcher, 1991.

Richard Grossinger, *Homeopathy: An Introduction for Beginners and Skeptics*. Berkeley: North Atlantic, 1994.

Randolph M. Nesse and George C. Williams, *Why We Get Sick*. New York: Times, 1995.

Rajan Sankaran, *The Spirit of Homeopathy*. Bombay: Homeopathic Medical, 1991.

Dana Ullman, *Discovering Homeopathy*. Berkeley: North Atlantic, 1991.

Dana Ullman, *An Introduction to Homeopathy* (a set of six cassettes). Boulder: Sounds True, 1995.

George Vithoulkas, *The Science of Homeopathy*. New York: Grove, 1980.

TWO

Healing Disease
Versus
Suppressing Symptoms

DEFINING HEALTH AND DISEASE

Defining health as the absence of disease is akin to defining wealth as
the absence of poverty. Health and wealth need to be defined by more
than their absence. Just because a person does not have symptoms certainly does not mean that he or she has vital health.

Symptoms may, in fact, be a good sign of vitality. Symptoms may
indicate that the body is responding to stress or infection and is now
working to defend itself from further illness. Being without symptoms
may even be a sign of ill health. Witness what happened to the survivors of Hiroshima and Nagasaki: many seemed to be in good health,
without symptoms after the bombings, but then died ten to twenty
years later of cancer. One could not say that they were "healthy" just
prior to the diagnosis of cancer. Also, it is a common phenomenon
that people with cancer claim that they had not had a cold or flu for

ten or more years. Perhaps the body's ability to inflame and to fight infection may be a sign of its strength rather than its weakness.

The paradox here is that being without symptoms does not necessarily mean that a person is healthy and having symptoms does not necessarily mean that a person is ill. Ultimately, health and sickness are relative. We are, in relative degrees, both healthy and sick. In order to fully understand and appreciate the homeopathic system of healing, one must understand the body's natural reactions to disease, such as the above-described paradox, as well as other phenomena discussed later in this chapter. It is also necessary to understand how homeopaths define health.

Homeopaths generally define health as a state of freedom from limitation on dynamic, interrelated physical, emotional, and mental levels.[1]

On the physical level, health is freedom from pain and from physical limitation, having as its basis an overall state of well-being.

On an emotional level, health is freedom *with* emotions, not freedom *from* emotions. A healthy person can and will feel varied emotions, but he or she does not dwell on them, is not overwhelmed by them, is not limited to the same recurring emotions, and is able to resolve them. Despite the emotions felt and experienced, the healthy person has an inner sense of calm, balance, and integration with others and the environment.

On a mental level, health is freedom from selfishness with the ability to think clearly, to understand competently, and to have a will that is strong, capable, flexible, creative, loving, and compassionate.

From this broader definition, health is a *process,* not simply a goal.

THE HEALING PROCESS

Physicians typically think of the healing process as the body's efforts to defend and heal itself. This is certainly true, but homeopaths and various natural healing specialists have discovered more detailed information about this process which has helped them support and augment it.

The human organism, like any living system, always seeks to survive and will go to great lengths to adapt to the various infections and stresses that it experiences. A part of its adaptation process is its ability to create a variety of symptoms as defenses. The human body will au-

tomatically create the best response it can, based on its present resources and on what it has learned in the past.

Constantine Hering, M.D., the father of American homeopathy,
and homeopaths since him have observed that there are three directions in which healing tends to progress (although homeopathic texts
usually refer to these directions as "Hering's laws of cure," it is more
accurate to consider them guidelines to evaluating the curative
process).[2]

1. *The healing process moves from the most vital to the least vital functions.*
With the recognition that some parts of the organism are more vital
for survival than others, Hering observed that the body externalizes
disease, pushing it from deeper, vital processes of the body to more superficial, less vital processes. The brain and heart will be protected as
the body externalizes disease to the soft tissue, connective tissue,
bones, and skin. From this point of view, skin symptoms are generally
not considered skin diseases; they are thought to be internal diseases
that are simply manifesting on the skin.

Inherent in this understanding of the healing process is also the
recognition that one's psychological state represents a deep and vital
process because of its influence on various important physiological
and immunological functions. And just as the body has deeper and
more superficial symptoms, so does the mind. A healing process on a
psychological level is thought to occur when deeper psychological problems evolve into more superficial ones. While recognizing
that the depth of a symptom depends on what it is and also its intensity, Greek homeopath George Vithoulkas theorizes the following
order of increasing depth of mental disease: absentmindedness, forgetfulness, lack of concentration, dullness, lethargy, delusions, paranoid
ideas, destructive delirium, and complete mental confusion.[3] Vithoulkas theorizes the following order of emotional disease: dissatis-
faction, irritability, anxiety, phobias, anguish, sadness, apathy, suicidal
depression.

Information on the physical, emotional, and mental levels becomes a part of the homeopath's comprehensive assessment of a person's health.

2. *The healing process moves from the top of the body to the bottom.* This
guideline is partially linked to the previous one because the most vital
organs are in the upper half of the body. For example, homeopaths ob-

serve that people with skin rashes or arthritis tend toward cure when their symptoms move down their body.

3. *The healing process may result in reexperiencing old symptoms that had been experienced earlier in one's life.* The organism maintains a memory of old symptoms and syndromes, and the body must sometimes reexperience them in order to resolve and heal them. Various natural physicians and healers, not just homeopaths, have also noticed this retracing of old symptoms as a sign that a deep healing is in process.

Homeopaths observe that people have different *layers* of illness. Each layer has a different pattern of physical and psychological symptoms, and as we add layers of illness, some symptoms disappear and are sublimated but are not "cured." In the healing process, as one layer is healed, the person may develop old symptoms from the previous sublimated layer.

The human body always strives to survive and will at times reduce certain superficial symptoms so that it can devote more energy to defending and healing more dangerous symptoms. For instance, a person may be suffering from a minor acute infection but is then seriously injured. In such instances, symptoms of the acute infection disappear or are greatly diminished as the body reacts to the injury. Once the body is out of danger from the injury, it is common for the person to reexperience his or her previous ailment.

An injury interceding an illness is but one example of this phenomenon; any serious illness can intercede into a less serious one. If and when an effective treatment is provided, a person may reexperience the earlier symptoms as a part of the healing process.

Homeopaths commonly refer to the healing process as "removing layers." They sometimes use the layers of an onion as a good visual analogy for the healing process, with a goal of getting to the core of the person without any encumbrances.

Homeopaths find Hering's guidelines to healing to be useful as a way to assess whether a person' s response to treatment is a real healing or is primarily a palliative or even a placebo response. Hering's guidelines help to assess not only if the person's health is improving but if it is getting worse. If, for instance, a person's primary symptoms disappear but new, more serious symptoms emerge, the homeopath would assume that the treatment was not successful and that the person's health is worsening. In comparison, a conventional physician would assume that the initial treatment was successful and that now a new disease, unrelated to the first, has emerged.

SUSCEPTIBILITY TO DISEASE

Contrary to common belief, one does not get sick simply as the result of infection or stress but also because of one's susceptibility (also called predisposition) to these pathological factors. American medical thinking has tended to neglect this essential co-factor to disease.

For instance, at this very moment, many people have streptococcus in their throat, pneumonococcus in their bronchial tubes, and cancer cells in different parts of their body, though this does not mean that they are suffering from any diseases. Our bodies are complex ecosystems in which the immune system does a remarkable job of keeping pathogenic agents from reproducing too rapidly. However, if our immune system is already overworked or is otherwise compromised, it may not be able to defend itself adequately against an infectious agent or stressful circumstance.

While exposure to cold does not "cause" a cold or sore throat, it can stress a person significantly enough that the bacteria or viruses that may already be resident in his or her body may be able to reproduce without adequate defense. On the other hand, exposure to cold at another time in the person's life will not result in any illness, due to some type of reserve that the body had at the time.

From minute to minute, the organism's susceptibility to illness changes.

We are all a little familiar with this concept of susceptibility. We know that only some people in our family may get a cold, cough, or flu, even though every member probably was exposed to the same sick person.

Susceptibility refers to the overall defenses of the human organism, and there are various factors that influence these defenses. A wide variety of internal and external factors in each person can either increase or decrease susceptibility. Dr. Claude Bernard, a nineteenth-century physician and physiologist who is considered the father of experimental physiology, acknowledged the importance of predisposition when he called it "the pivot of all experimental physiology and the real cause of most diseases."[4]

Ultimately, conventional medicine has focused its research and clinical attention primarily on developing treatments for specific symptoms, and yet it has done little to evaluate, assess, or predict susceptibility to illness. Such investigations are inherently more difficult because they require a holistic psychophysiological assessment of the person which is not as amenable to the reductionistic methods of science.

The confusing but intriguing point about susceptibility and illness is that people who get an infection may be sicker than those who don't, *or* they can actually be healthier. Sometimes, becoming ill from an infection suggests that a person's defenses were down at the time. On the other hand, a broader (and homeopathic) perspective is that a person may not get an infection because he or she is presently too sick to respond. For instance, people with schizophrenia rarely experience symptoms of infection during their psychotic episodes. Only after they are psychologically more stable are they "healthy" enough to experience a simple infection. Although one may think that a resistance to common acute infections is a sign of good health, it sometimes suggests that one is too sick to fight the infection.

While the inability to inflame against infection may suggest that a person is seriously ill, the other side of the equation is that it makes sense to let the body, when ill, create its symptoms of fever and inflammation, at least for a while. In fact, a growing number of pediatricians are today recognizing the value of not immediately treating a child who is suffering from certain infections, including strep throat. Some research has suggested that treating a strep throat too quickly may increase the chances of a recurrence.[5] Another study showed that children with strep throat who were treated with antibiotics immediately upon diagnosis had *eight times* the recurrence of strep throat of those children for whom treatment was delayed.[6]

Ellen Wald, M.D., medical director of Children's Hospital of Pittsburgh, has suggested that too early treatment with antibiotics may impair normal immunologic response and increase the chance of reinfection.[7] One can conjecture that a child's (and anyone's) body needs to inflame in order to learn how to fight infection successfully.

Similarly, research in the *Journal of the American Medical Association* has shown that childhood herpes may actually lower the adult's risk of genital herpes and even AIDS.[8] Although the reason why this is true is unknown, some homeopaths postulate that childhood infections may be important in challenging the immune system. Challenging and exercising the immune system may be essential for vitality and disease prevention.

The implications of this point of view are significant, especially in light of the perceived value of immunizations. Immunizations may provide some obvious benefits, but they may prevent people from experiencing some infections that may be important in building a strong immune system. While it may make sense to immunize against serious and potentially fatal infections such as tetanus, it makes less sense to immunize against mumps, measles, chicken pox, and whooping cough (this latter immunization is also questionably effective, with the majority of children who get the disease having been already immunized).

Once one realizes that symptoms of the body play an important role in its defenses, one must develop a new respect for the body's wisdom. When conventional physicians and scientists begin to appropriately honor the many miracles of the human body, they will inevitably start receiving insights into the healing process and avoid treatments that suppress disease.

Suppressing Symptoms

Symptoms of illness not only represent a sign of illness, they signify the body's best efforts to try to defend and heal itself. From this perspective, treatments like many conventional drugs that seek to stop, inhibit, or control these efforts are ignoring the body's inherent wisdom and suppressing its ability to heal itself.

Believe it or not, there are no such things as "side effects" from a drug. From a strictly pharmacological perspective, drugs only have "effects," and we arbitrarily differentiate those effects we like from those we don't like (calling the latter "side effects"). From a homeopathic perspective, side effects are primarily the result of suppressing the body's symptoms.

The fact that suppressing symptoms leads to new and often more serious symptoms, however, is almost totally foreign to conventional physicians and drug manufacturers today. They generally assume that new symptoms are simply new and usually unrelated symptoms.

The concept of suppressing symptoms is relatively simple. Fever, for instance, is now known to be an important defense of the body. Heightened temperature in the body increases the activity of the immune system's white blood cells and increases secretion of interferon, both of which help to fight infection. Although prolonged very high fevers can lead to serious neurological problems, fever itself is one of the methods the body deploys to defend itself from infection.

If a person with a fever is given a drug or treatment that reduces the fever, he or she will be less able to fight infection, which usually leads to a variety of new, sometimes dangerous symptoms. Children with fever who are given aspirin can, for instance, develop Reye's syndrome, a potentially fatal neurological disorder.

Homeopaths theorize that the reason why more chronic disease is affecting people at younger and younger ages is that conventional drugs are being used more frequently to treat common acute problems, and these drugs are effectively suppressing the body's abilities to defend and heal itself. A recent government report noted that "the proportion of children with limitation of activity [due to chronic conditions] has doubled since 1960."[9] Conditions such as asthma which were previously incapacitating but rarely a cause of death are now increasingly common fatal conditions. Death rates from asthma have doubled in the past decade.

Homeopaths also theorize that mental illnesses, cancers, and immune system disorders are affecting greater numbers of people in part because less serious physical illnesses are being suppressed to deeper levels of their being.

Psychiatrists and psychologists are intimately familiar with the concept of suppression, as they regularly see the effects of suppressing emotions. Mental health professionals note that suppressing emotions creates new, usually deeper problems which are not relieved until the original emotion is recognized, expressed, and resolved.

Homeopaths tend to be aware of and watchful for disease suppression because they interview their patients very thoroughly and often compare the totality of their symptoms before conventional medical treatment and afterward. By using Hering's guidelines, homeopaths commonly witness disease suppression and the emergence of increasingly serious ailments. Homeopaths also observe that people tend to reexperience old symptoms after homeopathic treatment, thus suggesting that these symptoms were either previously suppressed or at least left incompletely cured. The consistency with which homeopaths observe these phenomena provides evidence that disease suppression is real, and can and should be avoided unless a medical emergency exists.

Needless to say, research on disease suppression is not likely to receive funding from drug companies. Until governments, nonprofit organizations, and the public recognize the potential problems from certain medical interventions, it is safest for patients and their physicians to seek out therapies that augment the body's wisdom, rather than those that inhibit individual symptoms.

IMMUNOSUPPRESSIVE TREATMENTS VERSUS IMMUNOAUGMENTIVE TREATMENTS

The language of medicine today is fighting language. Physicians and drug companies pride themselves on developing and prescribing drugs that attack disease, battle illness, and kill microbes. They have created a "war on cancer," and like good generals, they commonly predict that victory is at hand, if only more money for research and armament is provided.

Even the types of action that drugs are purported to have take an antagonistic and fighting posture: anti-inflammatory, antihistamine, antibiotic, antispasmodic, and classically, painkilling. Although each of these actions may provide at least temporary relief to a sick person, they do not strengthen the body's immune system so that the body can heal itself, nor do they augment the body's defenses so that the condition does not return.

The reductionistic tendencies of medicine and science have limited their vision of what is possible in pharmacology. Few physicians and scientists have even looked for ways that the overall immune and defense system could be augmented. When researchers do study immunoaugmenting drugs, it is usually to evaluate specific effects on only one part of the immune system.

The good news is that since the emergence of AIDS, many physicians and researchers are beginning to understand the important role of the body's immune system. Despite the tragedy of the AIDS epidemic, it has encouraged greater understanding and respect for the vital functioning of our immune system.

In the most general terms, one can basically say that there are two types of treatments: those that tend to augment the body's defenses and those that tend to suppress them. A given treatment does not necessarily fit into one category or the other, though future research will probably clarify which treatments do what and to what degree. Just because a treatment is suppressive, however, does not necessarily mean that it isn't useful, valuable, or even curative. Although a treatment may have some mildly suppressive effects, the temporary relief that is provided may give the body's defenses some time to rest and gather themselves to deal effectively with the original source of the problem.

However, many people may not respond well to even mildly suppressive treatment. Infants whose immune systems are in development, the elderly whose immune systems are already severely challenged, and people who are immunocompromised in some way may be harmed by such treatment.

The common cough is a classic ailment in which one can compare suppressive and curative treatments. According to standard textbooks on pathology, the cough is an important protective mechanism of the body. It is a vital defense of the organism in its effort to expel foreign or irritating material so that the person can breathe. And yet there are many over-the-counter drugs that are marketed as "cough suppressants." While such drugs provide temporary relief, they do not cure the underlying condition and may even delay its resolution. In comparison, homeopathic and various other natural therapies are prescribed to either soothe or strengthen the bronchials so that the person can more effectively eliminate whatever may be irritating him.

It is no coincidence that immunizations and allergy treatments, two of the few conventional medical treatments that do something to augment the body's immune system, are based on the homeopathic principle of similars. Immunizations utilize small doses of microbes that cause a particular illness in order to augment the immune system's creation of antibodies against them, and allergy treatments are based on using small doses of what a person is allergic to in order to help the person develop less sensitivity to that substance.

Homeopathic medicines do not work simply by stimulating the body's immune system; some diseases, in fact, are the result of an overactive immune response. These diseases are called autoimmune disorders, and they are the result of the body attacking itself. Rheumatoid arthritis, one of the autoimmune diseases, is a condition that homeopaths commonly find treatable. One study showed that 82 percent of patients with rheumatoid arthritis received some degree of relief from a homeopathic medicine, while only 21 percent of those given a placebo received a similar degree of relief.[10]

Besides being used to reduce an overly active immune system, as seen in the above research on rheumatoid arthritis, homeopathic medicines have also been shown to stimulate immune response when such effects are necessary for healing. One study published in the *European Journal of Pharmacology* showed that a homeopathic medicine, *Silicea*, stimulated macrophrages by as much as 64 percent (macrophrages are an important part of the body's immune system).[11]

There have also been several laboratory studies showing that homeopathic microdoses can have immunomodulatory effects (effects in which the immune system is stimulated or reduced whenever each effect is necessary for healing).[12] This field of scientific inquiry is very ripe for future exploration.

As physicians and scientists recognize the importance of the immune system, they will inevitably begin to investigate the potential for homeopathic medicines in helping to heal the numerous ailments in which the body's immune system plays a role.

HOMEOPATHIC UNDERSTANDING OF CHRONIC DISEASE

Chronic disease may be akin to natural cataclysms like earthquakes. Earthquakes are predisposed to occur on previous faults. They result from a complex assortment of stresses to the geologic plates that lie under the surface. And they occur as the result of a pressure exerted from either close or distant stresses.

Likewise, chronic disease arises from certain predispositions, some of which may have occurred in a person's lifetime and some of which may be from a distant genetic source. Some chronic diseases may be buried deeply in a person and may not manifest until or unless the person experiences significant stresses, while other chronic diseases may lie just below the surface and will erupt from minor stresses.

Even though an individual may look extremely healthy, there is always the chance that he or she may be at the edge of a serious chronic illness and even death. And the opposite is also true: even though a person may look ill and may even have a chronic disease, he may be able to nurse his chronic illness into a ripe old age. The low-grade chronic symptoms may simply be the efficient way the organism is "letting off steam" in order to diminish the chances of one larger cataclysmic change. Perhaps this is why Sir William Osler, the father of modern medicine, once said, "The secret of longevity is to get a chronic disease and take care of it."

While it may sometimes seem that chronic disease and death attack arbitrarily, there are ways to reduce the risk of an early-onset chronic illness and delay premature death. Treatment with homeopathic medicines is one of the lesser-known ways to do so. Not only does homeopathy offer a valuable way of treating chronic ailments, it also has a way of understanding them.

Chronic disease does not simply appear out of thin air. It develops for a long time, not just in one's own lifetime but also through genetic predisposition.

Even though Gregor Mendel postulated his laws of heredity in 1865, homeopathy's founder, Dr. Samuel Hahnemann, recognized the important role that genetics played in disease as early as 1810. Hahnemann believed not only that certain diseases are inherited but that certain patterns of symptoms are too. In other words, two people in a family may develop two completely different diseases (one, colitis; one, Parkinson's disease), but they may both have recurrent canker sores and/or ulcerations of various sorts, significant aggravations of their symptoms at night, oily and/or thinning hair, hypersensitivity to extremes of temperature, self-destructive tendencies, and violent propensities. Even though these two people suffer from different diseases, they have a similar pattern of symptoms.

While conventional medicine has focused only on genetically based diseases, homeopathy has included and surpassed this inquiry with more detailed observations of genetic symptoms, syndromes, and tendencies. Homeopaths have developed an elaborate and somewhat complicated theory of chronic diseases called miasms, which are considered the underlying conditions that predispose individuals to the various acute, chronic, and hereditary ailments that they have and that they pass on to their heirs.[13]

Miasms are both genetic and acquired, and they create a susceptibility to certain patterns of symptoms. Because of their different miasms, three people who work together may experience a similar degree of stress but one develops a deep anxiety, another develops an ulcer, and another develops a tumor.

Hahnemann originally developed miasmatic theory after some of his patients received only temporary improvement from his individualized homeopathic prescriptions. He assumed that there was something underlying the person's state of health that was blocking the progress of further healing. Initially, he theorized the presence of three chronic miasms: psora, syphilitic, and sycotic.

The word "psora" is derived from the Hebrew word *tsorat,* which means "groove" or "deficiency." It makes reference to the primary predisposition, a weakened or deficient state that causes the human organism to become susceptible to infection and stress. Because every human has some predisposition to these factors, Hahnemann considered psora to be "the mother of chronic disease."

Laid on top of this miasm are the syphilitic and sycotic miasms. The syphilitic miasm is related to syphilitic infection, not necessarily acquired in this life but from one's genetic heritage. Thus, a person with a syphilitic miasm does not have syphilis, but someone in the family had syphilis and passed on the genetic influence from it.

The sycotic miasm is related to gonorrhea. Once again, people with the sycotic miasm (also called sycosis) do not have gonorrhea, but instead suffer from the influence of someone in their genetic history who had it.

While this theory of chronic disease may initially seem unlikely, present understanding of genetics actually supports the observations of two centuries of homeopaths. It is very real that people in previous centuries had these infectious diseases, and they lived and even procreated while suffering from them. While these diseases are not passed on genetically, it is known and accepted today that viruses can be incorporated into the genetic material of cells. Homeopaths' clinical observations are influenced by the theory that people's genes are affected by the infection of their progenitors.

Later in his life, Hahnemann asserted the existence of a fourth miasm, tuberculosis, though some modern homeopaths theorize that there are considerably more miasms than three or four. They believe that any infection can possibly lead to a miasm. Others go on to theorize that exposure to heavy metals, pesticides, radiation, and various toxic chemicals can also create a layer of illness that adds to the stress load of a person and goes on to influence genetic endowment. It may be that any infection or stress that the organism has not completely resolved creates a layer or miasm which can create present or future symptoms and syndromes.

Each of the above-described miasms leads to a constellation of symptoms that homeopaths consider when prescribing, especially when the traditionally individualized remedy is not working deeply or rapidly enough.

HOMEOPATHIC CONSTITUTIONAL CARE

Various schools of thought in psychology recognize the existence of certain psychological types, and various schools of thought in exercise physiology and in massage and body work therapy theorize the presence of certain body types. In homeopathy people fit certain bodymind types, commonly called "constitutional types." Each constitutional type is referred to by the medicine that fits the body and mind syndrome that it cures. For instance, a person may be a *Sulphur* type, a *Phosphorus* type, or a *Natrum muriaticum* type. Various books describe these bodymind types in ways that are often poetic and quite insightful to the human condition. (See the resources section on page 353 for a list of some of the better books on this subject.)

Homeopathic constitutional care refers to the homeopath's treatment of a person's totality of symptoms, past and present. A prescription of a constitutional medicine is made after a detailed analysis of the person's genetic history, personal health history, body type, and present status of all physical, emotional, and mental symptoms. This approach to homeopathic care is considerably more profound than treating a specific disease.

Homeopathic constitutional care is discussed in this chapter about the healing process because the homeopathic constitutional approach to healing represents a vital and integral part of homeopathic care, and it represents a distinctively different approach than the symptom-specific and disease-specific treatment common in Western medicine and in many alternative therapies as well.

When professionally and competently provided, constitutional care has the capacity to elicit a profound healing response. By strengthening the underlying defense processes of the organism, the correct constitutional medicine can enact a true cure, not just amelioration of symptoms or suppression of disease. The analysis of a true cure is determined not only by the reduction of pain or discomfort but by a systemic improvement in the totality of physical, emotional, and mental health, and a progression of the healing process over time; Hering's guidelines to cure, which were described earlier in this chapter, are carefully reviewed.

Just because a constitutional medicine can provide such profound therapeutic effect does not mean that a homeopath will immediately prescribe it to a patient. Sometimes a less deep-acting medicine is needed beforehand. Without it, a constitutional medicine can cause a healing crisis in which a person experiences a temporary exacerbation of symptoms prior to improvement. Because the homeopaths' ideal of cure is one that is slow and gentle, they try to avoid powerful healing crises.

If a patient is experiencing an acute condition, the homeopath will usually prescribe a remedy for this acute state before prescribing a constitutional remedy. Because acute ailments often have a cleansing and healing effect on people when they are effectively cured, homeopaths prefer prescribing a constitutional remedy shortly after a person has gotten over an acute illness.

If and when the homeopath prescribes what he or she thinks is the person's correct constitutional remedy and it doesn't work, the homeopath then seeks to ascertain if anything has possibly antidoted the remedy (see Chapter 12) or if a miasmatic remedy is indicated.

RESOURCES

Hans Reckeweg, *Homotoxicology*. Albuquerque: Biological Homeopathic Industries, 1981.

Andre Saine, "Hering's Law: Law, Rule or Dogma," *Simillimum*, Winter 1993, 6, 4:34–52.

Rajan Sankaran, *The Spirit of Homeopathy,* Bombay: Homeopathic Medical, 1991.

Dana Ullman, *Discovering Homeopathy*. Berkeley: North Atlantic, 1991.

George Vithoulkas, *A New Model of Health and Disease*. Berkeley: North Atlantic, 1991.

George Vithoulkas, *The Science of Homeopathy*. New York: Grove, 1980.

Andrew Weil, *Spontaneous Healing*. New York: Knopf, 1995.

Some of the better books that describe the homeopathic constitutional types are:

Philip Bailey, *Homeopathic Psychology: Personality Profiles of the Major Constitutional Remedies*. Berkeley: North Atlantic, 1995.

Catherine Coulter, *Portraits of Homeopathic Medicines* (2 volumes). Berkeley: North Atlantic, 1986, 1988.

Paul Herscu, *The Homeopathic Treatment of Children: Pediatric Constitutional Types*. Berkeley: North Atlantic, 1991.

Leon Vannier, *Typology in Homoeopathy*. Beaconsfield (England): Beaconsfield, 1992.

Edward C. Whitmont, *Psyche and Substance: Essays on Homeopathy in the Light of Jungian Psychology*. Berkeley: North Atlantic, 1991.

THREE

The Homeopathic Renaissance

HOMEOPATHY IN NORTH AMERICA, THEN AND NOW

Homeopathy is not widely known throughout the United States, but this lack of awareness is an exception to the rule. Homeopathy is very popular in Europe, especially France, Germany, and England, as well as in Asia, especially India. In fact, it is so popular in other parts of the world that it would be inappropriate to consider homeopathy an "alternative medicine" there.

Many Americans tend to maintain an attitude of medical chauvinism, in which they assume that conventional medicine is the only "true" medical system. This attitude is a historical and geographical anomaly; throughout history and throughout the world there has been a healthy respect for different approaches to healing.

Most Americans don't know that this country has an impressive history of experience with homeopathy, and in fact, at the turn of the century, this medical system was more popular in America than anywhere else in the world. At the time there were twenty-two homeopathic medical schools, over a hundred homeopathic hospitals, and over a thousand homeopathic pharmacies, and at least 15 percent of American physicians practiced homeopathy.[1] The medical schools that taught homeopathy included Boston University, the University of Michigan, New York Medical College, the University of Minnesota, the University of Iowa, Hahnemann Medical College, and Stanford University.

Many of America's literary greats were advocates of homeopathy, including Mark Twain, William James, Louisa May Alcott, Harriet Beecher Stowe, Henry Wadsworth Longfellow, and Henry Thoreau. Homeopathy was particularly popular amongst leading abolitionists such as William Lloyd Garrison and Zabina Eastman; leaders of the women's movement, including Susan B. Anthony and Elizabeth Cady Stanton; presidents, including James Garfield and William McKinley; progressive politicians such as William Seward and Daniel Webster; and successful entrepreneurs, including John D. Rockefeller and William Wrigley.[2]

Because homeopaths graduated from conventional medical schools, they could not be criticized as being uneducated. Homeopaths critiqued conventional medicines for being more dangerous than therapeutic, and they offered a different approach to healing that gave conventional physicians stiff competition. Because of this, homeopaths and homeopathy were frequently attacked by orthodox physicians. The American Medical Association in conjunction with drug manufacturers conspired to commit dirty tricks, political shenanigans, and various and sundry efforts to suppress the development and growth of homeopathy.

From the 1860s until the early 1900s, the AMA's code of ethics specified that it was unethical for AMA members to simply consult with homeopathic physicians on the health care of any patient. Even though most ethical guidelines for doctors were not enforced at that time, having any interaction with a homeopath was one of the few strictly forbidden ethical violations. In 1883 the entire New York State Medical Society was expelled from the AMA because they chose to include in their membership *all* properly graduated doctors, including members who used homeopathic medicines.[3] This incident and innumerable others suggest that the antagonism to homeopathy was based not on scientific issues but on personal ones.

These efforts to suppress homeopathy were not the only factors that ultimately led to its decline. The influence of the Industrial Revolution with its assembly line mind-set and mechanistic thinking gave credence to the conventional medical model. This model sought to treat every person with the same disease in the same way, as distinct

from the homeopathic approach, which was based on highly individualized treatments—an approach that seemed idiosyncratic and in-
consistent. The development of new conventional drugs, initially
painkillers and later antibiotics, gave the public the impression that
conventional medicine could rapidly and directly improve health. The
fact that these drugs also created various side effects or addictive states
wasn't known for many years to come.

Besides these influences, infighting among homeopaths also weakened the movement. Because there are many different ways to practice
homeopathy, some using high-potency medicines, some low potencies, some using frequent and others infrequent repetition, there has
been a tendency among homeopaths (as among virtually every group
of people) to believe that one school of thought is better than another.
It was common for homeopaths of one school of thought to fight
other schools of thought and sometimes to consider the other homeopaths to be "nonhomeopaths."

As a result of the various factors internal and external to the
homeopathic movement, homeopathy almost died out in America.
By 1950, there were only one hundred or so practitioners in the
United States.

In the 1960s, 1970s, and 1980s, the back-to-the-earth movement,
the growing interest in natural foods, the influence of the women's
movement on self-care, and the spiritual revolution led to more interest in alternative healing and homeopathy.

In the 1980s, several major European homeopathic companies established offices in America. Through their efforts to educate consumers and health professionals about homeopathy, along with
increased efforts to market homeopathic medicines into the mainstream, homeopathy began growing more substantially. According to
the Food and Drug Administration, sales of homeopathic medicines
grew by 1,000 percent from the late 1970s to the early 1980s.[4]

In the 1990s, homeopathic medicines have become a $250-million-
per-year industry, with an annual growth rate of 20 to 25 percent.[5] Although the size of this industry is relatively small by most American
standards, its growth rate is considered significant. Homeopathy is no
longer invisible, and it is becoming more mainstream every day. In
1994, more than 75 percent of the chain drugstores sold some homeopathic medicines, with this number expecting to increase. A survey of
American pharmacists discovered that 27 percent consider homeopathic medicines "useful," while only 18 percent consider them "use-

less."[6] While over half of American pharmacists didn't know enough about homeopathy to have an opinion, this survey showed that of those who do know enough about it to have an opinion, many more consider homeopathic medicines beneficial.

There are no formal statistics about the current number of practicing homeopaths in the United States, though it has been estimated that there are 1,000 to 2,000 medical doctors and osteopaths who practice homeopathy, 750 to 1,000 naturopathic physicians, 500 veterinarians, 300 to 500 dentists, and several thousand chiropractors.

Homeopathy in Canada has a slightly higher degree of acceptance. In Canada approximately 70 percent of the sales of homeopathic medicines are in pharmacies, 10 percent in health food stores, and 20 percent by practitioners.[7] In contrast, the vast majority of sales of homeopathic medicines in America are through health food stores, though this is rapidly changing.

The Medical Society of Nova Scotia was the first medical society to establish a "Complementary Medicine Section" as a part of the Canadian Medical Association ("complementary medicine" is a term popularized by Prince Charles as preferred over "alternative medicine"). The recognition of this medical specialty is evidence of a growing respect in the medical community for alternatives, including homeopathy.

Homeopathy is particularly popular among Canadian families. A recent survey in *Pediatrics* discovered that 11 percent of parents in Montreal brought their children to alternative practitioners, and 25 percent of those parents sought the care of a homeopath.[8] Because this survey was conducted in a hospital clinic, these numbers are probably lower than what is actually the case, because some parents who use alternative medicine do not visit such clinics or at least may not do so as often. The survey also showed that parents of these children tended to be better educated than those who did not seek alternative care, and further, that parents who sought out alternatives were more likely to be health professionals themselves. The researchers, who themselves were not partial to alternative health care, had to admit, "[These parents] had more access, more information, they knew more people, and they had a more questioning attitude."

In Mexico, homeopathy is even more popular than it is in the United States or Canada. There are two homeopathic medical schools in Mexico City, one of which typically has eight hundred students enrolled, and there are several postgraduate homeopathic courses for physicians throughout Mexico. Many pharmacies throughout Mexico, especially in the Yucatán peninsula, sell homeopathic remedies alongside conventional drugs.

HOMEOPATHY IN EUROPE

The entire field of complementary medicine is growing by leaps and bounds in Europe. According to a market survey, the field of complementary medicine was second only to the computer industry for growth during the 1980s.[9]

Homeopathy is particularly popular in France, where it is the leading alternative therapy. In 1982, 16 percent of the population used homeopathic medicine, rising to 29 percent in 1987, and to 36 percent in 1992.[10]

Homeopathy is popular not only among the French public but also among the French medical community. As many as 70 percent of physicians are receptive to homeopathy and consider it effective. Homeopathy is taught in at least seven medical schools—Besançon, Bordeaux, Lille, Limoges, Marseilles, Paris-Nord, and Poitiers—and there are numerous postgraduate training programs. Courses in homeopathy are taught in twenty-one of France's twenty-four schools of pharmacy, and also in two dental schools, two veterinary medical schools, and three schools of midwivery.

Homeopathic medicines are fully reimbursed by the national health care system. They are sold in virtually every pharmacy in the country. To get a good sense of the degree to which homeopathy has captured the French public, one can simply take note of the fact that the most popular cold and flu medicine sold in France is a homeopathic remedy, which has a remarkable 50 percent market share.

Earlier this century homeopathy was primarily kept alive in Great Britain as the result of support and patronage from the royal family. During the past decade, however, it has been living, breathing, and growing on its own. Homeopathy is the most popular postgraduate course of any discipline in Great Britain. There are five homeopathic hospitals working within the National Health Service, some of them with a two-year waiting list for nonemergency visits to a homeopath.

The respect accorded homeopathy and homeopathic practice by British physicians is evidenced by a 1986 survey in the *British Medical Journal* which showed that 42 percent of physicians referred patients to homeopathic doctors.[11] Other evidence of support from health professionals was a 1990 survey of British pharmacists which found that 55 percent considered homeopathic medicines "useful," while only 14 percent considered them "useless."[12] The normally conservative British Pharmaceutical Association held a debate in 1992 to decide whether pharmacists should promote homeopathic medicines. They concluded by a large majority that they should.[13]

The field of complementary medicine has gained much support in the 1990s. In 1993 the British Medical Association published a book entitled *Complementary Medicine: New Approaches to Good Practice*.[14] Britain's health minister, Dr. Brian Mawhinney, recently stated, "Complementary medicine has generally proved popular with patients, and a recent survey found that 81 percent of patients are satisfied with the treatment they received."[15] Another health minister stated that 80 percent of general practitioners want training in complementary therapies; 75 percent now refer patients to complementary therapists.

Of special interest was a survey of general practitioners which showed that over 30 percent have already received some training in complementary therapies, with 15 to 42 percent wanting further training,[16] and 80 percent of the younger physicians wanting such training.[17]

The German people are so supportive of complementary medicine that the German government mandated that all medical school curricula include information about complementary medicines. Approximately 10 percent of German doctors specialize in homeopathy, with approximately 10 percent more prescribing homeopathic remedies on occasion. In Germany there are eleven thousand natural health practitioners, called *Heilpraktiker,* three thousand of whom specialize in homeopathy.[18]

Sales of homeopathic medicines in Germany were approximately $428 million in 1991, growing at a rate of about 10 percent per year. Evidence of the significant support from the German medical community is the fact that 85 percent of these sales are prescriptions from physicians. Surveys indicate that 98 percent of pharmacies sell homeopathic medicines.

Other European countries in which homeopathy has a relatively strong presence include Switzerland, where different surveys have suggested that somewhere between 11 and 27 percent of general practitioners and internists prescribe homeopathic medicines; Italy, where 9

percent of medical doctors prescribe homeopathic remedies sometimes; and the Netherlands, where 45 percent of physicians consider
homeopathic medicines effective and 47 percent of medical doctors
use one or more complementary therapies, with homeopathy (40 percent of these select doctors) being the most popular.[19]

When the Iron Curtain was up, Hungary, Czechoslovakia, and
East Germany banned homeopathy, but this medical iron curtain fell
with communism. Homeopathy holds a unique place in Russia,
where it has been widely accepted, but is not sanctioned by the state
medical bureaucracy. Thus, homeopathic care is not free and has been
a part of the new Russian economy where fees are paid for health
services. Demand for homeopathic care is so great that Russians prefer to pay for homeopathic care than to receive free conventional
medical care.

Some skeptics have asserted that homeopathy and natural medicines are becoming increasingly popular in Russia because "real
medicine" is either unavailable or too expensive.[20] However, this assumption has been disproven, because the trend toward homeopathic
and natural medicine is particularly popular among those Russians
who are more educated and are in higher economic classes. Journalists
and skeptics tend to assume that homeopathic medicines simply do
not work, and thus they create fanciful theories about why the use of
homeopathy is increasing.

In Hungary, homeopathic literature was banned for forty years
until 1990. Homeopathy has now been accepted and integrated into
regular medical education and is taught in two medical schools. The
Hungarian Homeopathic Medical Association started with 11 members in 1990, grew to 75 after eighteen months, and grew further to
302 members in 1994.

After the fall of communism in Czechoslovakia, a homeopathic
organization in the Czech Republic was established in November
1990, and it was immediately accepted and integrated within the
larger, conventional medical society. Within a year, the Ministry of
Health officially recognized homeopathy as a medical specialty.

The last homeopathic pharmacy in Slovakia was closed in 1964,
and the last homeopathic physician died in 1967. And yet, by 1993,
the homeopathic medical organization in this country already had
800 members.[21]

Homeopathy Throughout the World

Although homeopathy is quite popular throughout Europe, it is considerably more so in India, where there are over 120 four- and five-year homeopathic colleges, and over 100,000 homeopathic doctors. Acknowledging the widespread popularity of homeopathy, a World Health Organization publication noted that "in the Indian subcontinent the legal position of the practitioners of homeopathy has been elevated to a professional level similar to that of a medical practitioner."[22]

The *Jerusalem Post* stated that training programs in Israel for complementary therapies are "sprouting like mushrooms after rain."[23] Homeopathy is being practiced in small medical clinics throughout Israel as well as in large hospitals such as Hadassah in Jerusalem. Because of the growing interest, a government commission spent three years reviewing the issue, and its report encouraged liberalization of medicine, allowing non-M.D.s to treat patients. However, the report created a hostile reaction from the Israel Medical Association, and as a result, the Israeli health ministry has shelved the report.

Homeopathy is relatively popular in South America, with its greatest popularity in Brazil and Argentina. It is formally recognized by the Brazilian government, and there are a dozen or so training programs for physicians. Homeopathy in Argentina is tolerated but not officially recognized, even though approximately 10 percent of the population uses these natural medicines. Because San Martín, the "George Washington of Argentina," who liberated Argentina from Spain, was an advocate of homeopathy, many of the country's citizens have a special appreciation for this medical system.

Homeopathy is experiencing a worldwide renaissance. Interest in homeopathy by both consumers and health professionals is growing at a significant rate, and there is no sign of this interest leveling off or slowing. It is now time for governmental bodies to begin listening to the needs and interests of people involved in homeopathy so that laws do not thwart the growth of this safe and effective system of natural medicine. It is now time for all health professionals, even those who may not be interested in practicing homeopathy, to at least learn something about it so that they can refer appropriate patients to homeopathic specialists.

With increasing numbers of people wanting to take a greater role in their own health and increasing numbers of people recognizing the limitations of conventional medicine, homeopathy will continue to grow. Homeopathy cannot cure everyone or everything, but its capacity to provide safe, effective, and cost-effective health care will lead to its playing an important role in health care in the nineties and in the twenty-first century.

FOUR

Scientific Evidence for Homeopathic Medicine

Most people who purchase this book will have no doubt that homeopathy works, though inevitably they will have some family members, friends, neighbors, and physicians who will be skeptical about it. One way to deal with these people's skepticism is to become familiar with research on the efficacy of homeopathic medicines (see also Chapter 5 for a discussion on how to respond to skeptics' remarks). There is actually considerably more laboratory and clinical research on homeopathic medicine than most people realize. That said, it must also be recognized that more research is certainly needed, not simply to answer the questions of skeptics but to help homeopaths optimize their use of these powerful natural medicines.

Some skeptics insist that research on homeopathy is mandatory since the exceptionally small doses used do not make sense and there is no known mechanism for action for these drugs. While it is true that homeopaths presently do not know precisely how the homeopathic microdoses work, there are some compelling theories about their mechanism of action (see the discussion in Chapter 1, "The Wisdom and Wonder of Small Doses," page 11). More important, there is compelling evidence that they do work, as this chapter will show. And although homeopaths may not understand how their medicines work, keep in mind that leading contemporary pharmacologists readily acknowledge that there are many commonly prescribed drugs today whose mechanism of action is partially or significantly not understood, but this gap in knowledge has yet to stop physicians from prescribing them.

Many conventional physicians express doubt about the efficacy of homeopathy, asserting that they will "believe it when they see it." It may be more appropriate for them to acknowledge that they will "see it when they will believe it." This is not meant as a criticism of conventional physicians as much as of conventional medical thinking. The biomedical paradigm has narrowed the view of, the thinking about, and the practice of medicine to the treatment of specific disease entities with supposedly symptom-specific drugs and procedures. An integral aspect of this approach to medicine is the assumption that the larger the dose of a drug, the stronger will be its effects. While this seems to make sense on the surface, knowledgeable physicians and pharmacologists know that it isn't true. There is a recognized principle in pharmacology called the biphasic response of drugs.[1] Rather than a drug simply having increased effects as its dose becomes larger, research has consistently shown that exceedingly small doses of a substance will have the opposite effects of large doses.

The two phases of a drug's action (thus the name "biphasic") are dose-dependent. For instance, it is widely recognized that normal medical doses of atropine block the parasympathetic nerves, causing mucous membranes to dry up, while exceedingly small doses of atropine cause *increased* secretions to mucous membranes.

This pharmacological principle was concurrently discovered in the 1870s by two separate researchers, Hugo Schulz, a conventional scientist, and Rudolf Arndt, a psychiatrist and homeopath. Initially called the Arndt-Schulz law, this principle is still widely recognized, as witnessed by the fact that it is commonly listed in medical dictionaries under the definition of "law."

More specifically, these researchers discovered that weak stimuli accelerate physiological activity, medium stimuli inhibit physiological activity, and strong stimuli halt physiological activity. For example, very weak concentrations of iodine, bromine, mercuric chloride, and arsenious acid will stimulate yeast growth, medium doses of these substances will inhibit yeast growth, and large doses will kill the yeast.

In the 1920s, conventional scientists who tested and verified this biphasic response termed the phenomenon "hormesis," and dozens of studies were published in a wide variety of fields to confirm this biological principle.[2]

In the past two decades there has again been a resurgence of interest in this pharmacological law, and now hundreds of studies in numerous areas of scientific investigation have verified it.[3] Because these studies have been performed by conventional scientists who are typically unfamiliar with homeopathic medicine, they have not tested or even considered testing the ultrahigh dilutions commonly used in homeopathy. However, their research has consistently shown very significant effects from such small microdoses that even the researchers express confusion and surprise.

Reference to this research on the Arndt-Schulz law and hormesis is important for validating homeopathic research because it demonstrates the evidence for the important biphasic responses and microdose effects that lie at the heart of homeopathy. This research is readily available to physicians and scientists yet is often ignored or not understood.

The amount of research on homeopathic medicines is growing, and it is becoming increasingly difficult to ignore these studies, because they are now appearing in many of the most respected medical and scientific journals in the world. This chapter is not meant to be exhaustive (that would require a book or two of its own). It will include many of the best studies, most of which have been published in conventional medical and scientific journals. Some of the studies are discussed because of the impressive results they showed, and others are included for their implications for better understanding homeopathy and the healing process. The review of research is not simply to provide evidence of the efficacy of homeopathic medicine but also to enlighten readers on how to evaluate homeopathic research, whether positive or negative results are obtained.

To best understand the remaining part of this chapter, some definitions are helpful: *Double-blind trials* refer to experiments in which neither the experimenter nor the subjects know whether a specific treatment was prescribed or a placebo (a "fake" medicine that looks and tastes like a homeopathic medicine). *Randomized trials* are those in which subjects of an experiment are randomly placed either in treatment groups or in placebo groups. The researchers attempt to place people with similar characteristics in equal numbers in treatment and in placebo groups. *Crossover studies* refer to experiments in which half of the subjects of a study are given a placebo during one phase of a study and then given the active treatment during the second phase, while the other half begin with the active treatment and then receive the placebo during the second phase. Crossover studies sometimes do not test a placebo and instead compare one type of treatment with another type of treatment.

Modern research is designed to evaluate the results of a therapy as compared to a placebo and/or another therapy. This type of study is valuable because many patients respond very well to placebos, and this "treatment" is so safe and inexpensive it is generally assumed that "real treatments" should have considerably better results than placebo medicine. One should note that placebo effects can be significant, and clinically, these effects can be very positive (some people think of them as a type of self-healing).

Double-blinding an experiment is important to research because experimenters tend to treat people who are getting the real treatment differently or better than those given a placebo, thus throwing off the results of the experiment. Research is randomized so that those people treated with the real medicine and those treated with the placebo are as similar as possible, making a comparison between real treatment and placebo treatment more accurate. Crossover studies allow researchers to compare the separate effects of a placebo and a treatment on all subjects in an experiment.

Statistics obviously are an important part of research. A treatment is thought to be considered better than a placebo if the results, according to statistical analysis, have no more than a 5 percent possibility of happening at random (the notation of this statistical probability is: $P = .05$). A study with a small number of patients (for example, thirty or less) must show a large difference between treatment and nontreatment groups for it to become statistically significant. A study with a large number of patients (for example, several hundred) needs to have only a small but consistent difference to obtain a similar statistical significance. This information is provided so that readers will know that all the studies described in this chapter are statistically significant, except when otherwise noted.

CLINICAL RESEARCH

People are often confused by research, not only because it can be overly technical but because some studies show that a therapy works and other studies shows that it doesn't. To solve this problem, a recent development in research is used, called a meta-analysis, which is a systematic review of a body of research that evaluates the overall results of experiments.

In 1991, three professors of medicine from the Netherlands, none of them homeopaths, performed a meta-analysis of twenty-five years of clinical studies using homeopathic medicines and published their results in the *British Medical Journal*.[4] This meta-analysis covered 107 controlled trials, of which 81 showed that homeopathic medicines were effective, 24 showed they were ineffective, and 2 were inconclusive.

The professors concluded, "The amount of positive results came as a surprise to us." Specifically, they found that:

- 13 of 19 trials showed successful treatment of respiratory infections,
- 6 of 7 trials showed positive results in treating other infections,
- 5 of 7 trials showed improvement in diseases of the digestive system,
- 5 of 5 showed successful treatment of hay fever,
- 5 of 7 showed faster recovery after abdominal surgery,
- 4 of 6 promoted healing in rheumatological disease,
- 18 of 20 showed benefit in addressing pain or trauma,
- 8 of 10 showed positive results in relieving mental or psychological problems, and
- 13 of 15 showed benefit from miscellaneous diagnoses.

Despite the high percentage of studies that provided evidence of success with homeopathic medicine, most of these studies were flawed in some way or another. Still, the researchers found 22 high-caliber studies, 15 of which showed that homeopathic medicines were effective. Of further interest, they found that 11 of the best 15 studies showed efficacy of these natural medicines, suggesting that the better the designed and performed the studies were, the higher the likelihood that the medicines were found to be effective. (Although people unfamiliar with research may be surprised to learn that most of the studies on homeopathy were flawed in one significant way or another,[5] research in conventional medicine during the past twenty-five years has had a similar percentage of flawed studies.)

With this knowledge, the researchers of the meta-analysis on homeopathy concluded, "The evidence presented in this review would probably be sufficient for establishing homeopathy as a regular treatment for certain indications."

There are different types of homeopathic clinical research, some of which provide individualization of remedies—which is the hallmark of the homeopathic methodology—some of which give a commonly prescribed remedy to all people with a similar ailment, and some of which give a combination of homeopathic medicines to people with a similar condition. While one can perform good research using any of these methods, there are certain issues that researchers have to be aware of and sensitive to in order to obtain the best objective results.

For instance, if a study does not individualize a homeopathic medicine to people suffering from a specific ailment and the results of the study show that there was no difference between those given this remedy and those given a placebo, the study does not disprove homeopathy; it simply proves that this one remedy is not effective in treating every person suffering from that ailment, each of whom may have a unique pattern of symptoms that requires an individual prescription.

In describing specifics of the following studies using homeopathic medicines, differentiation has been made between studies that allowed for individualization of medicines and those that did not.

Clinical Research with Individualized Care

Some people incorrectly assume that research using homeopathic medicines is impossibly complicated because each medicine must be individualized to the patient. The following studies disprove this simplistic belief.

A recent clinical trial evaluating homeopathic medicine was a unique study of the treatment of asthma.[6] Researchers at the University of Glasgow used conventional allergy testing to discover which substances these asthma patients were most allergic to. Once this was determined, the subjects were randomized into treatment and placebo groups. Those patients chosen for treatment were given the 30c potency of the substance to which they were most allergic (the most common substance was house dust mite). The researchers called this unique method of individualizing remedies "homeopathic immuno-therapy" (homeopathic medicines are usually prescribed based on the patient's idiosyncratic symptoms, not on laboratory analysis or diagnostic categories). Subjects in this experiment were evaluated by both homeopathic and conventional physicians.

This study showed that 82 percent of the patients given a homeopathic medicine improved, while only 38 percent of patients given a placebo experienced a similar degree of relief. When asked if they felt the patient received the homeopathic medicine or the placebo, both the patients and the doctors tended to guess correctly.

The experiment was relatively small, with only 24 patients. As noted, for statistically significant results, small experiments must show a large difference between those treated with a medicine and those given a placebo. Such was the case in this study.

Along with this recent asthma study, the authors performed a meta-analysis reviewing all the data from three studies they performed on allergic conditions, which totaled 202 subjects. The researchers found a similar pattern in the three studies. Improvement began within the first week and continued through to the end of the trial four weeks later. The result of this meta-analysis were so substantial (P = .0004) that the authors concluded that either homeopathic medicines work or controlled clinical trials do not. Because modern science is based on controlled clinical trials, it is a more likely conclusion that homeopathic medicines are effective.

Another recent study, published in the American journal *Pediatrics*, tested homeopathic medicine for the treatment of a condition recognized to be the most serious public health problem today, childhood diarrhea.[7] Over 5 million children die each year as the result of diarrhea, mostly in nonindustrialized countries. Conventional physicians prescribe oral rehydration therapy (ORT, a salt solution that helps children maintain fluid balance), but this treatment does not fight the infection that underlies the diarrhea.

Conducted in Nicaragua in association with the University of Washington and the University of Guadalajara, this randomized double-blind, placebo-controlled study of 81 children showed that an individually chosen remedy provided statistically significant improvement of the children's diarrhea as compared to a placebo. Children given the homeopathic remedy were cured of their infection 20 percent faster than those given a placebo, and the sicker children responded most dramatically to the homeopathic treatment. A total of eighteen different remedies were used in this trial, individually chosen based on each child's symptoms.

A study of the homeopathic treatment of migraine headache was conducted in Italy.[8] Sixty patients were randomized and entered into a double-blind, placebo-controlled trial. Patients regularly filled out a questionnaire on the frequency, intensity, and characteristics of their head pain. They were prescribed a single dose of a 30c remedy at four separate times over two-week intervals. Eight remedies were considered, and prescribers were allowed to use any two with a patient. While only 17 percent of patients given a placebo experienced relief of their migraine pain, an impressive 93 percent of patients given an individualized homeopathic medicine experienced good results.

A randomized double-blind, placebo-controlled trial was performed on 175 Dutch children suffering from recurrent upper-respiratory-tract infections.[9] Children in the treatment group were prescribed a constitutional medicine for their overall health as well as acute medicines to treat the acute respiratory infections they developed. The study found that the children given homeopathic medicines had a 16 percent better daily symptom score than children given a placebo.

This study also found that the number of children given a placebo who had to undergo adenoidectomy was 24 percent higher than for the children given homeopathic remedies. A 54.8 percent reduction in the use of antibiotics in the children given homeopathic medicines was reported, while the children who received a placebo experienced a 37.7 percent reduction in antibiotic use. (This reduction in both groups was determined to be the result of the normal growth and development of the child, dietary changes—the study provided written nutritional advice to the parents—and the change in expectations as the result of being under medical care.)

The statistical possibility of these results happening by chance was 6 percent ($P = .06$). Because statistical significance in science is recognized when there is a 5 percent or less chance of results happening at random, the researchers concluded that homeopathic medicine seems to add little to the treatment of upper-respiratory-tract infections. This more conservative conclusion appeared to be influenced by the fact that the authors sought and received publication of their study in the *British Medical Journal*. They should have more accurately said that homeopathic medicines provided benefit to children with upper respiratory infections, but there is a small chance (6 percent) that these good results happened at random.

Considering the closeness of these results to 5 percent, considering the other improvements in the homeopathic group's health, and considering the increasingly widespread desire to avoid antibiotics, it makes sense for physicians and parents to consider seeking homeopathic care for children's upper respiratory infections.

Another study that involved individualized homeopathic care was in the treatment of rheumatoid arthritis.[10] The study involved 46 patients. Two homeopathic physicians prescribed individually chosen medicines to each patient, though only half of them were given the real remedy, while the other half were given a placebo. The study found that 82 percent of those given an individualized homeopathic remedy experienced some relief of symptoms, while 21 percent of those given a placebo experienced a similar degree of relief.

One other very interesting trial that utilized semi-individualization of care was in the treatment of primary fibromyalgia (also called fibrositis).[11] Patients with fibrositis were admitted into a trial in which homeopathic physicians chose between three possible remedies, *Arnica, Rhus tox,* and *Bryonia.* Half of the patients were given one of these remedies, and the other half were given a placebo. There was no discernible difference between these groups. However, as an integral part of the experiment's design, a panel of homeopaths evaluated the accuracy of each prescription. This analysis found that those patients whom the panel considered to have received the correct remedy experienced a statistically significant improvement in symptoms as compared to those patients given the "incorrect" remedy or the placebo.

These same researchers next conducted a more sophisticated trial in the treatment of primary fibromyalgia.[12] This double-blind, placebo-controlled, crossover trial admitted only those patients who fit the symptoms of *Rhus tox.* The researchers found that this constituted 42 percent of the patients interviewed. One half of these 30 patients were given *Rhus tox 6c* during the first phase of the experiment, while the other half were given a placebo. During the second phase, those patients initially given the medicine were given a placebo, and those patients initially given a placebo were now given the homeopathic remedy. Researchers determined at the beginning of the experiment that improvement in pain and sleeplessness were the outcome measures most important in evaluating the results of this trial, and the results showed that 25 percent more of the patients experienced pain relief when taking the homeopathic remedy compared to when they were given a placebo and almost twice as many had improved sleep when taking the remedy.

This type of crossover design is considered a sophisticated type of research because it compares each person when using a treatment with the same person when using a placebo. Most other research compares two supposedly similar groups of people, but researchers commonly acknowledge that it is difficult and perhaps impossible to get two exactly similar groups of people. The limitation of the crossover design for homeopathic treatment, however, is that most homeopathic medicines provide long-term benefits, so that once a person stops taking a homeopathic remedy he or she may still continue to improve, even in the placebo stage of the trial. Low-potency medicines, such as the 6c used in the above-described experiment, generally have short-acting effects, while higher-potency medicines generally have increasingly longer-term effects.

Clinical Research with Nonindividualized Care

In addition to the studies on homeopathy in which individualized remedies are prescribed, there is also a body of research testing single remedies to people given in a nonindividualized manner. Such research is potentially problematic because homeopaths acknowledge that the remedies require some degree of individualization to be effective. The results of a nonindividualized study, either positive or negative, can be misunderstood by people who do not know basic principles of the homeopathic method.

One study using nonindividualized homeopathic treatment was sponsored by the British government during World War II and was conducted in 1941–42 on volunteers whose skin was burned with mustard gas.[13] The study showed the efficacy of *Mustard gas 30c* as a preventive or *Rhus tox 30c* and *Kali bichromicum 30c* as therapy. The study was double-blind, placebo-controlled, and was conducted at two centers (London and Glasgow), both showing similarly positive results. A more recent analysis of the data further substantiated the statistical significance of this study.[14]

It should, however, be mentioned that the researchers also tested the efficacy of *Opium 30c, Cantharis 30c,* and *Variolinium 30c,* none of which provided any noticeable benefit. If this trial had tested only these medicines, the researchers might have concluded that homeopathic medicines were ineffective in treating mustard gas burns. Finding the correct remedy is the key to making homeopathy work.

Some skeptics and journalists inaccurately report that homeopathy is primarily used to treat minor health problems. Homeopaths today primarily treat various chronic ailments for which conventional medicine has not provided effective treatment. One example of a chronic and serious problem shown by a controlled study to be effectively treated by homeopathy is diabetic retinitis[15] (retinitis is a common complication of diabetes in which there is an inflammation of the retina causing impairment of sight, perversion of vision, swelling, discharge from the eye, and sometimes hemorrhages into the retina). This double-blind, randomized, placebo–controlled study on 60 patients used *Arnica 5c.* The results of the study showed that 47 percent of patients given *Arnica 5c* experienced improvement in central blood flow to the eye, while only 1 percent of patients given the placebo experienced this improvement. Further, 52 percent of patients given *Arnica 5c* experienced improvement in blood flow to other parts of the eye, while only 1.5 percent of those given the placebo experienced a similar degree of improvement.

The best-selling flu remedy in France is actually a homeopathic medicine. *Anas barbariae 200c,* commonly marketed under the trade name *Oscillococcinum,* is also popular in the United States and is effective primarily at the first signs of influenza. A double-blind, placebo-controlled study with 478 patients suffering from influenza was conducted, making this the largest trial yet performed testing a homeopathic medicine.[16] This trial showed that almost twice as many people who took the homeopathic remedy got over the flu after forty-eight hours as compared to those given a placebo.

Although this remedy was found to work for all age groups, it was considerably more effective for people under thirty than for those over thirty. However, it was not found to be effective when subjects had severe flu symptoms. In severe cases of the flu, a more individualized homeopathic remedy may be indicated.

In addition to various studies on human health, there have also been some animal studies. British researchers have conducted trials showing that homeopathic medicines, specifically *Caulophyllum 30c,* could lower the rate of stillbirths in pigs.[17] Pigs given a placebo had 103 births and 27 stillbirths (20.8 percent), while those given *Caulophyllum 30c* had 104 births and 12 stillbirths (10.3 percent).

Not all studies show efficacy of homeopathic medicines, not because they don't work but mostly because the studies were poorly designed. One such study tested a single homeopathic medicine in the treatment of osteoarthritis.[18] This study consisted of 36 patients, of whom one third were given *Rhus tox 6c,* one third were given a conventional drug (fenoprofen, a nonsteroidal anti-inflammatory drug), and one third were given a placebo. Those patients given the conventional drug experienced some relief of symptoms, but those given the homeopathic remedy and the placebo had a similar lack of response to treatment. While some people would erroneously conclude that homeopathic medicines are ineffective in the treatment of osteoarthritis, it would be more appropriate and accurate to conclude that *Rhus tox 6c* is an ineffective remedy when given without individualization to people with osteoarthritis.

One of the confounding variables from this trial was that 2 of the 12 patients given the homeopathic medicine were withdrawn from the trial because they experienced an aggravation of symptoms after taking the medicine. Because homeopathic medicines sometimes cause a temporary increase in chronic symptoms before significant improvement, it was disappointing that the researchers did not follow their status. Because this trial lasted only two weeks, it did not allow time for the homeopathic remedy to be adequately evaluated. If, for instance, these 2 patients experienced the significant relief that is common after an initial aggravation of symptoms, the results of the trial would have been different.

Further, it is unfair to compare a fast-acting conventional drug that has side effects with a slower-acting homeopathic medicine that is considerably safer. Finally and of great significance is the fact that while *Rhus tox* is a common remedy for rheumatoid arthritis, it is less common for osteoarthritis.

Clinical Research with Homeopathic Combination Remedies

Homeopathic combination remedies are formulas in which several homeopathic substances are mixed together into one remedy. This untraditional approach to using homeopathic medicine is commercially popular in many countries. While these remedies are not thought by homeopaths to be as effective as individually chosen medicines, they do work and research has verified this. Yet homeopaths consistently find that single homeopathic medicines have the potential to truly cure a person's disease, while combination medicines at best provide safe but temporary relief of symptoms.

The same researchers who conducted the study on asthma described earlier also performed a study on the treatment of hay fever.[19] This double-blind, placebo-controlled study prescribed a 30c potency of a combination remedy made from twelve common pollens. The results showed that those subjects taking the homeopathic remedy had six times fewer symptoms than those given the placebo. Both groups of subjects were allowed to use an "escape" medicine (an antihistamine) if their remedy didn't work adequately. The study showed that homeopathic subjects needed this medicine half as often as did those given the placebo.

Another example of significant results from a homeopathic combination remedy was in the treatment of women in their ninth month of pregnancy.[20] Ninety women were given the 5c potency of the following remedies: *Caulophyllum, Arnica, Cimicifuga, Pulsatilla,* and *Gelsemium.* They were given doses of this combination remedy twice daily during the ninth month. This double-blind, placebo-controlled study showed that women given the homeopathic medicines experienced a 40 percent (!) shorter labor than those given a placebo. Also, the women given the placebo had four times (!) as many complications of labor as those given the homeopathic medicines.

One of the limitations of research on combination remedies is that the results do not reveal whether the effective treatment came from one specific medicine or from the unique combination of remedies. A recent study of 22 healthy women in their first pregnancies tested *Caulophyllum,* one of the medicines used in the study cited above, which was administered in the 7c potency during the active phase of labor (one dose per hour repeated for a maximum of four hours). The time of labor for those women given the homeopathic medicine was 38 percent shorter than for women given a placebo.[21] This trial was not double-blind; however, the researchers recently completed a double-blind trial and confirmed their earlier results.[22]

A popular homeopathic external application marketed as *Traumeel* has been studied for its efficacy in the treatment of sprained ankles.[23] This combination of fourteen remedies in 2x to 6x potencies was given to subjects with sprained ankles. After ten days, 24 of the 33 patients who were given the homeopathic medicine were pain-free, while 13 of 36 patients given a placebo experienced a similar degree of relief. This same medicine was also used in the treatment of traumatic hemarthrosis (joint swelling) and was shown to significantly reduce healing time as compared to a placebo. Objective measurements of joint swelling and movement and evaluation of the synovial fluid at injury were assessed.[24]

A study of 61 patients with varicose veins was performed double-blind and placebo-controlled.[25] Three doses of a popular German combination of eight homeopathic medicines were given daily for twenty-four days. Measures were venous filling time, leg volume, and subjective symptoms. The study found that venous filling time improved in those given the homeopathic medicines by 44 percent, while it deteriorated in the placebo group by 18 percent. Other measures also had significant differences.

In addition to the various clinical studies on humans, there has also been some research using homeopathic medicines to improve the health of animals. German researchers have shown that dairy cows given *Sepia 200c* experienced significantly fewer complications of birth than those given a placebo.[26] Low-potency (1x to 6x) combinations of *Lachesis, Pulsatilla,* and *Sabina,* or *Lachesis, Echinacea,* and *Pyrogenium,* along with *Caulophyllum,* given to pigs had preventive and therapeutic effects on infections (inflammation of the breasts and the uterus) as well as on diarrhea in the piglets.[27]

Not all clinical studies on homeopathic combination medicines find efficacy of treatment, but there are often important factors that explain the failure. A Canadian study on the treatment of plantar warts is one such example.[28] This randomized double-blind, placebo-controlled trial with 162 patients prescribed three medicines to each patient. (Because the trial did not mix the remedies together, it is not completely accurate to call the use of these remedies a combination. It is more precise to consider its polypharmacy, the use of several medicines.) The remedies used were *Thuja 30c, Antimonium crud 7c,* and *Nitric acid 7c. Thuja* was taken once a week, and the other two remedies were taken once a day. The trial lasted six weeks. The results showed that there was no noticeable difference between those subjects given the homeopathic medicines and those given a placebo.

Many homeopaths may be initially surprised at the result of this trial because they consider these remedies commonly effective in the treatment of warts. But while the remedies may be effective for treating warts, they are not necessarily effective for *all* types of warts or in *all* people. A recent study of homeopathic treatment for various types of warts found that 18 of 19 people with plantar warts were cured, on average, in 2.2 months.[29] The most common remedy was *Ruta,* prescribed to 12 of the 19 patients. *Thuja* was prescribed for only 3 patients, and *Antimonium crud* was prescribed for 2 patients.

This study teaches us that individualization and the use of well-chosen remedies are necessary for most effective treatment.

One additional note about research using homeopathic combination medicines: The homeopathic literature refers to the fact that some remedies are antidoted by other remedies. While the medicines in the Canadian trial are not known to antidote each other, homeopaths acknowledge that our understanding of which remedies antidote each other is somewhat primitive (for a listing of which remedies antidote each other, see the appendix in Kent's *Repertory* or in the Indian edition of Boericke's *Pocket Manual of Materia Medica with Repertory,* noted in bibliography, page 360). Homeopathic research must, therefore, be aware of this possibility so that conclusions from research are not overstated.

LABORATORY RESEARCH

As valuable as clinical studies are, laboratory research is able to show biological activity of homeopathic medicines that cannot be explained as a placebo response, a common accusation of skeptics. Laboratory research is also capable of shedding some light on how the homeopathic medicines may work.

Distinct from clinical research which seeks to measure improvement in the health of a person or an animal, laboratory research seeks to assess changes in biological systems (cells, tissues, organs, viruses, etc.). Typically, animal research can fit under either clinical or laboratory research, depending on the goal of the study. If the study seeks to test the efficacy of a treatment on the health of an animal, it can be considered an animal clinical study. If the study seeks to test the effects of a treatment on animals so that researchers can apply the information for human health or to understand biological phenomena, it can be considered a laboratory study.

Admittedly, while some of the animal studies discussed here are humane, others are not. Reference to these studies is not meant to suggest that this author condones all such research. Rather, discussion of these studies is intended to verify the benefits of homeopathic medicines, both to animals and to humans, and to encourage wider use of homeopathic remedies.

Some of this section is somewhat technical, though an effort has been made to describe the studies in a user-friendly manner.

Earlier in this chapter, reference was made to some important double-blind clinical research with homeopathic medicines conducted as far back as 1941. There were also some high-quality scientific laboratory studies investigating homeopathic microdoses at that time. One extensive and meticulously controlled study was performed in 1941–42 by a Scottish homeopath/scientist, W. E. Boyd.[30] This work showed that microdoses of mercuric chloride had statistically significant effects of diastase activity (diastase is an enzyme produced during the germination of seeds). This research was so well designed and performed that an associate dean of an American medical school commented, "The precision of [Boyd's] technique exemplifies a scientific study at its highest level."[31]

There have been over a hundred studies evaluating the prophylactic and therapeutic effects of homeopathic doses of normally toxic substances. A collaborative effort of scientists from German research institutions and from America's Walter Reed Hospital performed a meta-analysis of these studies.[32] Like the meta-analysis described earlier on clinical trials using homeopathic medicines, most of the studies were flawed in some way. However, of the high-quality studies, positive results were found 50 percent more often than negative results. What was particularly intriguing was that researchers who tested doses in the submolecular range (potencies greater than 24x) were found to have the best-designed studies and more frequently found statistically significant results from these microdoses.

Specifically, several researchers gave, usually to rats, crude doses of arsenic, bismuth, cadmium, mercury chloride, or lead. The research showed that animals who were pretreated with homeopathic doses of these substances and then given repeated homeopathic doses after exposure to the crude substance, excreted more of these toxic substances through urine, feces, and sweat than did those animals given a placebo.

Several studies noted that pretreatment and treatment with potentized doses of substances different from those to which the animal was being exposed did not provide any benefit.

As horrible as this research may be for the animals tested, animal researchers claim that it can have considerable benefit for treating animals and humans exposed to toxic substances. Such studies cannot be performed humanely on human subjects, and because of the newness of the research, no computer models to simulate the effects of homeopathic medicines are presently possible. While public health measures must primarily focus on preventing exposure to toxic substances, medical treatment must be developed for healing if and when exposure takes place. The research suggests that homeopathic medicine may play a significant role in the treatment of toxicological exposure.

Homeopathic research has also explored the benefits of homeopathic medicines to protect against radiation.[33] Albino mice were exposed to 100 to 200 rad of X-rays (sublethal doses) and then evaluated after twenty-four, forty-eight, and seventy-two hours. *Ginseng 6x, 30x,* and *200x* and *Ruta graveolens 30x* and *200x* were administered before and after exposure. When compared with mice given a placebo as treatment, mice given any of the above homeopathic medicines experienced significantly less chromosomal or cellular damage.

Albino guinea pigs were exposed to small doses of X-ray that cause reddening of the skin. Studies showed that *Apis mellifica 7c* or *9c* had a protective effect and a roughly 50 percent curative effect on X-ray–induced redness of the skin.[34] *Apis mellifica* (honeybee) is a homeopathic medicine for redness, swelling, and itching, common symptoms of bee venom.

In one very intriguing study, *Thyroxine 30x* (thyroid hormone) was placed in the water of tadpoles.[35] When compared to tadpoles who were given a placebo, the study showed, morphogenesis of the tadpoles into frogs was slowed for those who were exposed to the homeopathic doses. Because thyroid hormone in crude doses is known to speed up morphogenesis, it makes sense from a homeopathic perspective that homeopathic doses would slow it down.

What makes this study more interesting is that additional investigations resulted in the same effect when a glass bottle of the homeopathic doses of thyroid hormone was simply suspended in the water with the lip of the bottle above the water line. This research was replicated at several laboratories, and results were consistent.

The implications of this study are somewhat significant, not only for verifying biological effects of homeopathic doses but for showing that these medicines have some type of radiational effect through glass. Some types of unconventional approaches to homeopathy have been developed over the past decades in which pupil reflex, pulse, muscle strength, and skin conductance have been changed as the result of simply holding on to a bottle of an individually indicated homeopathic medicine. While this approach may seem strange to classically oriented homeopaths, the above research provides some basis for its application.

One other interesting experiment dealing with water is worthy of mention. This study used nuclear magnetic resonance (NMR), also called magnetic resonance imaging (MRI), to determine whether high potencies of homeopathic medicines placed in water had any measurable effects.[36] Without getting into the details of this highly technical study, the researchers found that high potencies of *Silicea* did, in fact, show a distinct difference as compared with placebo-treated water.

There have been several studies investigating very high dilutions of histamine (above 30x) on isolated guinea pig hearts, showing that this remedy increases blood flow through the heart. What is particularly interesting about these studies was that this effect was completely neutralized if the very high dilutions were exposed to 70 degrees Centigrade for thirty minutes or exposed to magnetic fields of 50 Hz for fifteen minutes.[37]

Needless to say, it is unlikely that these microdoses could have only a placebo effect when known physical stresses to the medicine can halt its activity.

A professor of hematology at the School of Pharmacy of Bordeaux has carried out eight years of research on the effects of acetylsalicylic acid (the active ingredient in aspirin) on blood.[38] It is known that crude doses of aspirin cause increased bleeding, while this research showed that homeopathic doses of acetylsalicylic acid shorten bleeding time in healthy subjects.

Two Dutch professors of molecular cell biology recently completed a significant body of experimentation which not only provided evidence of the effects of homeopathic microdoses on cell cultures but that also suggested that these microdoses are only effective when homeopathy's principle of similars is followed.[39] Specific reference to the body of studies cannot be provided in this chapter, both due to the space necessary to describe this work and due to its highly technical nature.

A now famous study by respected French physician and immunologist Jacques Benveniste tested highly diluted doses of an antibody on a type of white blood cells called basophils (basophils increase in number when exposed to substances such as antibodies which cause an allergic reaction). This work was replicated at six different laboratories at four different universities (the University of Paris South, the University of Toronto, Hebrew University, and the University of Milan). Although the prestigious journal *Nature* published this study,[40] it also published concurrently an editorial stating that they did not believe the results.[41] The editor insisted on going to the primary researcher's laboratory at the University of Paris South to observe the experiment conducted in his presence, along with two known experts in scientific fraud (one of whom was a magician).

The details of what followed require more detail and technical information than is appropriate for this book. In summary, the experiment did not show significant results, leading the *Nature* editor to pronounce in his journal that the original study was a fraud.[42] The problem, however, was that the editor and the fraud experts were not immunologists, and thus, they did not seem aware that many studies in immunology require considerably more replication than could be done in the couple of days that the *Nature* team visited.

Another problem was in the study itself, which was very difficult to do. The researchers later simplified it, provided even greater scientific controls, and found significant results. *Nature,* however, chose not to publish these results, and this study was published instead in the *Journal of the French Academy of Sciences.*[43]

Evidence of the bias that "defenders of science" have against homeopathy is their refusal to publish or even comment on the increasing body of research accruing to homeopathic medicine.

Science is supposed to be objective, though both physicists and psychologists teach us that objectivity is impossible. Science's long-term antagonism to homeopathy is slowly breaking down but not without significant reaction, fear, anxiety, and sometimes downright attack against homeopaths.

Change is difficult, and significant change is even more difficult. Even though science grows from new knowledge, it tends to be resistant, often very resistant, to perspectives and knowledge that do not fit contemporary paradigms and scientific theories. The information presented in this chapter and in this book is not meant to overthrow science but to enlarge its perspective so that it more broadly and accurately describes and accepts many presently unexplainable phenomena of nature.

IN SUMMARY

This review of research is not meant to be complete. Readers are encouraged to review the books listed in the resources section of this chapter for access to many other clinical and laboratory studies as well as to theoretical foundations of homeopathic microdoses.

Despite the now strong evidence that homeopathic medicines promote biological activity and clinical efficacy, there is still great resistance to them. Recently, the *Lancet* published the research on the homeopathic treatment of asthma.[44] In a press release announcing this research, they emphasized that although homeopathic medicines may provide some benefit to people with asthma, conventional medicines offer greater benefit.

This was a strange statement for two reasons. First, the study didn't compare homeopathic and conventional medicine; it only compared homeopathic medicine with a placebo. Any other conjecture was not founded on the data presented. Second, the *Lancet* refused to openly acknowledge that homeopathic medicines may work after all.

One can't help but wonder whether if a man flew and science proved that he flew, the editors of some medical journals would remark: "But he doesn't fly as high or as fast as a jet plane!"

Despite the resistance to change in general and to homeopathy specifically, it is getting increasingly difficult for physicians and scientists to doubt the benefits that homeopathic medicines offer.

Italian hematologist Paolo Bellavite and Italian homeopath Andrea Signorini's *Homeopathy: A Frontier in Medical Science* is presently the most comprehensive resource of controlled studies on homeopathy. The authors conclude, "The sum of the clinical observations and experimental findings is beginning to prove so extensive and intrinsically consistent that it is no longer possible to dodge the issue by acting as if this body of evidence simply did not exist."[45]

They go on to say, "To reject everything *en bloc*, as many are tempted to do, means throwing out the observations along with the interpretations, an operation which may be the line of least resistance, but which is not scientific because unexplained observations have always been the main hive of ideas for research."

To ignore the body of experimental data that presently exists on homeopathic medicines and to deny the body of clinical experience of homeopaths and homeopathic patients, one would have to be virtually blind. One can only assume that this blindness is a temporary affliction, one that will soon be cured.

Resources

Paolo Bellavite and Andrea Signorini, *Homeopathy: A Frontier in Medical Science*. Berkeley: North Atlantic, 1995.

Harris L. Coulter, *Homeopathic Science and Modern Medicine: The Physics of Healing with Microdoses*. Berkeley: North Atlantic, 1980.

P. C. Endler and J. Schulte (eds.), *Ultra High Dilution*. Dordrecht: Kluwer Academic, 1994.

M. Doutremepuich (ed.), *Ultra-Low Doses,* Washington, D.C./London: Taylor and Francis, 1991.

Gerhard Resch and Viktor Gutmann, *Scientific Foundations of Homoeopathy*. Munich: Bartel and Bartel, 1987.

A. M. Scofield, "Experimental Research in Homoeopathy: A Critical Review," *British Homoeopathic Journal,* July–October 1984, 73, 3–4: 161–80, 211–26.

Dana Ullman (ed.), *Monograph on Homeopathic Research,* volumes 1 and 2, 1981, 1986.

Roeland van Wijk and Fred A. C. Wiegant, *Cultured Mammalian Cells in Homeopathy Research: The Similia Principle in Self-Recovery*. Utrecht, University of Utrecht, 1994.

British Homoeopathic Journal (2 Powis Place, Great Ormond Street, London WC1N 3HT, England).

FIVE

What Skeptics Say
and How to Respond to Them

It's good to have an open mind, but not so open that your brains fall out. On the other hand, a too skeptical mind is one that isn't open, even to the truth.

When skepticism leads one to inquire more about a subject to determine its veracity, such skepticism is invaluable. The father of American homeopathy, Dr. Constantine Hering, was introduced to homeopathy by a publisher who had hired him to write a negative critique about it. In his research for the book he became convinced that it was an invaluable medical system.

This chapter will provide you with specific information to enable you to respond to skeptics' questions and their doubts. The skeptic may be a physician or a scientist, a husband or an in-law, a neighbor, or even yourself.

Most skeptics of homeopathy are unfamiliar with the field. They commonly scoff at it, even though they don't really know what it is. They believe that the medicines don't work, and they inaccurately presume that there isn't any research to verify its efficacy. They assume that homeopathy must be quackery because they incorrectly believe that it isn't taught in medical schools. Having very limited knowledge of homeopathy does not hinder many skeptics from providing misinformation about homeopathy. For example, it is common for physicians in medical advice columns in newspapers and magazines to denigrate homeopathy, despite being underinformed and usually unaware of homeopathy's body of research.

Ironically, most skeptics of homeopathy have an uninformed and emotionally laden point of view about the subject which is not consistent with the scientific approach they may espouse. It may be helpful to remind the person who is expressing skepticism that the goal of a good scientist is to have impartial objectivity. The ideal scientist asks questions and is seriously interested in the answers as they truly are, not in whether they fit what is presently known or not. Because the attitudes of scientists on a specific subject have significant impact on the general public's view of the subject, people can benefit from understanding the limitations of contemporary science.

In his seminal book *Towards a Psychology of Science,* Abraham Maslow stated, "Before all else, science must be comprehensive and all-inclusive. . . . It must describe and accept the 'way things are,' the actual world as it is, understandable or not, meaningful or not, explainable or not."[1]

Scientists do not often achieve this high goal for which they strive. Rather than being comprehensive and all-inclusive, scientists develop experiments in which a single treatment is measured for its effect on a single or small group of parameters. The scientific process is commonly called the reductionistic method because it reduces the whole to parts, which are assumed, not always correctly, to act like the whole. The inherent narrow focus of the reductionistic method ignores a variety of effects, limiting the value of its results.

Scientists are also limited by their own technological instruments and are therefore unable to measure a variety of subtle factors and interrelated effects. They are not always able to describe "the way things are" because they are able to know only that which can be seen or that which their instruments can measure. Prior to the development of the microscope, for instance, scientists assumed that microorganisms didn't exist, and they considered theories about their existence to be unscientific and described proponents of such theories as quacks.

Scientists must accept real phenomena whether or not they understand how or why they work. Probably more than anything else, the factor that leads scientists to assume that new ideas or phenomena are wrong is their tendency to deny the validity of something primarily because it does not fit within their paradigm of what is real.[2]

For instance, acupuncture is based on concepts of energy flowing through the body, and acupuncturists have developed a sophisticated and integrated healing system based on their clinical experience. However, a great number of scientists not only believe that this energy does not exist, they *insist* that it does not exist. Modern scientific concepts of the human body as an elaborate physiochemical machine do not allow conceptual room for bioenergetic phenomena.

Good scientists are humble, for they recognize the limitations of their own tools and of the scientific method. Although the microdoses that homeopaths use cannot presently be measured, who is to say that a major technological advance will not be developed tomorrow that *can* measure them?

Good scientists may not believe that homeopathy, acupuncture, or other unconventional therapies work, but they are open to the *possibility* that they are wrong. Because these methods have not been disproven, real scientists maintain a dispassionate attitude, rather than an antagonistic one.

Homeopathic medicine does raise some serious questions. Admittedly, it is difficult to understand how such small doses can have any effect, and it is additionally confusing to learn that homeopathic medicines become stronger the more they are sequentially diluted and shaken.

A certain degree of skepticism is expected when homeopathic pharmacology is explained, and such skepticism can be healthy when it leads people to ask more questions and even to experiment themselves as to homeopathy's validity. A blind skepticism that simply assumes it is impossible for homeopathic medicines to have any effect does not provide the opportunity to expand the discussion for mutual benefit.

Ultimately, homeopathy is either a sophisticated method of stimulating a placebo response, or it is a powerful but mysterious way to augment the healing process. Either way, the homeopathic phenomenon is worthy of further investigation.

"It can't work because the doses are too small."

Homeopaths readily acknowledge that some homeopathic remedies are so diluted that they may not contain any of the molecules of the original substance, but that a holographic imprint or template remains which has powerful clinical effects when correctly prescribed in this submolecular dose.

Skeptics who have only a little knowledge about homeopathic medicine assume that these remedies do not work because the doses of active ingredient are too small to have any biochemical action. They believe that homeopathic medicines act simply as placebos. The primary question then becomes: Can all the phenomena that surround the effective use of homeopathic medicines be explained only as a placebo response? Homeopaths, like other practitioners or scientists, recognize the power and value of placebos, but they have found that there is much more to these microdoses than simply the power of suggestion.

Those people who assert that homeopathy is quackery because homeopathic medicines are so small are showing an unscientific attitude. It is as though they are saying that these medicines can't work because they don't fit our present paradigm of medicine and physics. These people are usually unfamiliar with the controlled studies or the wide body of clinical experience with homeopathic medicine in the homeopathic and conventional medical literature.

Typical of the attitude of many skeptics is *Consumer Reports* editor Joel Gurin's. In an article on homeopathy in the *New York Times Sunday Magazine,* Gurin expressed his astonishment that homeopaths expect people to believe that their small doses could have any effect, especially when homeopathy is only based on the observations of "one lone German physician a couple hundred years ago."[3]

What is astonishing here is that Gurin, like many skeptics of homeopathy, is so ill informed about homeopathy. Although Hahnemann founded this system of healing, he was simply one of *hundreds of thousands of physicians* since then who have observed similar phenomena. Gurin totally ignored the following facts:

1. Historical records indicate that homeopathy gained its greatest popularity in the United States and Europe during the 1800s due to its successes in treating the infectious disease epidemics that raged during that time, including ty-

phoid, cholera, yellow fever, scarlet fever, and pneumonia. Records show that death rates in homeopathic hospitals, as well as in mental institutions and prisons supervised by homeopathic physicians, were one half to as little as one eighth of those in conventional hospitals. Could a placebo effect be an adequate explanation for this?

2. There are large numbers of medical doctors who use homeopathic medicines today, including 39 percent of French family physicians,[4] 20 percent of German physicians,[5] and 10 percent of Italian physicians.[6] Further, 42 percent of British physicians refer patients to homeopathic physicians,[7] and 45 percent of Dutch physicians consider homeopathic medicines to be effective.[8] Are skeptics willing to call this large number of physicians "quacks"?

3. Millions of people worldwide rely upon homeopathic medicines to treat common ailments for themselves, as well as for newborns and infants. Parents commonly notice that teething and colicky babies stop crying within seconds after a homeopathic medicine is given. Could this effect be explained as a placebo response?

4. There are large numbers of veterinarians successfully using homeopathic medicines in the treatment of cats, dogs, horses, goats, birds, and cows. Is it possible for a placebo to be the primary effect here?

5. Homeopaths perform provings of their medicines to determine what they cause in overdose. These experiments commonly either use the crude dose or the submolecular potentized doses (30x or higher) of the substance. If homeopathic medicines are not supposed to have any biological activity, why then can they *cause* symptoms if taken in repetitive doses? And further, how can even higher potencies of a substance (i.e., more diluted) help to get rid of the symptoms that a proving medicine causes?

6. Numerous laboratory studies have shown that homeopathic medicines do have biological activity, and yet if a homeopathic remedy is exposed to high temperatures or certain magnetic fields, its ability to stimulate biological activity is abolished (see page 58). Is it possible for a

placebo's action to be wiped out if it is exposed to heat and magnetism?

7. Three of the five largest medical libraries in the United States at the turn of the century were in homeopathic medical schools. There were twenty-nine different homeopathic medical journals at that time. Were the thousands of volumes of clinical experience with homeopathic medicines simply delusional?

When one considers these facts as well as the body of research that demonstrates that homeopathic medicines have biological effects and clinical efficacy, one realizes that trying to explain these varied phenomena as simply a placebo response is inadequate. In fact, skeptics who think this way are demonstrating an extreme faith in mind over matter. To believe that the mind can effect a cure of so many of the normally fatal infectious diseases and that animals and infants can be cured of both acute and chronic ailments through placebos is quite a metaphysical notion.

Further evidence of homeopathy's clinical effects which cannot be explained as the placebo effect comes from the day-to-day practice of homeopaths throughout the world. One homeopathic clinic in Albany, California, called the Hahnemann Clinic, is staffed by three medical doctors, two physician assistants, and a nurse practitioner. It is common for these homeopaths to treat their patients with only homeopathic medicines. These practitioners maintain a family practice and heal patients suffering from strep throat, pneumonia, ear infection, asthma, epilepsy, and a wide variety of other ailments. I personally challenge any skeptic of homeopathy to have a single conventional physician prescribe only placebos for one week to see how effective they are. Ultimately, anyone who takes me up on this challenge will quickly learn that using placebos may be considerably safer than conventional drugs but their use is at best inadequate in treating the common ailments experienced in a family medical practice.

"IT'S WITHOUT ANY SCIENTIFIC FOUNDATION."

One of the common notions that skeptics tend to have about the field of homeopathy is that there is no scientific foundation for it. To make matters worse, many skeptics and scientists are not interested in homeopathic research because they already "know" that the medicines cannot work. When the scientific attitude does not respect systematic inquiry, it imbues itself with an arrogance that diminishes its own scientific standards.

When the controlled, double-blind study on the homeopathic treatment of hay fever described in Chapter 4 was published in the Lancet,[9] some physicians wrote letters saying that double-blind studies using homeopathic medicines were useless because they were simply testing one placebo against another placebo.[10] Because double-blind studies were developed to help differentiate placebo from therapeutic effects, this criticism is ultimately an attack on the scientific method. Since these physicians think of themselves as the defenders of science, one must ask why they aren't defending themselves against their own unscientific attitudes. (For more details about other studies on homeopathic medicines, also see Chapter 4.)

Commonly, scientists assert that homeopathic medicines are not based on any known laws of pharmacology. Although this may seem on the surface to be true, a little knowledge of some specialty areas in pharmacology uncovers serious interest in the effects of microdoses.

Pharmacologists have long recognized the power of microdoses. As noted, recognition of the power of small doses is significant enough that this basic principle is included in most medical dictionaries. Under the word "law" is the Arndt-Schulz law, which states: "Weak stimuli increase physiologic activity and very strong stimuli inhibit or abolish activity."

Today, as noted, the phenomenon of microdose effects is called hormesis, and the journal Health Physics has devoted an entire issue to the subject.[11] Hundreds of studies are referred to in this issue, and the researchers commonly noticed that exceedingly small doses of certain substances were having a more significant effect than larger doses. Although these experiments tested exceptionally small doses of substances and found unpredictably large effects, none of the trials tested submolecular doses of substances. It seems as though these scientists' own paradigm was being stretched by their work, and yet they did not consider going farther to test submolecular doses of substances.

There are, of course, still many mysteries about how homeopathic medicines work. However, the present gaps in knowledge in homeopathy do not mean that a scientific foundation is lacking. It simply means that people are unfamiliar with its foundation, either as a result of ignorance or because their own limited paradigm of science blinds them.

"It's not taught in medical schools.
It must be quackery."

A common knee-jerk belief about homeopathy is that it must be quackery because it isn't taught in medical schools. Besides the fact that homeopathy *is* taught in medical schools around the world, one must keep in mind that American medical schools are notoriously narrow-minded in their concepts of healing.

For instance, despite all the advances in nutritional science today, only a few medical schools have developed significant training in this important preventive and therapeutic method. According to the World Health Organization, 80 percent of the world's population relies on various traditional healing methods, especially herbs, and yet, despite this widespread and long-term use, botanical medicine is not widely taught in medical schools. There are many other examples of the tendency of medical schools to ignore effective treatments that do not fit the classic biomedical model.

Homeopathy is actually taught in many medical schools throughout the world, especially in Europe. In Germany, medical students are *required* to take course work in homeopathy and are tested on it in their basic sciences examination. In France, as mentioned previously, seven medical schools have homeopathic training programs and numerous other schools have postgraduate training programs for physicians. Homeopathy is presently the most popular postgraduate course of *any* discipline in the United Kingdom.

While it may be true that homeopathic and alternative medicines have not been taught in American medical schools in the past, this is no longer the case. A survey in 1994 revealed that approximately twenty-seven medical schools offer at least one course in alternative medicine, most of which include information about homeopathy.[12] Some of the schools that have such course work include Harvard, Yale, the University of California at San Francisco, Tufts, Georgetown, and Columbia, which are among the best medical schools in the country. Further, the American Medical Students Association considers alternative medicine so important that they devoted their 1995 conference to this topic.

While basic principles of alternative medicine are beginning to be taught, medical schools still have a long way to go before students are adequately taught to integrate natural therapies into standard medical practice.

"CONSUMERS NEED TO BE PROTECTED FROM QUACKERY."

Skeptics of homeopathy sometimes consider their opposing point of view as an effort to protect consumers from quackery. They assert that homeopaths exploit ill people who may not be in the best position to make intelligent and rational decisions. Some leaders in the American "antiquackery" movement recommend that laws be passed and enforced which make homeopathic medicines illegal and prevent people from going to the health practitioner of their choice. These same leaders have even encouraged state medical boards to revoke the licenses of medical doctors who "are not practicing in accordance with community standards of medical practice."

Ultimately, what these quack busters are recommending is a virtual "doctatorship." In North Carolina, for instance, Dr. George Guess, a family practice physician who specializes in homeopathy, had his state medical license revoked by the North Carolina medical board simply because he practiced homeopathy. Not a single one of his patients had complained about him; the only complaint against him was from a conventional physician who considered homeopathy to be quackery.

Although one court determined that the medical board's action was "arbitrary and capricious" and an appeal court likewise disagreed with the medical board's actions, the North Carolina Supreme Court ruled that the medical board can determine what type of medicine physicians can and should practice. Shortly after this decision, however, the people of North Carolina rose up and lobbied their representatives, and a law was passed that stipulates that the medical board cannot discipline any physician who practices alternative therapies unless the board proves that this doctor is harming patients.

Sadly, by the time the law was passed, Dr. Guess had left North Carolina and established a practice in Virginia. The people of North Carolina were deprived of the quality natural health care they worked hard to protect.

In the classic book *The Brothers Karamazov,* Feodor Dostoevsky includes a story within the story about the Grand Inquisitor. This chapter tells of a powerful ruler who maintains strict and comprehensive control over the lives of the citizenry. He decides who works where and when, who marries whom and when, and who lives where, and controls innumerable other basic day-to-day decisions in the lives of his people. This ruler considers his job a difficult but essential responsibility because, as he says, people cannot make these decisions better than he can.

While we might all recognize that the government does indeed have an important role in consumer protection, the American constitution acknowledges that there are certain basic rights which are "personal and important" to each individual and in which the government should not intervene. A strict paternalism and a dictatorship that discourages and disallows safe methods like homeopathic medicines have no place in countries where individual freedoms are honored.

While it is certainly true that quackery does exist today, there is no evidence that people who practice alternative forms of healing are using more unsafe or ineffective methods than are conventional physicians. In fact, there is a significant body of evidence to suggest that many conventional therapies are not safe or effective,[13] and it is obvious that if alternative treatments, at worst, may not always be effective, they are generally considerably safer.

The best strategy to prevent quackery, by those who practice conventional as well as those who practice unconventional treatments, is to educate people. As Thomas Jefferson said in 1820, "I know of no safe depository of the ultimate powers of the society but the people themselves; and if we think them not enlightened enough to exercise their control with a wholesome discretion, the remedy is not to take it from them, but to inform their discretion."

Surveys have shown that people who seek homeopathic care tend to be considerably more educated than those who do not.[14] Despite this, no one involved in homeopathic medicine has ever said that those people who seek conventional medical care are not competent in making their own health care decisions.

Consumers should know that many leading skeptics and skeptics' organizations derive funding from drug manufacturers, medical device companies, (junk) food industries, and health insurers. *Dirty Medicine,*[15] a book by investigative journalist Martin Walker, has uncovered some of these ties.

Skeptics assert that consumers of homeopathy are wasting their money on useless cures. Advocates of homeopathic medicines, on the other hand, do not consider homeopathic medicines to be useless, but even if a specific homeopathic medicine did not work, who should decide what consumers spend their money on? And considering how often conventional medical treatments are found to be ineffective and dangerous, even deadly, does this mean that consumers of conventional medical care should not be allowed to make their own health care decisions?

WHAT DOES IT TAKE TO CHANGE THE MIND OF A SKEPTIC?

A double standard exists in medicine. The U.S. Congressional Office of Technology Assessment has stated that only 10 to 20 percent of medical procedures have been proven in controlled clinical studies.[16] Contrary to popular belief, most physicians do not use specific drugs or medical procedures because of scientific proof of their efficacy, but because of their own or a colleague's positive clinical experiences with the treatment. The vast majority of surgical procedures, for instance, have not been proven in double-blind studies, and yet few surgeons consider their work to be unscientific.

Physician and author Larry Dossey notes that physicians tend to consider case histories in medical journals valid when they like the story and when it fits their paradigm of medical thinking, but they consider it a useless anecdote when it does not fit their medical paradigm.

Although there is a body of laboratory and clinical research on homeopathic medicine (see Chapter 4) and there is a considerably larger body of clinical evidence of its efficacy, skeptics generally diminish this material. Part of the reason why some skeptics deny the possibility of the efficacy of homeopathic medicines is that this medical system does not fit their paradigm of medicine. They assume that the larger the dose, the larger the effect, and they ignore the growing body of evidence that suggests that exceedingly small doses of certain substances can have profound biological and clinical effects.

Skeptics assert that repeated research by independent investigators must be done. While it is uncertain if this repeated research will change the point of view of some of the closed-minded skeptics, it will probably sway the vast majority of serious scientists. Homeopaths likewise recognize that repeated research by independent investigators is an important and worthy goal. However, a catch-22 exists here. Numerous physicians and scientists have been personally and professionally attacked simply for expressing an interest in researching homeopathic medicine, and many institutions have refused access to patients for trials using homeopathic remedies.

A lack of financial resources to fund research has also limited homeopathic research. Because some European homeopathic manufacturers are large enough to fund research, there are presently many research projects in development in Europe. Because most American homeopathic companies are quite small, and homeopathic medicines themselves are so inexpensive (usually $3 to $8 per bottle), corporate funds available for research in America are limited.

The U.S. National Institutes of Health has finally developed an Office of Alternative Medicine, for which it was initially given $2 million and in 1995 $5 million to fund research in the field. However, $5 million is but a homeopathic dose of money, especially when this small amount has to be spread across the very broad area of alternative medicine.

After this small amount was granted for research on alternative medicine, several leading skeptics went on record calling it a waste of money and actively lobbied to have the money withdrawn. These efforts to thwart research epitomize an emotional rather than rational state of mind and have no place among those truly interested in scientific inquiry.

It should be noted that research alone is not enough to change the mind or practice of skeptical physicians. Dr. David Reilly, a professor at the University of Glasgow, surveyed physicians and medical students and asked them what kind of validation was necessary before they would accept an alternative therapy as useful for their patients. Ranked almost as high as research was their own clinical experiences and that of their colleagues.[17] Perhaps one of the reasons why homeopathy is so popular in Europe is because the number of physicians who are actively sharing their knowledge and experience with one another has hit a critical mass.

The Changing Face of Medicine

One must realize that science should be considered as verbs, not nouns. Medicine and science are ever changing, ever evolving, and (hopefully) ever improving upon themselves. What is conventional medicine today may be tomorrow's quackery, and what is considered quackery today may be tomorrow's orthodoxy. This is not a prediction; this is the natural evolution of medicine. It is thus our job to try to learn which presently emerging unconventional therapies are valuable contributions to the science and art of healing, and which are not.

Homeopathy's founder, Samuel Hahnemann, is buried in the famous Paris cemetery Père-Lachaise, where on his tombstone are the Latin words *"Aude sapere."* These words mean "dare to taste, to understand." This was Hahnemann's challenge to his fellow doctors and to everyone. Dare to try homeopathy, experience it, and then decide for yourself. This is a worthy goal, whether one is skeptical of homeopathy or not.

The Interface Between Homeopathy and Conventional Medicine

The American health care system is presently sick. It is not even a "system," but rather an unintegrated, uncoordinated conglomeration of services, and one can equally argue that its services provide disease care, not health care.

An effort to reform health care is presently under way in the United States. However, initial efforts at health care reform have tended to be limited to changing how health care is financed, not significantly changing how it is actually practiced. Until and unless health care reform includes homeopathic and other natural medical treatments as an integral part of primary care and also encourages significantly increased self-care, the American health care system will continue to provide expensive, inadequately effective disease care.

Ideally, medicine of the twenty-first century will be an integration of high-tech and "high-natural" medicine. The high-tech side of medicine will focus on the diagnosis and treatment of problems in specific physiochemical structures of the body and will be particularly effective in emergency care and in providing care to people in the advanced stages of illness. In comparison, high-natural medicine refers to various therapeutic measures that, when systematically and individually applied, augment immune response and stimulate the inherent healing capacities of an individual. Such therapies are particularly effective in treating chronic illnesses because of the ability of these healing methods to strengthen the body's own defenses. And because these therapies are considerably safer and less costly than high-tech strategies, it makes sense for high-natural methods to be utilized as the first treatment of choice in primary care.

When a truly comprehensive medical system integrates these two important approaches to healing, a more effective and more cost-effective health care system will be created. This collaborative model of medicine will utilize normally disparate healing methods, including:

- laser surgery and laser acupuncture
- low doses of electrical currents and the laying on of hands to stimulate healing
- elaborate diagnostic equipment and intuitive assessment
- antioxidant multivitamins and antioxidant botanical remedies
- sophisticated intravenous feeding equipment and fresh, nutrient-rich foods served in hospitals
- genetically engineered drugs and homeopathic medicines

Despite the unquestionable progress that conventional medicine has made in the past century, despite the regular airing of major breakthroughs in the treatment of one disease or another, and despite the sophisticated diagnostic capabilities that are presently available, we must admit that there are major gaps of knowledge and clinical effectiveness in the conventional treatment of common acute, chronic, and genetic disorders.

There are also limits to what homeopathic medicine offers, but the difference is that people involved in homeopathy tend to know and respect the benefits of conventional medicine, while those involved in conventional medicine remain unaware of and sometimes even antagonistic to homeopathy.

People who seek out homeopathic and other natural health care do not necessarily turn their backs on conventional medicine. Surveys have shown that two thirds of the people who utilized alternative treatments had previously received conventional medical treatment for their conditions, though they experienced little or no positive result. Over 20 percent reported seeing their conventional physician as recently as two weeks before the survey, and 18 percent were using conventional and alternative treatment concurrently.[1]

WHEN INTEGRATIVE MEDICINE IS POSSIBLE

An integrative approach in which conventional treatments and homeopathic medicines are used can be highly beneficial in the treatment of numerous conditions.

Childbirth presents many opportunities for integrative medicine. There are numerous homeopathic remedies that can prevent complications of pregnancy and labor, and when some type of medical intervention is necessary, whether it be cesarean section, episiotomy, or any other emergency procedure, there are homeopathic medicines that can aid in the healing from these interventions.

While the use of homeopathic medicines can sometimes prevent the need for surgery, homeopaths acknowledge that surgery is sometimes necessary. When surgery is medically indicated, using homeopathic medicines before, during, and after the procedure can help the patient recover more rapidly.

One classic example of the successful integration of conventional and homeopathic treatment was demonstrated in the study on Nicaraguan children suffering from diarrhea[2] (see page 47). The children were given oral rehydration therapy, a special salt solution which keeps children from dying by helping them retain water, but does not cure the underlying infection of which the diarrhea is a symptom. The study showed that the administration of individually chosen homeopathic medicines sped up the underlying healing process.

Some areas in which homeopathic and conventional therapies can be integrated have great potential but have not yet been adequately tested. Specifically, some homeopaths claim that homeopathically prepared doses of chemotherapeutic drugs can reduce the side effects of these drugs. Also, at least two studies in rats have shown that *Ruta 30x* and *200x* and *Ginseng 6x, 30x,* and *200x* can reduce the side effects of radiation,[3] suggesting that these remedies should be tested as a way to reduce the problems associated with radiation treatment in cancer patients. Some homeopaths also recommend the use of *X-ray 30* just before and after getting X rays.

One of the more obvious ways that conventional and homeopathic approaches are already being integrated is in the field of diagnosis. Homeopaths presently use conventional medical technologies to diagnose a person's disease, though their treatment is based on a homeopathic assessment of their totality of symptoms. Homeopathy may be particularly useful after diagnosis when the physician and the patient wish to seek safer, natural methods first and when there are no known medicines for the patient's unique ailment. Also, the homeopathic approach which utilizes the totality of symptoms, including subtle symptoms, helps to prevent more serious conditions from developing in the future.

An integrative approach can be helpful in the treatment of asthma. A study published in the *Lancet* showed that conventional allergy testing was useful in selecting a homeopathic medicine that provided benefit[4] (see page 46). Researchers used conventional allergy testing to determine what substance people with asthma were most allergic to. They then gave this substance in homeopathic doses to the subjects, and these subjects had significantly fewer symptoms of asthma than those subjects given a placebo. The researchers called this approach "homeopathic immunotherapy."

An integrative approach may sometimes mean that homeopathic medicines are used first, and then, only if they were ineffective, would conventional therapies be used. The reverse approach is also possible and is presently more common; most people have already used many conventional treatments without adequate success and are now seeking homeopathic care for their conditions. As people become increasingly familiar with homeopathy, it is likely that they will use these natural and safer medicines prior to the more risky therapeutic interventions offered by conventional physicians.

Part of the trick to making either homeopathic or conventional treatments work is to seek the care of well-trained professionals and to give their treatments reasonable time to act.

Sometimes a person is in severe pain, and while it may be possible to find the correct homeopathic remedy, he or she wants a higher degree of certainty that relief will be rapid. In such instances, it makes sense to use conventional medicines at least temporarily, while homeopathic medicines are recommended after the acute crisis is diminished or over. Sometimes a person may receive both homeopathic and conventional medical care for a chronic ailment and not experience any relief. After six months of ineffective treatment, it may be necessary to get another opinion from another homeopath or conventional physician, or perhaps to seek another form of alternative care.

Homeopaths commonly refer patients to various conventional specialists when they feel a specific diagnosis and/or treatment is important. And yet there are relatively few referrals to homeopaths from conventional physicians. Considering how many patients do not receive appropriate diagnoses or effective treatments for their ailments despite long-term conventional care, it is unfortunate that there aren't more referrals to homeopaths. A significant obstacle to a more cooperative relationship between homeopathic and conventional physicians is conventional physicians' lack of knowledge of homeopathy.

When Integrative Medicine Isn't Possible

Although the concept of integrative medicine makes sense, one should not have a Pollyannish viewpoint about the subject. It is not always easy or therapeutically effective to use homeopathic and conventional therapies concurrently or even in sequence.

Certain powerful conventional interventions, such as steroidal medications, are immunosuppressive, and while they provide valuable short-term relief of symptoms, over time they tend to weaken immune competence and reduce the possibilities of creating significant health improvement through homeopathic treatment.

Other conventional medications may be so effective in suppressing a person's symptoms that they mask them, making it very difficult for the homeopath to find the correct individualized remedy. In such instances, patients must decide which treatment they prefer to start with and which they would like to consider secondarily. Physicians should not be the decision makers here, but instead should inform patients of the risks and benefits associated with either decision.

THE DEMAND FOR ALTERNATIVE/ COMPLEMENTARY HEALTH CARE

The increasing demand for alternative medicine has led some people to question whether the word "alternative" is appropriate. As noted, Prince Charles popularized the term "complementary medicine" as a less offensive description and one that suggests that these therapies should be an integral part of health care.

Even the conservative British Medical Association has openly acknowledged the growing importance of alternative therapies with the publication of their book *Complementary Medicine: New Approaches to Good Practice.* This book notes that one of the primary reasons for the current upsurge of "official" interest in unconventional medicine is the rapidly increasing number of people who are seeking help from such practitioners. This growing popularity has prompted the Council of Europe to state: "It is not possible to consider this phenomenon as a medical side-issue. It must reflect a genuine public need which is in urgent need of definition and analysis."[5]

The British health minister, Dr. Brian Mawhinney, said, "Complementary medicine has generally proved popular with patients, and a recent survey found that 81 percent of patients are satisfied with the treatment they received."[6] American and British citizens are walking with their feet and their wallets. They are seeking the care of unconventional practitioners, and their interest is so significant that they seek these services even though they often have to pay out of their own pocket rather than rely on government or insurance reimbursement.

In April 1994, the Committee on the Environment, Public Health, and Consumer Protection of the European Parliament adopted a proposal on complementary medicine which called for incorporation of complementary therapies within social security systems, integration of complementary medicines within the European pharmacopeia, and an end to prosecutions against non-medically-qualified practitioners until a pan-European regulatory system is established. The European Parliament also voted for a $7.5-million-per-year budget for funding research projects in complementary medicine. Although this homeopathic dose of money is not adequate to investigate the many important issues in the broad field of complementary medicine, it is a start, and hopefully will generate more significant support in the near future.

A *New England Journal of Medicine* study showed that 34 percent of Americans utilized one or more alternative therapies in the year 1990 alone.[7] One important but little-known statistic from this study indicated that 70 percent of people who used alternative treatments did not tell their physicians about it. This fact suggests that the American public is not being up-front with their doctors, in part because they know that their doctors have an antagonistic attitude toward alternative treatments.

Physicians could improve relations with patients by listening more carefully to their concerns and interests in alternative medicine. Becoming more familiar with alternative treatments would be a positive step in this direction. Recognizing the problem, the British Medical Association has gone on record saying, "Whether or not doctors wish to practice different techniques themselves, it is clear that there is a definite need among doctors for better *information* in the use and practice of non-conventional therapies, which is not presently being met."[8] Sadly, the American Medical Association has thus far tended to ignore this subject or, even worse, to publish articles and books that continue to express antagonism toward alternative therapies.

REDUCING HEALTH CARE COSTS

Now that governments are more concerned than ever with the costs of health care, there is some serious interest in homeopathic and complementary medicine. According to a survey conducted by the French government, the average annual cost for the services rendered by a homeopathic physician was approximately *one half* the cost of the services rendered by a conventional doctor.[9] This report also noted that the cost of homeopathic medicines, on average, is less than one third the price of conventional drugs.

The Bristol Homoeopathic Hospital in Great Britain provides care for three thousand patients a year, five hundred of them new patients. The total pharmacy costs for one year were only $23,000. The average price of a prescription was $5.13, which *included* the cost of employing the pharmacist or dispenser.[10] The actual cost of the medicine was $2.50. These figures are at least 40 percent less than those for any other medical specialty in Britain.

Not only will the use of homeopathic medicines reduce the costs of going to a doctor, it will commonly reduce the need to go to a doctor at all. Consumers can easily learn to use certain homeopathic medicines at home for common ailments. Even conservative medical texts acknowledge that medical care is not necessary for many common conditions, and if consumers can learn to treat these ailments themselves with homeopathic medicines, substantial savings can be attained. Such self-care is not meant to take the place of proper medical care, only to reduce the need for it in the treatment of self-limiting ailments.

In Summary

In the recent past, "comprehensive health care" was a term used to refer to prevention through immunization, regular medical checkups, early medical diagnosis, and access to various specialty medical services. We know today that truly comprehensive health care is so much more than this. It involves more activated patients who are aware of the effects of nutrition, exercise, stress, and psychological states on their health. It involves interaction with various health specialists who can provide individualized and sophisticated treatment programs used either alone or in conjunction with other therapies in order to nurture, nourish, and augment a person's inherent defenses.

We are entering a new era in healing, an era when high-tech instruments will help assess the therapeutic benefits of old and new healing methods. As we approach the twenty-first century, it is time to consider integrating the best of scientific medicine and the best of natural medicine. To do this, we must consider using safer methods *first* (and sometimes even *second*) before resorting to more risky therapeutic measures. Such health care will not only be safer and less expensive, it will also encourage patients to play a greater role in their own health. This empowerment has its own therapeutic benefits.

Historians have commonly noted that history is always written by the victors, and the history of ideas is always written by those who maintain and defend the dominant conceptual paradigm. Because of this, homeopathy and various natural healing systems have been portrayed in medical history books as unproven and ineffective healing methods. History, however, will soon be rewritten.

Common Concerns of Consumers

SEVEN

Homeopathic Self-Care: When to Use It and How to Make It Work for You

WHEN SHOULD HOMEOPATHIC SELF-CARE BE CONSIDERED?

Taking care of yourself and your family is empowering and has therapeutic value that is healing in its own right. The fact of the matter is, health is too vital to each of our lives to simply rely upon someone else to take care of for us. While it is certainly valuable to call in the experts when they are needed, the vast majority of acute health problems are within the treatment abilities of us all.

No sane person questions the value of self-care. The primary question is when and what kind of self-care is appropriate. If people never treated themselves and only sought the care of a doctor for all their ills, the medical care system would be inundated (and our national debt would be unbelievable!).

Self-care has always been an integral part of the homeopathic tradition. Constantine Hering, M.D., the father of American homeopathy, was particularly known for writing *The Homeopathic Domestic Physician,* a homeopathic guidebook that was so successful that homeopathy's popularity in the nineteenth century was thought, in part, to be the result of this self-care text.

Today, there are numerous self-care texts available, and the resources section in Part IV of this book provides readers with a wide variety of such source material. Most of these books teach people how to treat many common acute ailments, and for better and worse, others go a step farther and provide instruction on how to treat chronic and potentially serious ailments.

It is widely recognized in homeopathic circles that people should generally limit homeopathic treatment of themselves and their families to acute ailments, and leave the treatment of chronic or life-threatening conditions to professionals. Acute ailments refer to conditions of a short-term and basically self-limiting nature. Self-limiting conditions are those which tend to resolve themselves, though with homeopathic care they usually resolve considerably faster than when left untreated. Colds, coughs, sore throats, flus, allergies, sinus conditions, headaches, and PMS are some examples of such self-limiting conditions.

However, ailments do not always fit neatly into simple categories. While the above-listed conditions generally resolve themselves quickly, many of them resolve only temporarily and then return, occasionally with other minor symptoms and sometimes accompanied by serious ones.

For instance, a simple cough may be an acute condition, but when people get recurrent coughs, it suggests an underlying susceptibility and weakened condition that could benefit from professional homeopathic treatment. The common homeopathic remedies for the acute stage of the cough tend to relieve this short-term ailment, but other deeper-acting remedies must be considered to deal effectively with the underlying condition. It generally requires a professional level of understanding of which deep-acting homeopathic medicine to consider to effectively cure the deeper problem.

When people who are undergoing professional homeopathic care are given a homeopathic constitutional medicine to heal this deeper problem, it is generally recommended that they apply self-care for acute ailments only in consultation with their homeopath. Because a constitutional remedy sometimes initiates a healing crisis in which old or underlying symptoms temporarily manifest, homeopaths prefer that people avoid treating themselves, for these symptoms may be part of

the healing process (see "The Healing Process" in Chapter 2 for further discussion on this topic). One exception to this general rule is
when a person under constitutional care is physically injured, at which
time self-treatment presents no problem.

Self-treatment of nonserious chronic ailments, though not recommended, may make sense when professional homeopathic care is
not readily accessible, either because of the distance to a good homeopath or because of financial barriers to obtaining professional care.
These nonserious chronic ailments include but are not limited to
arthritis, insomnia, back pain, and sinusitis.

Self-treatment for medical emergencies is an exception to the
general rule of not treating potentially serious conditions oneself,
since it can be extremely valuable to provide immediate homeopathic
care on the way to the doctor or hospital. This is particularly indicated
in accidents, heart attacks, or appendicitis (the chapters on injuries,
heart disease and pre- and postsurgical treatment will be of particular
benefit in such cases).

Self-care with homeopathic medicines can be used concurrent with
conventional medical treatment. However, some conventional treatments, by suppressing symptoms, make it more difficult to find the
correct homeopathic medicine, and sometimes conventional treatment suppresses the person's defenses in a significant enough way that
effective homeopathic care is not as easy to achieve.

Self-care with homeopathic medicines is considerably easier and
more effective when used with other natural therapies than with conventional medications because natural therapies tend to nourish and
nurture the body's own defenses and do not disrupt the delicate balance of the body as significantly as do conventional drugs. While
many natural therapies, such as nutrition, herbal remedies, meditation,
and relaxation methods, gently augment the body's defenses and
slowly help the person heal, homeopathic medicines offer the unique
benefit of often having more rapid effects when used for the treatment of acute conditions. When homeopathic and other natural therapies are used together, health is often reestablished even faster and
more deeply.

Various natural therapies can augment the effects of homeopathic
medicine in treating many acute problems. For instance, one can consider taking the herb feverfew for migraine headaches concurrent with
taking a homeopathic medicine. Studies have found that feverfew is

effective in preventing and treating headaches; however, it has to be taken for several weeks before noticeable results occur. In such instances, it makes sense to use homeopathic medicines to treat the acute stage of the headache and to also use feverfew to prevent future onsets of the condition.

Besides herbal treatment, one can concurrently use nutrition, massage, yoga, meditation, visualization, stress management, and numerous other self-care modalities along with homeopathic medicine. These natural therapies provide rest, relaxation, and nourishment to the body so that it can most effectively work its self-healing wonders.

One of the problems that concurrent treatment of ailments creates is that one is never certain if the homeopathic medicine provided the relief or it was one of or a mixture of the other treatments. While there may be certain benefits in knowing this information so that one can use a specific treatment again, most people simply want relief, and it is not essential for them to know the precise method that was most therapeutic.

Another possible problem is that natural therapies may, on occasion, antidote the action of a homeopathic medicine. Homeopaths have found, for instance, that some herbs can slow down or stop the effects of a homeopathic medicine. At present, there is little data on this potential situation, though it is generally considered by practicing homeopaths to be a rare rather than a regular observation.

HOW TO FIND THE CORRECT HOMEOPATHIC MEDICINE

Finding the correct individualized homeopathic medicine is akin to being a medical detective. Whether you are treating yourself, a family member, a close friend, or even your pet, you need to investigate the situation. You need to figure out the who, what, why, where, and when of the case. In other words, you need to find out everything you can about what the person is experiencing: what type of pain or discomfort he has, what other major and minor symptoms he is experiencing, what unusual symptoms he has, what makes his pain and any other symptoms feel better or worse, and what he is feeling emotionally and mentally (also see page 124 in Chapter 9: "What Information Will the Homeopath Want about My Personal Health History?").

Every symptom that a person experiences is a clue to finding the correct remedy. While conventional physicians tend to use only those "clues" that fit specific disease categories and ignore the rest, homeopaths make use of every physical, emotional, and mental symptom the person is experiencing.

Homeopaths classify people's symptoms into simple, distinct classifications. As you will note, these terms are nontechnical and easy to understand.

Common symptoms are those which are common to a specific diagnosis. These are the symptoms upon which conventional physicians focus. Because they do not help you or the homeopath determine an individualized remedy, they tend to be the least valuable of all symptoms. Examples of common symptoms are pain in the joints in people with arthritis and lack of appetite in people with hepatitis.

Particular symptoms are symptoms localized to specific places on the body. Head pain, weak ankles, and nasal discharge are examples of these symptoms. To get more useful detailed and individualizing symptoms, ask probing questions to determine the unique nature of a person's condition.

General symptoms are those symptoms which are felt by one's entire being. While weak ankles is a particular symptom, overall fatigue is a general symptom because the whole person feels tired. General symptoms are not only of a physical nature; all emotional and mental complaints are considered general symptoms because the whole person feels them (one cannot feel depression just in the lungs).

One trick for differentiating particular symptoms from general ones is that people tend to use the construction "my (head, stomach, joints)" when making reference to a particular symptom, and they say "I am (tired, hungry, irritable)" when making reference to a general symptom.

General symptoms are usually of greater value than common or particular symptoms in determining the correct homeopathic medicine because they represent the entire body's response to illness, not just a localized response.

Strange, rare, and peculiar symptoms are just what they sound like. These unusual symptoms are often the most valuable because their uniqueness helps you to find the correct remedy faster. Some examples include flaring or flapping of the nostrils while breathing or a ticking sound in the ear as if from a distant watch.

Modalities are characteristics that make a person's symptoms better or worse. For instance, head pain is a particular symptom, but when the person says that the pain is worse upon waking and/or is relieved by motion, these characteristics are the modalities of the head pain. Modalities help provide more detailed and individualizing symptoms of an ailment.

Once you have written down all your symptoms (or those of someone else), you can use this book and other homeopathic self-care texts to find the individualized remedy. There are different strategies for finding the correct medicine in self-care situations, usually based on the other homeopathic texts you may have. If this is your only homeopathic book, simply turn to the chapter on your complaint, review the remedies described, and find the remedy that most closely matches your symptoms. This process is sometimes extremely easy, and at other times extremely difficult.

It is often helpful to have several books, because no single book in homeopathy is complete. Read the information on the various remedies recommended for the specific ailment in whatever books you have. Besides books like this one which list specific ailments, it is extremely useful to have a *materia medica* and a repertory. One book that includes both a *materia medica* and a repertory is the *Pocket Manual of Materia Medica with Repertory* by William Boericke, M.D. This book and other *materia medica* and repertories are not often available in bookstores today but generally must be obtained from a mail order homeopathic resource center (see Part IV).

As noted in Chapter 1, a *materia medica* (derived from Latin words which mean "materials of medicine") is a listing of homeopathic medicines and the specific symptoms that each substance has been found to cause in overdose and cure in homeopathic dose. After reviewing other books to determine the potentially correct remedies, using a *materia medica* can help you to be more precise.

Complementary to a *materia medica* is a repertory, which is a book listing almost every symptom you can imagine. A repertory has chapters on the mind, the head, the eyes, ear, and nose, and the rest of the body. After each symptom is a list of substances that have been found to cause the symptom in overdose and cure it in homeopathic dose. Once you have looked up in a repertory the numerous unique symptoms a person has, you create a chart that compares the medicines listed under each symptom.

Repertories list medicines for each symptom in plain type, italics, or boldface, representing a remedy's increasing order of importance. Medicines listed in plain type are those which occasionally cause and cure the specific symptom. Medicines listed in italics are those which frequently cause and cure the specific symptom. And the medicines in bold face are those which very frequently cause and cure the specific symptom.

Make a chart listing the symptoms you or another sick person is experiencing on one axis, and the medicines from the symptoms recorded in the repertory on the other axis. Give medicines listed in plain type 1 point, those listed in italics 2 points, and those listed in boldface 3 points. One key to improving the accuracy of your selection of remedies is to double this point score when the symptom is either a *general* symptom or a *strange, rare, and peculiar* symptom, or if the symptom is extremely strong.

After scoring all the medicines, read in a *materia medica* the chapters on the five top-scoring medicines. The medicine that best matches your or the sick person's symptoms is the correct remedy. The remedy you ultimately prescribe will not necessarily be the medicine that gets the highest score or that has the most number of symptoms, though these scores often lead to the best choice, especially the medicine that covers the greatest number of symptoms. You can feel confident that you have found the correct remedy when a medicine within the five top-scoring remedies covers the strongest and the most individual symptoms you or the sick person has.

It is not always necessary to have a *materia medica* or a repertory to use homeopathic medicine effectively for acute care. Using this book and other homeopathic self-care books, you can choose homeopathic remedies successfully. Having a *materia medica* and a repertory will simply improve the accuracy of your remedy selection.

The medicine that is the most similar to the person's symptoms is called the simillimum. This does not mean that other remedies will not help the person. In fact, many remedies can often provide some benefit, though the simillimum usually acts the fastest, longest, and deepest. If an incorrect remedy is taken, generally nothing happens, though sometimes a medicine may have enough characteristics similar to the sick person's that the individual experiences a partial relief of symptoms.

Those of you who wish to take the easiest road can consider using one of the homeopathic combination medicines which contain two to eight of the remedies commonly used in treating a specific ailment (see Chapter 10 for discussion on the benefits and limitations of combination medicines). Although an individualized remedy tends to work faster and more deeply than a combination product, it is recommended that you consider using a formula if the single remedy you need is not immediately available or if you cannot figure out which remedy is indicated for your acute complaint.

How to Select the Best Potency and Dosage

After you have carefully figured out what the correct medicine is for your particular ailment, the choices are not over. When you go to the health food store or pharmacy to get your remedy, you may be initially confused to find that each remedy is manufactured in various potencies (the different kinds of potencies are discussed in "The Small Doses of Homeopathic Medicines" in Chapter 1 as well as later in this section).

Although some people experience great anxiety about figuring out the best potency, there is general agreement in homeopathic circles that finding the best potency is not nearly as important as finding the correct individualized remedy. Once one finds the correct remedy, most potencies of it will have a beneficial effect, with the best potency simply having a deeper and/or faster result. There are individual instances when one potency of a medicine doesn't seem to work and then another potency of the same medicine has a significant effect, but these experiences are more the exception than the rule.

There are varying opinions on how to choose the best potency. Some schools of thought in homeopathic practice primarily recommend the low potencies (1x or 1c to 12x or 12c), some primarily utilize the high potencies (200 and higher), and some utilize the entire range of strengths.

Whatever the different opinions, there is general consensus that nonhomeopaths should not use potencies higher than the 30th, except in selected instances, such as *Arnica 200* for shock of injury or *Ignatia 200* immediately after an acute grief. There are two primary reasons for this cautionary advice:

1. The higher the potency, the more accurate the remedy must be. Thus, people who are not expert homeopaths

and who use higher potencies may not experience effective results.

2. The higher potencies are more apt to initiate a healing crisis, during which some symptoms are initially aggravated in the process of cure. Because this exacerbation of symptoms can be anxiety-producing and even frightening to the patient and to the prescriber, it is prudent for nonexperts to avoid using high-potency medicines.

The "c" potencies tend to be slightly more dilute and more powerful than the "x" potencies ("x" potencies refer to remedies that were diluted 1:10; "c" potencies were diluted 1:100), which means that people have to be more accurate in prescribing them to benefit from their increased strength. Because there are certain benefits from using both types of potencies, medicines in this book are recommended by their potency number, without reference to their "x" or "c" strength.

One simple rule for selecting potencies is use lower potencies when you are less certain about the accuracy of the remedy. For instance, use the 3 or 6th potency when you are not confident that you know the correct medicine, use the 12th potency if you are relatively confident, and use the 30th potency when you are extremely confident about your selection.

Other factors that you can consider when choosing the correct potency include the following:

> *When the person's general symptoms fit a specific remedy,* the 30th potency is preferred (general symptoms refer to psychological and whole-body symptoms; see page 89 for more details about general symptoms).

> *If the onset of symptoms is rapid,* it suggests using a higher potency (the 30th) rather than a lower potency (the 6th).

> *If a remedy has a clear indication of a factor that occurred just prior to an ailment,* consider the 30th potency. (For instance, if a person gets a cold or cough shortly after being exposed to cold or wet weather, consider *Aconitum 30* because this remedy is known to benefit people who develop their acute symptoms after exposure to cold or wet weather.)

If a person has many allergies, his or her hypersensitive state sometimes extends to homeopathic medicines, too. Lower potencies should be given to such people because they may experience a proving of a higher-potency remedy (a proving is the experience of symptoms that a substance is known to cause; further discussion of provings is provided in Chapter 1, page 7).

If a person is taking or being exposed to substances that tend to antidote homeopathic medicine (see Chapter 12, pages 147– 64), it is generally recommended to use lower potencies in frequent repetition (every two to four hours).

In addition to learning how to choose the correct potency, one must also learn how to determine the correct dosage.

The cardinal rule of the proper dosage of a homeopathic medicine is "the minimum dose." What this means is that one should take as few doses as necessary to catalyze a healing response. Sometimes a person may need only a single dose, especially when a 30th or higher potency is taken. Once noticeable improvement has begun, no more doses are necessary unless improvement levels off or reverses, at which time one should repeat taking the medicine, as long as the medicine still fits the pattern of symptoms. If not, find the remedy that fits the new pattern of symptoms and begin taking it.

Generally, the more intense a person's symptoms, the more frequent dosages tend to be necessary. For instance, one may need to take a remedy every thirty minutes immediately after a wrenching injury or during a high fever, while one may need only three or four doses in a day in which minor discomfort is experienced. In any case, stop taking the remedy once significant improvement has begun. You may have some symptoms remaining, but no more doses are necessary if the remedy has obviously begun a healing response. Once the healing response has begun, rest assured that the symptoms will soon (or eventually) disappear.

If you are improving slowly rather than rapidly, continue to take the remedy, either until no discomfort is felt or until the symptoms change in a way that suggests that another remedy may be indicated. Although there are exceptions, it is rare to need to take a remedy for more than seventy-two hours.

The number of homeopathic pills, globules, pellets, or drops to take per dose is generally not considered as vital to a therapeutic response as is the correct remedy, potency, and frequency of repetition. It is common to recommend simply a single pill per dose when the medicine is aspirin-size (though usually not as thick). If the remedies are globules (round pellet-sized pills), two to four globules are generally recommended per dose. If the pills are the size of cake sprinkles, five to fifteen pills are recommended. If the medicine is in liquid form, five to fifteen drops are recommended.

Labels on homeopathic medicines commonly list the recommended number of pills or drops as well as the recommended frequency of dosage. While consumers can benefit from knowing the manufacturer's recommended number of pills or drops per dose, the frequency of dosage is better determined by individualized factors as discussed in this chapter.

WHAT TO DO IF A HOMEOPATHIC MEDICINE DOESN'T WORK

It is generally necessary to allow at least one night's rest to evaluate the effectiveness of a homeopathic medicine in treating an acute ailment (one should allow more time in the professional homeopath's treatment of chronic ailments). However, there are exceptions to this rule, especially in the treatment of people who have a high fever or intense pain. Homeopaths commonly find that homeopathic medicines work more rapidly when a person's symptoms have come on rapidly. When this happens, improvement in health is often noticeable within hours, sometimes even minutes.

To determine whether a homeopathic medicine has or has not worked, it is important to evaluate both the primary symptoms the person is experiencing and his or her general state of health. Sometimes, a headache is still hurting, but overall energy is considerably better. Improvement in one's general state of health is a good sign and suggests that the person will shortly experience a reduction in head pain and/or other acute symptoms.

It is useful to know that there are certain conditions such as fevers, coughs, and earaches, especially in children, which without treatment tend to improve in the day and get worse at night. In such cases, one cannot determine until nighttime whether improvement from the remedy has actually taken place.

As noted, homeopathic medicines sometimes create a healing crisis—that is, they catalyze a healing response which causes a temporary exacerbation of certain symptoms prior to a healing. It can be difficult determining whether the remedy has caused these symptoms, or whether the new symptoms simply mean the person is getting sicker. A healing process is thought to be occurring if:

- the new symptoms are externalizations of some sort (skin discharges, expectoration, diarrhea, vomiting, early or profuse menstruation),
- overall energy and psychological state are better,
- the person experiences old symptoms that he or she hasn't had in a long time.

Recognizing a healing crisis is helpful so that people do not try to treat it, because treatment can slow or stop this important process.

If it is determined that the remedy is not working, it is useful to reevaluate the person's symptoms to assess whether the correct remedy was given. If you are extremely confident that it was, you must consider factors that may be antidoting its action (see in Chapter 12), or you may want to try a different potency.

If another remedy is indicated, give it. If you are not certain about which remedy to give, you can either wait for the symptoms to change further and become clearer, or consider using a homeopathic combination product if one is available for the condition in question.

It is generally recommended that you avoid prescribing too many remedies during a single bout of illness. Try not to use more than two or three remedies per bout.

If several homeopathic medicines have been prescribed without adequate results, there are numerous natural healing modalities that should be considered. One should not be a "homeopathic chauvinist" and assume that homeopathy is the only way. In fact, one can consider using supplements, herbs, massage and various physical therapies, stress management strategies, and acupuncture concurrent with homeopathic medicines.

Although some of these therapies may in rare instances antidote the effect of homeopathic medicine (see Chapter 12), there is obviously no problem in using them when homeopathic medicines are clearly not being effective.

One should also avoid being a "natural therapy chauvinist." There may be times when some type of conventional therapy is indicated. The intent of this book is not to discourage people from using conventional therapies, but simply to educate them about what homeopathy has to offer as a first and safer mode of treatment. Such prudent health care brings the potential dividend of a healthier, happier life.

RESOURCES

Elizabeth Wright Hubbard, *A Brief Study Course in Homoeopathy*. St. Louis: Formur, 1977.

P. S. Rawat, *Select Your Dose and Potency*. New Delhi: B. Jain, 1992.

George Vithoulkas, *The Science of Homeopathy*. New York: Grove, 1980.

EIGHT

Seeking Professional Homeopathic Care

WHAT PROFESSIONAL HOMEOPATHIC CARE OFFERS

A distant cousin of mine from Argentina came to visit our family for the first time in 1982. Although we were adults, we had never met or corresponded. When I told him my professional field was homeopathic medicine, his eyes lit up and he said that his entire family sought the care of homeopaths. After I told him that there were very few homeopathic physicians in the United States, he looked at me greatly puzzled and asked, "Then what do people do?"

He told me that he and his family went to conventional physicians only for diagnosis and always went to homeopaths for treatment. Although he had thought that Americans were educated and sophisticated, he was shocked to learn that they primarily and almost exclusively seek the care of conventional doctors.

Just as it is standard practice to have a personal physician, hopefully it will one day soon be standard practice in America to have a homeopath (actually, it is already standard practice to seek homeopathic care in many countries, as was detailed in Chapter 3). Ideally, it is best to have one's physician and one's homeopath be the same person, though it is not always possible to find M.D.s who are also good homeopaths. If a doctor who specializes in homeopathy is not available, there are often other types of professionals who also do so, many of them being exceptional practitioners.

The reason why professional homeopathic care should become the standard for care is that homeopaths offer people significant health benefits that are not available through conventional medical practice. Professional homeopathic treatment usually emphasizes "constitutional care," which may be the most profound way to augment a person's immune and defense system. Constitutional care refers to treatment of a person's totality of present physical and psychological symptoms, in the light of a detailed analysis of his or her genetic history, personal health history, and body type. This level of care provides substantial benefits for those who are ill as well as for people who wish to stay healthy.

While conventional medicine and even most alternative therapies provide treatment for specific complaints, homeopathic constitutional care is unique because it offers a profound way to strengthen a person's overall state of health. There are few people who cannot benefit from this care.

Professional homeopathic care is primarily known for its benefits in treating people with chronic ailments. What is not as well known is its value in treating those with subclinical conditions: ailments that include discomforting and debilitating symptoms which may be very bothersome but do not fit known diagnostic categories.

A subclinical condition may include symptoms such as unrefreshed sleep; being easily fatigued; a tendency to be easily chilled; hypersensitivity to noise, light, or weather; increased emotional vulnerability; decreased or increased appetite; constipation or diarrhea; and many others. If a person with such complaints seeks medical treatment for his symptoms, the physician will commonly order laboratory tests, but these tests often show no noticeable abnormality or obvious disease, leading the doctor to shrug his shoulders and suggest that the patient come back when he is sicker.

Just because a physician cannot find a specific pathology does not mean that the person isn't sick; it simply suggests that conventional medical diagnostic tests are not adequately sensitive to many early symptoms of imbalance and disease.

Homeopaths make great use of these subtle symptoms to find a remedy that fits the person. In fact, homeopaths feast on such symptoms and usually systematically ask questions to uncover other subtle symptoms their patients experience but may not have thought about consciously.

Inevitably, through the prescription of a constitutional medicine, homeopaths prevent untold chronic ailments without even knowing the depth or breadth of the problem. They may know only that they successfully helped a person, and that the person no longer experiences any problems, even minor ones.

Finally, the professional homeopath is knowledgeable about little-known homeopathic remedies which may be indicated in the condition you or a family member has. Not only is this knowledge sometimes vital, but most homeopaths also have a large homeopathic pharmacy in their office which contains many of these rare medicines, plus varying potencies of the common remedies. Because health food stores and pharmacies usually have relatively small collections of homeopathic medicine and a limited choice of potencies, seeking care from a homeopath also has the advantage of providing immediate access to the right remedy.

WHEN IS PROFESSIONAL HOMEOPATHIC CARE APPROPRIATE?

Most homeopaths encourage self-care for common acute ailments and injuries. However, there are times when it is best to get professional homeopathic care.

For example, although self-treatment of acute stages of chronic conditions is possible and some relief can be obtained from it, a layperson will rarely be lucky enough to find the right constitutional medicine and follow-up remedies to elicit a deep and powerful cure of the chronic condition underlying acute and chronic symptoms.

A true cure of chronic and even some genetic disease can be achieved with homeopathic medicines, though it requires expert attention and it often requires time. Professional care is necessary because deep-acting, curative remedies require a significant knowledge of homeopathic *materia medica* and the various miasms (see "Homeopathic Understanding of Chronic Disease" in Chapter 2 for details about miasms).

Because the correct homeopathic constitutional medicines can so deeply improve a person's overall state of health, professional homeo-pathic care makes sense for virtually any person at least sometime in his life. There are, in particular, seven primary indications for seeking professional homeopathic care:

1. Disease prevention and health promotion
2. Genetic disorders
3. Prepregnancy and during pregnancy
4. Recurrent subtle symptoms
5. Serious acute symptoms
6. Recurrent injuries
7. Chronic ailments

1) Disease Prevention and Health Promotion

Even if people are relatively healthy, professional homeopaths can often find remedies that can strengthen them even further. By careful review of a person's genetic endowment and personal health history, and by systematic assessment of his or her various subtle symptoms and predispositions, the homeopath is able to find a constitutional remedy or a series of remedies that can chip away at layers of underlying im-balances which would, if unchecked, lead to disease in the future.

There is a tendency among many physicians and consumers to ap-preciate the value of disease prevention but ignore the value of pro-moting high levels of health. There is a real difference between being without symptoms and being vitally and vibrantly healthy. Homeopa-thy and other natural healing methods help people attain and maintain this latter high state of health.

2) Genetic Disorders

People with genetic illnesses are generally taught that they must learn to live with their condition. Although homeopathic medicines cannot "cure" such illness, homeopaths commonly notice that their patients with genetic disorders do not tend to experience the various compli-cations of their ailment as often as people not under homeopathic treatment. For instance, the homeopathic treatment of a child with Down's syndrome will not cure his genetic condition, but this child will not experience as many infections as other mongoloid children, and he will tend to achieve a higher degree of intelligence.

A person with diabetes who is under homeopathic treatment may still have diabetes, but may not require the same amount of insulin or the same strict diet as diabetics not under homeopathic care, and may not experience as many complications of diabetes. People with insulin-dependent diabetes who undergo homeopathic treatment require ongoing careful measurement of their insulin because homeopathic remedies can sometimes improve pancreatic function, which means that the person should then adjust their insulin intake. Some cases of adult-onset non-insulin-dependent diabetes are actually curable with homeopathic medicines.

Homeopaths have observed that we have many more genetic tendencies than are commonly recognized by conventional physicians. While conventional doctors acknowledge the existence of a relatively small number of genetic diseases, such as mongoloidism, sickle cell anemia, and Turner's syndrome, homeopaths have commonly observed that we all inherit certain predispositions (as discussed in greater detail in Chapter 2). For instance, physicians do not consider stomach ulcers to originate from a genetic defect, but homeopaths find that a person with ulcers may have inherited this disposition from someone in his or her family tree who had an ulcerlike disease such as syphilis.

People with genetic disorders generally require a series of remedies over time to slowly lift off the layers of disease. By prescribing a homeopathic medicine based on a person's genetic history and personal health history, homeopaths are able to reduce the impact of genetic disease on the person's health.

Homeopathic care cannot do the impossible, but it commonly surprises both practitioners and patients with powerful healing responses that grant greater health.

3) Prepregnancy and During Pregnancy

Physicians today recognize the importance of healthy living during pregnancy, but it makes sense to begin healthy habits prior to pregnancy as well. Not only can this lead to a quicker conception, it can reduce the chances of miscarriage or other complications of pregnancy. Homeopathic medicines, especially constitutional remedies prescribed by professional homeopaths, can also help create a healthy pregnancy.

Homeopaths have long noticed that pregnant women respond particularly well to homeopathic medicines, and because improved health of the mother tends to lead to better health of the fetus, it is worthwhile to consider using homeopathic remedies during pregnancy. Whether the woman experiences common symptoms of pregnancy such as nausea, fatigue, and hemorrhoids or has her own unique symptoms, homeopathic remedies can provide effective and safe relief.

Not only can these remedies be effective in treating the various symptoms that pregnant women tend to experience, the use of constitutional medicines, as individually selected by professional homeopaths, has the potential of significantly raising their overall health status, which tends to prevent complications of pregnancy and labor.

4) Recurrent Subtle Symptoms

Many people who think they are healthy actually have numerous subtle and even not so subtle symptoms that diminish their physical and psychological potential. Although conventional physicians may declare such individuals "healthy," homeopaths tend to apply considerably higher standards for their definition of health.

A person may not have any clearly diagnosable condition but may not be as healthy as he could be. For instance, he may wake up feeling unrefreshed and be low in energy in the late afternoon. He may have a tendency to constipation, be sensitive to cold, and be easily startled by noise. He may occasionally get a headache, experience a recurring sore throat, and have dry skin.

Conventional physicians would generally assume that this person is basically healthy, with no noticeable abnormalities according to standard laboratory reports. They would not consider him worth treating.

However, many people know that they can and should have a higher state of health, and homeopaths agree. They, unlike conventional physicians, can do something with these vague and seemingly disparate symptoms; there is no need for people to suffer with them. With more detailed questioning the homeopath obtains the idiosyncratic information about the person's overall state of health, and ultimately, a constitutional remedy is prescribed to raise his or her health and eliminate these recurrent symptoms.

5) Serious Acute Symptoms

Conventional medicine is at its best in treating serious acute symptoms, whether it be a heart attack, a fast-moving infection, or an injury. However, just because conventional medicine is effective in dealing with these conditions does not mean that homeopathic medicine isn't also useful. In fact, homeopathic medicines can often complement and sometimes replace some of these conventional medical treatments.

As noted, homeopathy actually achieved its greatest popularity in Europe and the United States because of its success in treating the infectious disease epidemics that raged during the nineteenth century. Homeopathic remedies are likewise effective in treating contemporary infectious conditions.

Besides infectious conditions, homeopathy can be effective in treating many types of serious acute ailments. Acute attacks of asthma, epilepsy, and colitis are commonly relieved by the prescription of a homeopath. Because the treatment for these and other serious acute conditions often require the use of remedies not readily available in stores or home homeopathic kits, professional homeopathic care is vital.

There are, however, certain risks in using these medicines without concurrent conventional therapies (as there are other risks in using conventional medicines without concurrent homeopathic treatment). Because homeopathic medicines require individualization and because a seriously ill person needs to have a high degree of certainty that the therapy will work, it is risky to use homeopathic medicines alone. Serious circumstances may call for using both conventional and homeopathic medicines.

6) Recurrent Injuries

Recurrent injuries refer to situations in which people easily reinjure themselves in the same place, even several months or years after the initial injury.

Conventional medicine is excellent at controlling pain from injuries, setting bones, and preventing or reducing infections associated with injuries, but little is offered to actually augment the healing of the injury itself. Letting nature take its course will generally lead to a healing, but homeopathic medicines can speed up the healing process and make the healing more complete.

People can easily treat themselves with homeopathic medicines for common injuries (see the chapter on injuries in Part III), though standard practices of first aid should also be followed (treatment for shock, application of pressure to inhibit bleeding, etc.). When people experience recurrent injuries, professional homeopathic care may be indicated because often a more highly individualized remedy is needed than can usually be found from self-care. While frequent injuries may simply indicate that a person is being reckless, it may also mean that the person has an internal weakness which makes him or her susceptible to easy injury. Such individuals can benefit from professional homeopathic care.

7) Chronic Ailments

Today homeopathy is gaining its greatest reputation in the successful treatment of chronic ailments. While conventional medicine is weak in the treatment of the chronically ill, homeopathy provides useful and often effective medicines.

According to a study by Jennifer Jacobs, M.D., some of the ailments for which people most commonly seek care from a homeopathic physician are chronic conditions such as asthma, depression, migraine headache, eczema, arthritis, and hypertension.[1] Conventional medications may palliate these conditions, but often create side effects which can be more aggravating than the original disease. Research in the *New England Journal of Medicine* on the use of alternative medicines noted that people suffering from heart disease who used alternatives to conventional medicine most often sought the care of a homeopathic practitioner.[2]

One of the additional benefits of professional homeopathic care is that homeopaths prescribe their medicines based on the totality of a person's symptoms. People with chronic ailments commonly have multiple symptoms, sometimes concurrent and sometimes alternating with other symptoms, and homeopaths have a method of systematically treating the various and seemingly disparate conditions. Homeopaths commonly prescribe a single remedy that fits the person's overall pattern of symptoms, distinct from the conventional medical approach in which one drug is prescribed for one symptom and another drug for another, and so on, each with its own side effects along with unknown effects from the synergy of all the drugs together.

Who Exactly are Homeopaths?

There is some confusion and ignorance in this country about who and what homeopaths are. This is understandable because they fall into so many different categories. Some are medical doctors, some are naturopathic doctors, some are various other types of health professionals, and a small number are lay homeopaths. Also, some of these practitioners specialize in homeopathy and use these remedies as their primary practice, while others use homeopathy in conjunction with various other alternative and conventional therapeutics.

Homeopaths are primarily conventionally licensed health professionals who have added training in homeopathic medicine to their education. Internationally, the vast majority of practicing homeopaths are medical doctors (M.D.s) who have developed a specialty in homeopathy after completing medical school. The exception to this is in India and Pakistan, where there are over 120 five-year homeopathic medical colleges. While the graduates of these colleges are considered homeopathic doctors, they are not considered medical doctors.

The largest professional group of homeopaths in North America are medical doctors, most of whom are general practitioners and family physicians, while a smaller number are specialists such as cardiologists, obstetrician/gynecologists, pediatricians, psychiatrists, neurologists, and surgeons. There are also a variety of other homeopaths who have been trained in other specialties, including osteopaths, dentists, podiatrists, physician assistants, nurses, midwives, chiropractors, naturopaths, and even veterinarians. There may presently be more chiropractors who actually use homeopathic medicines than any other health professionals, but only a small number consider themselves homeopaths, since they do not specialize in its practice.

There is also a large and growing number of naturopathic physicians who specialize in homeopathic care. Due to their rigorous education in the basic sciences as well as in the natural healing disciplines, the schools of naturopathic medicine represent some of the best training programs in the country to be a real healer. (Please note, however, that there is at least one active mail order school that offers a naturopathic degree, but because this training is significantly less than that of accredited naturopathic schools, graduates from mail order programs cannot get licenses to practice in the nine states in the United States that presently recognize naturopathic physicians.)

In part because there are so many different licensed professionals who practice homeopathy, the legal definition of a homeopath is vague and undefined. Part of the reason for this is that many of these professionals do not need separate or additional licensing in homeopathy to prescribe its medicines (most homeopathic medicines are legally considered over-the-counter drugs, and thus they do not require a prescription from a medical doctor). Three states (Connecticut, Arizona, and Nevada) have separate homeopathic medical boards which license medical doctors who specialize in homeopathy, but it is not necessary that a state have such a board for individuals to engage in homeopathic practice. Homeopathic medical boards are established primarily so that medical doctors who practice homeopathy cannot be disciplined by conventional medical doctors who may have disdain for the homeopathic specialty.

Another reason for some confusion about who is and is not a homeopath arises from the fact that just because health professionals prescribe homeopathic medicines does not necessarily mean that they think of themselves as homeopaths. Most often, health professionals think of themselves as homeopaths when they have specialized in the study of homeopathy to some degree. However, until national guidelines are established, there will be some confusion about who is a homeopath.

In America there is also a small but growing number of individuals who have seriously studied homeopathy and who engage in its practice, sometimes in a physician's office and sometimes in private practice, but are not licensed in any health profession. The legal questions about the lay practice of homeopathy remain unanswered. Because most homeopathic medicines do not require a doctor's prescription, it may not be illegal to give a homeopathic medicine to a friend or relative. Yet, because these substances are legally considered "drugs," some medical boards have determined that one must be properly licensed to prescribe them to sick individuals as a practice.

While some lay homeopaths are truly excellent practitioners, most are not adequately trained in medical diagnosis and pathology, and therefore they may not know when some type of immediate medical intervention is necessary. I personally predict that growing interest in homeopathy by the medical community may someday lead to lay homeopaths working in supervised medical practice. During this time they can help train medical personnel in homeopathy and be trained themselves in medical diagnosis and pathology.

In England, the four-year training of unlicensed practitioners is so sophisticated that graduates are not considered "lay practitioners" but "professional homeopaths" (this trend is also beginning in the United States, though it is probably a decade behind the developments in England). There is increasing acceptance of the place of these practitioners in a comprehensive health care system, and presently British government officials are seriously considering adding their care to the National Health Service (the National Health Service already covers the homeopathic care provided by medical doctors).

WHAT TRAINING DO HOMEOPATHS RECEIVE?

Dr. Franklin Cookingham graduated from a San Francisco homeopathic medical school in 1906 and practiced for seventy years. Upon his retirement, he flew to Athens, Greece, to study with a world-famous homeopath because he felt that he needed to learn more.

Needless to say, the study of homeopathic medicine is a lifelong endeavor. Teachers and students of homeopathy readily recognize that homeopathic schools are just the beginning of their training.

Presently, most homeopathic schools provide three-year programs, usually one weekend per month (some programs have four consecutive days per month). Classroom lectures, however, are only a small part of the study. The greatest amount of study is at home with a wide variety of books and assignments. Depending upon the training, students are expected to study between one and three hours a day.

Naturopathic medical schools also provide good training in homeopathy. These schools are four-year, full-time training programs. They require the same premed courses in undergraduate programs as do conventional medical schools. A significant amount of clinical instruction is also provided. Please note that there are four accredited naturopathic schools in North America (National College of Naturopathic Medicine in Portland, Oregon, Bastyr University in Seattle, Southwest College of Naturopathic Medicine in Scottsdale, Arizona, and Ontario College of Naturopathic Medicine in Toronto).

There are also some homeopathic correspondence courses available. Some of these programs are actually quite good, though as homeopathy develops greater popularity, one can expect some programs to excel and others to provide inadequate training. Correspondence courses integrate cassette lectures, books, written material, and homework. Some correspondence courses also integrate in-class course work in their program.

In addition to these formal programs, there are many informal training programs by homeopaths who provide apprenticeship, though the availability of such opportunities varies.

For a list of homeopathic training programs, see page 369.

For a list of homeopathic training programs, see page 369.

WHAT ARE THE DIFFERENT WAYS THAT HOMEOPATHY IS PRACTICED?

The practice of homeopathy has evolved from its inception, and there has never been simply one way to practice this system of medicine. Some homeopaths use primarily low-potency medicines, others use primarily high-potency remedies. Some use only a single dose of a remedy and expect the effects to last one to twelve months, while others recommend several doses daily for several weeks. Some recommend only a single remedy, while others prescribe several remedies at the same time. And there are variations on each of these approaches.

Basically, there are three primary ways to practice homeopathy: 1) the classical homeopathic approach, 2) the unconventional homeopathic approach, and 3) the use of homeopathic formulas.

Classical Homeopathy

"Classical homeopathy" has different definitions. Classical homeopathy originally was thought to define the way homeopathy was practiced by its founder, Dr. Samuel Hahnemann, and his closest followers. Classical homeopathy was therefore thought to be based on the following:

1. The prescription of a single remedy based on the totality of a person's symptoms

2. The prescription of a remedy based on clinical experience and on experiments called provings, which delineate the symptoms a substance causes in overdose and cures in microdose

3. The use of a minimum dose of medicine.

The strongest feature of what typically defines classical homeopathy has been the emphasis on using only a single medicine at a time. However, recent investigation by Rima Handley for her book *A Homeopathic Love Story* has shown that Hahnemann practiced differently from how he wrote.[3] By a careful review of his case reports during the last ten years of his life, Handley found that he prescribed two different remedies to virtually every patient. One remedy was primarily for the patient's acute symptoms, and one was for the underlying chronic ailment. Hahnemann recommended that one remedy be taken in the day and the other at night. Most contemporary homeopaths are not familiar with these recent discoveries of Hahnemann's practice.

Homeopaths who practice what they call classical homeopathy today usually use high-potency medicines (1M, 10M, 50M, and higher; "M" refers to the Roman numeral for 1,000, meaning that they were diluted either 1:10 or 1:100 one thousand times) more than low-potency remedies (3, 6, 12). And yet Hahnemann was found to have used high-potency remedies in only a small number of instances. During the first twenty years when Hahnemann was initially developing homeopathy, he primarily used medicines that were not potentized very much, usually 1c to 6c doses. As he and his colleagues experimented with higher potencies, they found that these higher-potency doses had even greater effects.

The clinical results from such small doses surprised these early homeopaths, including Hahnemann. However, because homeopathy was already ridiculed by conventional physicians for using small doses, Hahnemann actually discouraged his colleagues from using medicines more potentized than the 30c because he thought that such doses would open homeopathy to further derision. Ultimately—because Hahnemann was a serious researcher who sought the truth—even if these ultradiluted medicines didn't at first make sense, he relented on his criticism of the use of high potencies because he, too, found them effective.

James Tyler Kent, M.D., an American physician in the late 1800s and early 1900s, carried the torch of classical homeopathy into the twentieth century. He wrote several major homeopathic texts, was a leading professor of homeopathy, and edited a major homeopathic journal. However, as a result of a complicated incident which delayed the publication of Hahnemann's last writings about homeopathy until after Kent had died, Kent never had the opportunity to learn about Hahnemann's last ideas about homeopathic practice.

These last writings by Hahnemann emphasized his adoption of a new type of potency, called an LM potency. "LM" refers to the Roman numeral for 50,000. These medicines are made through a process of diluting one part of the original substance with 50,000 parts water (when one empties a two-dram vial, it is estimated that one drop adheres to the sides of the bottle and that this drop represents one in 50,000 drops which are then added to the bottle to continue the consecutive dilution).

This historical background is important because Kent's writings and teachings had a major influence on twentieth-century homeopathy, and when homeopaths today mention "classical homeopathy," they usually have reference to Kentian homeopathy. Kent prescribed only a single medicine at a time, would not prescribe a follow-up medicine until he was certain that the previous remedy was no longer working, and usually prescribed high-potency remedies.

One additional reason why Kent's contributions to homeopathy are so significant and why his type of practice has become almost synonymous with classical homeopathy is that he, more than any other homeopath before him, popularized the practice of prescribing constitutional remedies. Because constitutional prescribing places stronger emphasis on the person's psychological characteristics than homeopaths had done in the past, this type of practice fit the growing twentieth-century awareness of the importance of the mind and personality upon health.

Although Kentian homeopathy is one style of classical homeopathy, it is not the only classical method. It would be preposterous not to consider Hahnemann's method to be classical homeopathy also. Distinct from the Kentian method, Hahnemann prescribed two remedies to patients, as noted, gave them doses daily for several weeks at a time or until symptoms had changed, and often prescribed LM potencies.

Both Hahnemannian and Kentian homeopathy base the selection of remedies on the totality of symptoms as determined by careful and detailed case taking. This method of case taking is considerably different from some modern methods of determining the correct homeopathic medicines.

The various types of classical homeopathy represent the most common practice of homeopathy throughout the world. It is particularly popular in the United States, Great Britain, the Netherlands, India, Brazil, Argentina, and Mexico.

Unconventional Homeopathy

The term "unconventional homeopathy" primarily refers to the fact that the following methods of prescribing homeopathic medicine are different from those of the traditional practice—which is not meant to say or imply that they are "better," just different.

There are different types of unconventional homeopathy. One type utilizes several, usually three to five, homeopathic medicines concurrently, each of which is individually prescribed for the different symptoms a person is experiencing. This use of multiple homeopathic remedies is commonly practiced in France and Germany.

In another type of unconventional homeopathy, practitioners use various instrumentation or physical tests to find appropriate homeopathic medicines. One form of this type of unconventional homeopathy uses electronic testing devices in which an electrode measures skin conductance on an acupuncture point. Too much or too little skin conductance suggests a bodily imbalance which might benefit from a homeopathic medicine. Practitioners then ask the patient to hold on to a homeopathic medicine. The correct remedy will create a balanced reading.

Typically, the practitioner will find individual remedies for each imbalance point, sometimes leading to the prescription of fifteen to twenty different remedies. Some practitioners seek to find a smaller number of medicines—usually one, two, or three—which will aid the majority of imbalances.

Electronic homeopathy is most commonly practiced in America, Germany, and Italy, though it represents a small group of these countries' homeopaths.

Some practitioners of unconventional homeopathy use muscle testing, also known as "applied kinesiology." This type of testing measures the strength of certain muscle groupings which supposedly are representative of the person's overall health. Only a very small number of practitioners use muscle testing to find the correct remedy, though a larger number use this method to assess which potency to give.

Another form of unconventional homeopathy uses hand-held pendulums to help find the correct homeopathic medicines. A pendulum can be made from various metals or natural substances which are swung from a metal chain or a string. A remedy is placed in the patient's hand, and the pendulum will usually swing clockwise when it is a beneficial medicine for him or her. This method, like other methods of unconventional homeopathy, is quite subjective and tends to be as good as the practitioner's intuition.

An even more mystifying method of finding the correct homeopathic medicine is through an instrument called a radionics machine. Although radionic machines seem to be the epitome of quackery, an early 1900 version was developed by the Dean of Clinical Medicine at Stanford Medical School, Dr. Albert Abrams. A practitioner places a sample of a person's blood or sputum or even a photo of the individual onto a metal plate in the machine's panel, and then places different medicines near the sample, using a pendulum to determine which medicines are needed.

Consulting a practitioner of unconventional homeopathy makes sense when practitioners of classical homeopathy have not been effective in finding the proper remedies for a sick person, especially after a year of effort. Practitioners of unconventional homeopathy are sometimes able to find rare and unusual remedies which can be extremely effective. They also sometimes uncover unusual genetic tendencies or recent exposure to toxic substances which can be important in selecting the proper homeopathic remedy for the patient.

Although unconventional homeopathy does not tend to discover a person's constitutional medicine, it sometimes is able to uncover remedies which will enable a constitutional remedy to act in a powerful manner, when the seemingly correct constitutional remedy had little or no effect.

Good practitioners of unconventional homeopathy tend to be those who already know a lot about homeopathy and homeopathic medicines. They do not simply depend on their instruments or their testings to provide them with "the answers"; they use their knowledge to find a select number of remedies and then use their modern techniques to distinguish which is the best remedy and its best potency.

It has also been said that practitioners of unconventional homeopathy are as good as their intuition because the pendulum and other instruments may simply be tools to tap into their own subconscious. Although some practitioners take offense at this statement because they feel they are objectively testing patients, this striving for objectivity sometimes allows their intuition to flourish because their own preferences do not color their assessment. And because some practitioners are true healers who have strong intuitive senses, they are well suited to the methods of unconventional homeopathy that thrive in this sixth sense.

Formula Homeopathy

"Formula homeopathy" refers to mixtures of two to ten homeopathic medicines, all of which may be indicated for a similar type of ailment. Typically, these formulas are marketed for a specific complaint, such as allergy, sinusitis, migraine headache, PMS, sore throat, arthritis, etc. The assumption behind homeopathic formulas is that many sick people are likely to benefit from at least one of the remedies in the formula. The use of these formulas is a user-friendly method, since it does not require the same high level of individualization that is applied in all other forms of homeopathy.

Using a formula makes sense when the practitioner doesn't know how to find the individual remedy or when the remedy isn't obvious. Formulas are also indicated at the early stages of an acute ailment when there are few individualizing symptoms. Although homeopathic formulas do not "cure" the patient's chronic disease or underlying ailment, they often provide important temporary relief of his or her complaint.

Most classical practitioners do not use homeopathic formulas often because they rely upon their professional training to find individualized remedies for sick people. This doesn't mean that the formulas don't work; it simply suggests that the professional homeopath often aspires toward higher goals of a deep cure, a step beyond temporary relief of symptoms.

For further information about homeopathic formulas, see Chapter 10.

How Do I Find a Homeopath?

The National Center for Homeopathy publishes a directory of homeopaths in the United States and Canada. It is available from them as well as from Homeopathic Educational Services of Berkeley (addresses for these organizations are in the resources section, Part IV). In addition to listing homeopathic practitioners, it also lists several hundred homeopathic study groups. These groups of laypeople meet once or twice a month to learn homeopathy together. Homeopathic study groups are usually the best resource for learning about homeopathy and for getting recommendations for the best practitioners in the area.

This directory is by no means complete because every practitioner listed must be a member of the National Center for Homeopathy and must pay a small listing fee, and many good practitioners do not need or want additional publicity. For further recommendations of practitioners, consider checking out the following:

1. *Health food stores.* It is useful to go to local health food stores and ask the people who work in the homeopathic sections for recommendations. Some health food stores have personnel who are more knowledgeable than others, so you may have to check out a couple of stores.

2. *Homeopathic pharmacies.* Some pharmacies have begun to specialize in homeopathy. Such pharmacies are a great source for finding a homeopath.

3. *Conventional pharmacies that sell homeopathic medicines.* There are also a growing number of conventional pharmacies which sell a small number of homeopathic medicines. These pharmacies are usually relatively new to the field and may not know much about homeopathy. Still, it may be worth asking them.

4. *Health and medical professionals.* Health and medical professionals, especially those who utilize some natural therapies themselves, are sometimes aware of homeopaths in the area. Many conventional physicians still remain ill informed about homeopathy and homeopathic practitioners, though a select few have seen enough of their own patients improve under homeopathic care to refer patients to homeopaths.

5. *Alternative newspapers and magazines.* Newspapers and magazines that cover natural health and healing often have listings and advertisements for homeopaths.

6. *The Yellow Pages.* You may be able to find homeopaths by simply looking in your Yellow Pages. However, because many homeopaths do not know that they can obtain this separate listing, the number of homeopaths in the book is usually limited.

7. *The Internet.* There are now various alternative medicine/ holistic health forums with people discussing homeopathic

and natural medicine. The Internet is great for asking for what you need and getting it.

8. *Your friends.* One of the tried-and-true ways to find a homeopath is to ask a friend. You'd be surprised how many people assume that their friends aren't into "this homeopathic stuff," but once the question is broached, you may discover that they and their family have been using these medicines for a long time and may be aware of a good homeopath in the area.

How Do I Know If a Homeopath Is Good?

This may be a more difficult question than at first it seems. While it may be easy to compare mechanics, it is not so easy to compare homeopaths or other types of healers. Still, there are various specialty board certifications available, some of which are open only to those who have certain professional degrees. One can generally assume that practitioners who have received one of the following certifications are qualified homeopaths.

Medical doctors (M.D.s) and osteopathic physicians can obtain a doctorate in homeotherapeutics (D.Ht.) from the American Board of Homeotherapeutics.

Naturopathic physicians (N.D.s) can obtain doctoral certification (a D.H.A.N.P.) in homeopathy through the Homeopathic Academy of Naturopathic Physicians.

Recently, the Council of Homeopathic Certification was formed to provide certification to any individual, otherwise licensed or not. Despite the laxness of this qualification, the test for certification is considered one of the most challenging given by any certifying agency. The certification (C.C.H., Certificate in Classical Homeopathy) does not guarantee the legal right to practice homeopathy, though it does convey to the public that the holder is knowledgeable in homeopathy.

Another certifying agency is the National Board of Homeopathic Examiners. Originally started by and for chiropractic physicians, this board now certifies any graduate of an accredited homeopathic training program. It offers different certificates depending upon the practitioner's previous degree: a D.N.B.H.E., a diplomate with the board, is awarded as a first-level certification for medical doctors, osteopaths, dentists, and chiropractors; a Sr.D.N.B.H.E., or senior diplomate, is awarded as a second-level status; a R.N.B.H.E., a registrant with the board, is awarded for nonphysician health professionals such as nurses, nurse practitioners, physician assistants, and acupuncturists; a C.P.H.T., a certified practitioner of homeotherapeutics, is awarded to laypeople.

There are other certifying organizations in the United States, though as yet they have not established the same high standards as those listed above.

Because certification is not presently required to engage in homeopathic practice, many homeopaths have not sought to be certified. There are, however, some general guidelines which can help a consumer determine if a homeopath is good. You are more likely to know that the practitioner is a good homeopath if he or she:

- specializes in homeopathy as the primary therapy,
- prescribes constitutional medicines, not just remedies for acute or recurrent symptoms (see Chapter 2, page 30 for a discussion on constitutional homeopathy),
- asks you to describe each symptom that you have in exquisite detail,
- conducts a first interview at least one hour in length,
- devotes a significant part of the interview process to a detailed series of questions about your psychological state,
- uses a computer to help find the correct medicine,
- uses a book called a repertory in your presence (this may not be necessary if he or she has a computer).

It is important first to recognize that these guidelines are based on the premise that classical homeopathy—that is, the prescription of only a single medicine at a time—is the preferred method of prescribing homeopathic medicines. Although, as noted previously, there are different ways to practice homeopathy that are also effective, classical homeopathy is generally the preference of the greatest number of homeopaths throughout the world.

Because homeopathy is a deep system of medicine that requires many years of study and practice, a practitioner tends to be better at it when he or she specializes in this system. If a practitioner uses homeopathy, acupuncture, herbs, nutrition, and massage, it may suggest that he has not focused his learning on homeopathy. Please note that there are exceptions to this rule, because some practitioners may have seriously studied other disciplines prior to, during, or after their involvement in homeopathy. But unless these practitioners have been serious students of the healing arts for at least ten or twenty years, it is unlikely that they could have effectively mastered these various disciplines at the same time.

The best practitioners question you about each symptom in exquisite and sometimes infuriating detail. The first interview is at least one hour long, and many good practitioners will not prescribe a medicine at the end of this first interview because they still need more information about you and your symptoms.

A significant part of this first and most of the subsequent interviews should be devoted to detailed questions about your psychological state. This is essential because a person's psychological symptoms play an important, sometimes vital role in selecting the correct remedy, even when the ailment seems purely physical.

Another sign that the practitioner is good is if he or she uses a computer to help find the correct medicine. The most informed practitioners know that they cannot have information about every symptom and every medicine in their head. Computers now provide access to the incredibly large store of information accumulated on homeopathic medicines and help practitioners be more accurate in their prescribing.

Despite the value of using computers in homeopathic practice, it is important to acknowledge that there are many older and more experienced homeopaths who don't use computers but are excellent homeopaths. One of the most important criteria for measuring a good homeopath is decades of experience. It is, however, important to find out if the practitioner's experience was primarily in homeopathy or if it was dispersed among many types of treatment.

If a practitioner does not have a computer, he or she will often need to review the homeopathic resource books called repertories. Do not consider the practitioner ill informed if this takes place; it is a good sign that special effort is being made to individualize a remedy specifically for the patient.

Another strategy for determining whether the practitioner is good before you see him is to go to his office and talk to people in the waiting room. This strategy is not always viable because some people in the waiting room may be new patients and without experience, and it may be a bit uncomfortable "hanging out" in the waiting room to talk to them.

One other factor worth considering is how you feel intuitively about the homeopath. Do you *like* him, feel comfortable talking to him, and confident in his knowledge and skills?

An important final note is that people sometimes have to travel long distances to see a good homeopath. Although such efforts may have their downside, the special health benefits that accrue from quality homeopathic care make these efforts worth the extra cost and aggravation of traveling.

When Should I Consider Changing Homeopaths?

Ideally, it is best to stay with a homeopath for a long time. The longer you obtain care from a practitioner, the better he knows you and the better able he is to find the correct remedies for you. However, it can and should be readily admitted that some practitioners are unable to understand and effectively treat certain people. At other times, a homeopath may be effective at first but unable to continue the healing process to deeper levels. And sometimes, as with any type of health professional, a homeopath gets into a rut in prescribing for a patient and fails to consider some remedies that should be considered.

If your practitioner has not adequately helped improve your health, it is sometimes a good idea before moving on to request that he or she consult with a colleague about your case. In such instances, practitioners discuss your case over the phone.

At other times, you may feel you have developed good rapport with your original practitioner, but now want to get a second opinion and need to see another practitioner for a certain number of visits. If you express this desire to your homeopath, he or she can be helpful in suggesting a colleague.

You should not consider changing homeopaths unless you have not made much progress in your health for at least six months. Before changing practitioners it may be worthwhile to try to talk with your homeopath, even though it is difficult for some people to be so candid. There is actually a chance that the homeopath may help you acknowledge that there has been some progress in your health. There is a tendency for people to forget about the symptoms they once had when they are no longer experiencing them. A conversation with your practitioner may give you insight into yourself by helping you determine whether or not you have been in denial about your progress, or if you have been too impatient in seeking significant changes in a limited time. On the other hand, this conversation may further confirm your desire to move on.

Because there is always the chance that you will return to this practitioner at some time in the future, it is best to be up-front with him. Your change to another practitioner will inevitably come to his attention anyway, because you will want to have your files sent to the new practitioner so that she can benefit from knowing which remedies have or haven't worked for you.

If it is clear that no progress has been made and you sense that the homeopath is not adequately understanding you and your symptoms, it may be appropriate to seek not only another homeopath but a different type of homeopathic care. For uncertain reasons some people have conditions that do not seem to be easily treated with classical homeopathy. They may need a rare medicine that can more easily be discovered by a person practicing a more unconventional approach to homeopathy.

Since good healers recognize that there is no single way to heal people, they usually have an open mind to other methods, especially when their own has not been effective.

How Much Does Professional Homeopathic Care Cost?

The cost of homeopathic care varies considerably from one homeopath to another. Generally, medical doctors who practice homeopathy charge more than non-M.D.s, and the longer the practitioner has been practicing, the higher the fees tend to be.

The first visit to a homeopath usually lasts from sixty to ninety minutes. When seeking the care of an M.D. homeopath, you will find the fees for this visit comparable with other physician specialists, ranging from $100 to $300. Other homeopaths charge from $50 to $250. Follow-up visits last between fifteen and forty-five minutes; M.D.s charge from $50 to $100, while non-M.D.s charge from $30 to $80.

While fees for homeopathic care by homeopathic M.D.s are similar to conventional physicians', the amount of time that homeopaths spend with their patients tends to be significantly longer. Homeo-pathic physicians earn good incomes, though generally not as high as the average medical doctor.

The actual cost of the medicine itself is negligible. If only one med-icine is prescribed (as is most common), it costs between $4 and $10. Some homeopaths provide whatever they prescribe without charge.

The costs of homeopathic care, like the costs of all medical care, are high, but the costs of illness, especially chronic illness, are even higher. Some people may be tempted to treat themselves and avoid professional homeopaths, but such decisions can be more costly in the long run because it is highly unlikely that this care will be effective.

When one considers that homeopaths typically discourage fre-quent visits unless they are medically necessary, and that the time be-tween visits ranges from one to six months, the yearly cost of homeopathic care is considerably less than conventional medical care as well as most types of alternative medicine. This does not even take into account the further cost savings that accrue from the ability of homeopathic medicines to strengthen one's immune system and pre-vent future costly diseases.

While medically trained homeopaths will recommend laboratory analysis when indicated, they rarely need to run such tests to deter-mine the appropriate homeopathic medicine. Because of this, they tend to perform laboratory tests significantly less frequently than do conventional physicians,[4] further reducing costs. The absence of side effects from homeopathic medicines also reduces the cost of care, since side effects usually lead to the need for more medical treatment.

The French government compared all the costs associated with treatment from a homeopathic physician with that of a conventional physician and discovered that homeopathic care costs *one half* as much![5] Considering the growing concern about the cost of health care, let alone the concerns about the efficacy of therapies, homeo-pathic medicine again seems to provide significant advantages.

WILL INSURANCE COVER HOMEOPATHIC CARE?

Because the vast majority of professional homeopaths in the United States are licensed professionals such as medical doctors, osteopaths, chiropractors, acupuncturists, naturopaths, and others, most insurance companies pay for their care. Consumers are encouraged to review their own insurance to determine the coverage of chiropractors, acupuncturists, and naturopaths, because many policies allow only a limited number of visits and some do not cover any visits at all. If your policy does not cover the care you want, rather than immediately switch insurance companies, contact the company or your insurance broker and inform them of your interests. Only when consumers make their desires heard will the insurance market change. It is also good to know that there are now some insurance companies that specialize in coverage of alternative health care. Look for their advertisements in health magazines or consult an insurance broker.

When a homeopath is not a licensed professional, it is unlikely that an insurance company will cover his or her care, except in instances when a medical doctor prescribes homeopathic care and the insurance company agrees to pay for specialty care when prescribed by a medical doctor.

As mentioned earlier, the first interview with a homeopath usually lasts sixty to ninety minutes, and therefore homeopaths commonly charge more than the usual office visit fee for this lengthy interview. Some but not all insurance companies pay for these higher first visit fees. In such instances the patient may be required to pay a portion of the homeopath's fee.

Insurance companies will not cover the small expenses of homeopathic medicines because they tend to pay for prescription drugs only, and homeopathic remedies are primarily over-the-counter drugs.

NINE

Working with Your Homeopath

WHAT CAN I EXPECT WHEN VISITING A HOMEOPATH?

A visit to a homeopathic practitioner is a considerably different experience than going to a conventional doctor. Conventional doctors will inquire about your primary symptoms, may do a physical examination, and, when appropriate, will order laboratory tests. The homeopathic practitioner will perform an in-depth interview, asking questions that require you to describe in detail the various physical, emotional, and mental symptoms that you have. This interview will elicit not only the various symptoms experienced but also idiosyncratic factors that make each symptom better or worse. The homeopath may also perform a physical examination and may order lab tests, though the information accumulated from these analyses will be used primarily to establish a baseline level of health and to provide a conventional diagnosis, not a homeopathic prescription.

A homeopath is not interested simply in knowing what disease you have but in how your symptoms of this specific disease are unique to you. Homeopaths do not simply prescribe medicines for a specific disease but for the totality of your physical and psychological symptoms.

You can do a lot to help your homeopath find the best medicine for you. He or she will inevitably ask you a lot of questions about your family, your own personal health history, and your present health status. The more prepared you are, the more accurate and complete the information your homeopath will have.

A minority of homeopaths prefer patients to be totally unprepared so that the homeopaths' questions can be answered in a fresh, unrehearsed manner. Because this may be an appropriate concern, a good compromise would be to come prepared but without "rehearsal."

How Much Family History Will the Homeopath Want?

The homeopath will be interested primarily in your own health, but she will also benefit from knowing some key information about your family's health. (Please note that "family" refers to your immediate family, not in-laws.)

A homeopath will want to know:

- What physical or mental diseases tend to run in your family?
- If your parents or grandparents have passed away, what did they die of?
- If your siblings have passed away, what did they die of?
- What chronic ailments do your siblings have?
- What chronic ailments do your children have?
- Does alcohol or drug abuse run in the family?
- Are there behavioral traits that run in your family?

What Information Will the Homeopath Want about My Personal Health History?

The symptoms and diseases that you presently have did not come out of nowhere; they have evolved over time. Just as there is a healing process, there is a diseasing process which is a result of your genetics, your personal health history, your lifestyle, and the consequences of the various treatments you have used.

Homeopaths seek whatever patterns of symptoms and syndromes you have experienced in your life. They also seek out significant events, diseases, and emotional crises in your life which may have led to present symptoms and syndromes.

If you cannot answer all the questions, the homeopath will still be able to treat you effectively. The vast majority of homeopathic patients do not know all the answers to questions about their health history. Homeopaths simply rely upon other information that you can provide. The more information you provide, the easier it will be for the homeopath to help you.

Most homeopaths will begin talking about your health history with open-ended questions that allow you to give specific information on whatever you think is most important to you. The homeopath may simply ask you to tell her about your health as an infant or child. Depending on the answers you provide, she may follow up your responses with some specific questions, such as:

- Did anything particularly stressful occur during your mother's pregnancy or labor?

- How would you or your parents describe your health status as an infant? Give specifics.

- How would you or your parents describe your growth and development as an infant and child?

- If you had vaccinations, did you have any obvious reaction to any of them?

- Was your experience of the common childhood illnesses unique in any way or were any complications experienced?

- Did you have any recurrent conditions as a child, and how were you medically treated?

- Was puberty experienced early or late?

- Do you experience any allergies, and if so, to what and for how long have you had allergies?

- Are you sensitive to any medications?

What Does the Homeopath Want to Know about My Present Symptoms?

Homeopaths practice what I affectionately called *"Dragnet* medicine"*: Joe Friday, the lead detective on *Dragnet,* always said, "I just want the facts, ma'am." Homeopaths are not interested in theories about *why* the person has a symptom; they are interested in what specific and unique symptoms the person has.

As part of being a good homeopath (and a good detective), the practitioner seeks as much information as possible about the patient. Just as a good detective asks who, what, why, where, and when for each situation, so does a good homeopath. He or she will want to know where it hurts, when it hurts, what makes it worse, what makes it better, when it began, and why it exists. (This last question is not usually necessary, because the patient is forced to theorize about his symptoms, and homeopaths rely most on just the facts, ma'am. That said, how the patient theorizes about his illness does provide the homeopath with insight into the patient.)

By far the major part of an interview with a homeopath focuses on the symptoms you are presently experiencing. While some homeopaths prefer to ask first about your family history or your own personal health history, other practitioners prefer to engage you by eliciting information about your most immediate health concerns. It is sometimes helpful to begin keeping a journal two weeks or more prior to your first homeopathic consultation (see the following section). You should record what symptoms you are experiencing and what factors make them better or worse.

Each homeopath has his or her own style of interviewing patients. Some ask specific questions, some tend to be extremely quiet and let the patient describe his own symptoms, and some provide a combination of these two approaches.

The homeopath ultimately wants you to describe what concerns you most about your health. Even if your concerns may seem under- or overstated, the homeopath wants your honest and detailed description of your physical, emotional, and mental symptoms.

Because the job of the homeopath is to find the medicine that best fits your unique pattern of symptoms, she seeks to discover whatever common or unusual symptoms you may have. Although some people think that their practitioner may not be interested in their idiosyncratic symptoms, homeopaths actually thrive on them because they make finding the best remedy easier.

Homeopaths tend to ask open-ended questions so that the patient can take the question in whatever way he considers most important. One of the most common first questions that a homeopath asks is: "What are you most concerned about in your health?" After the patient finishes describing his concerns, the homeopath, in an almost psychiatric way, repeatedly asks him to elaborate further.

After it seems that the patient has described everything about these symptoms, she will ask him if there is anything that aggravates or ameliorates them. This question is not meant to inquire what therapies or treatments have worked or not worked. Rather, it seeks to uncover more information about the patient's unique experiences and the various factors that may affect his individual symptoms and overall health: Is there a time in which the symptoms are better or worse? Does temperature or weather affect the symptoms? Does motion or rest influence them? And so on. (See "Important Information Your Homeopath Will Want to Know" later in this chapter for more detailed information.)

After the patient has provided this information about his symptoms, the homeopath then asks, "What other symptoms are you concerned about?" She follows this question with a similar barrage of questions to uncover details about these additional health concerns. The homeopath continues this pattern of questioning to discover the entire constellation of symptoms the patient is experiencing.

After eliciting whatever primary symptoms you have, the homeopath asks questions about every part of your body, usually beginning in the head and moving down to your toes. This "body scan" is a way to help jar your memory about potential symptoms that you may occasionally have but may not have initially remembered.

The homeopath eventually will ask questions about your psychological state, if she hasn't done so already in the process of discussing your other symptoms. Homeopaths do not "psychoanalyze." They do not delve into the psyche to uncover why you are the way you are. Instead, homeopaths seek primarily to uncover how you react to events in your life and what physical and psychological symptoms you have experienced.

Again, in an almost psychiatric way, homeopaths often follow up your answers by encouraging you to tell them more. After they have obtained as much information as possible about your every physical symptom and psychological characteristic, they then do the homework necessary to find the correct remedy for you. Sometimes they use one or more books or some of the recently developed computer software programs that have been developed for homeopaths. At other times, the homeopath may feel confident that the correct remedy is obvious, and no other further investigation is needed.

Do *not* think that your practitioner is ill informed about homeopathy just because he is looking up things in books. In order to find the individualized remedy for a patient's unique symptoms, homeopaths review several books. Only in special instances when a practitioner is exceedingly confident that a patient fits a remedy does the homeopath not review homeopathic texts or software.

Is It Helpful to Keep a Journal?

Yes, it is helpful to keep a journal, both before seeking homeopathic care and during homeopathic care, but it is certainly not necessary.

We commonly experience subtle and even obvious symptoms that we tend to forget to mention to health professionals. Although we usually remember some of our most significant symptoms, we often do not remember some of the idiosyncratic factors that aggravate or ameliorate them. Because both minor and major symptoms can be important to a homeopath, keeping a journal helps by reminding you of what symptoms you have been experiencing.

The value in keeping a journal after taking a homeopathic medicine is twofold. First, homeopaths usually schedule appointments a month after prescribing a remedy in nonacute and nonemergency situations, and it is common for people to forget some symptom changes that occur during that time. By writing down their experiences after taking a homeopathic medicine, people are more apt to notice the subtle as well as obvious changes. Second, some people experience a profound healing after taking a homeopathic medicine, and during this time it is common for them to have unusual dreams and important insights which can help them better understand themselves.

Is It Useful to Have a Family Member or Friend Help You Describe Your Symptoms?

While it may be helpful to have a family member or friend remind you of your symptoms, it isn't necessary for them to do so. Still, because their input may be useful, there is no problem in seeking their feedback, though usually you need not bring them to the homeopath.

Family members and friends are sometimes able to remind you of common and not so common problems that you have. They can also be helpful in giving you honest feedback about your personality (though you may have to encourage them to be candid, and you may need to be open to hear what they have to say!).

It is often essential for homeopaths to interview parents of children, not only because children can't always articulate their symptoms but because they may tend to exaggerate or minimize them.

It is also useful to consider bringing a family member or friend into a homeopathic interview if and when your practitioner is having some difficulty finding the correct remedy for you. It may be best to ask your practitioner if she thinks it is a good idea to bring this person into the interview.

Important Information Your Homeopath Will Want to Know

A homeopath will generally need to know as much information as possible about your unique symptoms. He or she will want to know not only the type and kind of pain and discomfort you feel, but also when it began, if it began suddenly or gradually, where it is felt, if it extends up, down, or to one side, and if it is experienced with any other symptoms. The practitioner will also need to know if any local symptoms or your overall health are aggravated or ameliorated by any of the following factors:

- *time of day:* specific times when the symptoms are more noticeable
- *time of the year:* specific times of year in which the symptoms are more noticeable

- *weather:* cold, hot, rainy, foggy, snowy, windy, humid; thunderstorms; open air, changes in weather

- *temperature:* heat, warm rooms, warmth of bed, heat of stove or heater, stuffy rooms, cold, cold rooms, drafts, uncovering; changes in temperature

- *rest or motion:* slow or rapid motion, ascending or descending; upon first motion, upon continued motion, after exertion, from passive motion of a vehicle, rocking motion

- *position of the body:* lying down, lying on the back, abdomen, left or right side; rising from lying; lying with head up; sitting, sitting with legs crossed; rising from sitting, stooping, standing

- *external stimuli:* hot and cold applications, touch, pressure, rubbing, constriction, jarring, light, noise, odors, conversation, music

- *eating or drinking:* cold or hot food or drink; salty, sweet, or sour foods; milk or milk-based foods; meat, fish, bread, fatty or rich foods, spicy foods, alcohol

- *sleep:* before, during, or after sleep, during first part of sleep, upon waking

- *urination or defecation:* before, during, or after

- *sweat or other discharges:* before, during, or after

- *coition, continence, masturbation:* before, during, or after

- *emotions:* What psychological state was experienced before or during your symptoms? What emotions aggravate or ameliorate the symptoms experienced?

In addition to the above modalities, a homeopath will want to know about your general bodily functions:

- What time of day are you highest and lowest in energy?
- Is there any type of weather or temperature that makes you feel particularly good or bad?
- Describe your sleep and any problems that you have with it.

- Is there anything unusual about your stools or urine in terms of pain or discomfort, difficulty of elimination, position necessary to eliminate, or shape, size, or odor?

- Do you sweat too much or too little? What odor does your sweat have? Where on your body do you sweat?

- What food or drink cravings or aversions do you experience? Describe your appetite and thirst.

- For women: Do you experience any physical or psychological symptoms prior to, during, or after menstruation?

Your homeopath will also inquire into your emotional and mental characteristics, not only during an acute stage of illness but also as part of your "normal" personality tendencies. To determine a person's constitutional medicine, the homeopath places special emphasis on psychological characteristics, including but not limited to:

- anxieties
- fears
- sadness or weeping
- moodiness
- indifference
- introversion/extroversion
- openness/closeness
- indecision/opinionatedness
- stubbornness/flexibility
- quarrelsomeness
- impatience
- over-/underconfidence
- selfishness/generosity
- laziness/industriousness
- desire to be alone/with groups
- desire/aversion for sympathy
- fastidiousness/sloppiness

- mental dullness/acuity
- confusion
- delusions
- absent-mindedness
- obsessiveness
- suicidal thoughts or tendencies
- sense of self

The better prepared patients are when consulting with a homeopath, the better the chance he or she will find the best homeopathic remedy for them. The detailed interviews by homeopaths engage the patient in a more significant way than those done by conventional physicians. This interview process creates a partnership between the practitioner and the patient from which conventional physicians can certainly learn.

TEN

Combination Homeopathic Medicines: The Single-Remedy and the Multiple-Remedy Controversy

If you've ever browsed displays of homeopathic medicines in health food stores or pharmacies, you've probably seen remedies labeled to treat specific conditions such as colds, PMS, sinusitis, or injuries. Upon closer inspection you may have noticed that the contents list not just a single ingredient, as is common in classical homeopathy, but two to eight different low–potency remedies. Because homeopathy is based on individualizing a single remedy to each person's unique pattern of symptoms, some people are initially confused by these multi-remedy formulas.

These remedies are called homeopathic combination medicines, homeopathic formulas, or homeopathic complexes. Their various manufacturers select the medicines most commonly prescribed for a specific illness, based on the assumption that one ingredient or the combination of ingredients will help benefit a person's problem.

These combination medicines are popular in the United States and Europe because they often provide some relief and because they are so easy to prescribe.

When I first got involved in the field of homeopathic medicine in 1972, anyone who used or advocated the use of homeopathic combination medicines was considered to be committing blasphemy. Because the classical traditions of homeopathy emphasized strict individualization of the total person and prescribed a single remedy based on the totality of his or her physical and psychological symptoms, any method that oversimplified this arduous task was viewed with varying degrees of contempt and disdain.

At that time many of us were also taught that those who used lower-potency medicines (3, 6, 9, or 12th potencies) were wimps who were either afraid to use the powerful higher potencies or not educated to know how to use them. The "real" medicines, we thought, were the high potencies (200, 1M, 10M, 50M and higher).

Since those early days, I have grown beyond this homeopathic chauvinism and microdose machisimo which pervaded the first dozen years of my involvement in the field.

As someone who regularly lectures to thousands of laypeople and health professionals every year, I have had the opportunity to share my knowledge *and* to hear theirs. Initially, I was defensive about the classical method, until too many people told me of their successes with various nonclassical forms of homeopathy. I ultimately found that my own dogmatism somewhat resembled the dogmatism many physicians had toward homeopathy as a whole.

As much as I still honor the classical method and consider it the most effective way to change a person's health in a truly profound way, I also recognize and appreciate the various nonclassical methods that help improve health in perhaps less profound but still significant ways.

It is important to recognize the value of individualization that single-remedy homeopathy brings to healing. On the other hand, homeopathic formulas provide a user-friendly approach which helps provide easy access to some of the benefits that homeopathic medicines offer. Combination homeopathic remedies are considerably safer than conventional drugs, and people with access to these simple-to-use natural remedies will certainly be healthier for it.

It is helpful to note that Chinese medicine and virtually all herbal traditions commonly incorporate the use of formulas of two to eight ingredients. The use of these mixtures has consistently shown that there is a synergistic action when certain ingredients are mixed together which creates greater benefit than the use of single herbs. The herbalist may not know which individual ingredient was most significant in stimulating a healing response or if it was the unique combination of ingredients that provided the healing. However, it is not always as important to know which specific remedy was most useful in healing as it is to do everything possible to encourage healing to happen.

One can only wonder if the beneficial synergy that is created by mixing together three or more Chinese herbs might also be experienced by mixing together homeopathic medicines. Because of this possible synergy, homeopathic combinations may, in fact, be more effective than single remedies in relieving acute conditions. Only further research will determine this.

The Uses and Limitations of Combination Homeopathy

One of the primary reasons why some homeopaths do not like combination medicines is that their use resembles the allopathic (conventional medical) method: a specific medicine is prescribed for a specific condition without any individualization of the patient's symptoms, which is the hallmark of the classical homeopathic method. Whether the use of combination formulas resembles conventional medicine or not, it is important for us to assess treatment by results, not by personal biases. Observation of results is and must be the healer's, empiricist's, and scientist's credo.

The results of using combination remedies are not just empirical. There are now several controlled trials which have shown the efficacy of homeopathic formulas, including for the treatment of hay fever,[1] sprains,[2] labor and delivery,[3] postsurgical treatment,[4] and varicose veins.[5]

I have personally found that combination medicines are valuable remedies for many acute, non–life-threatening conditions. Their use makes sense to me particularly when the correct single medicine is not immediately available or when the person cannot determine with confidence which single medicine to take. Because it is not always easy to determine the correct homeopathic remedy in acute situations and because single homeopathic remedies are not as easily accessible as

homeopathic formula products, there is a place for combination remedies in healing.

Steven Subotnick, a homeopath, podiatrist, and sports physician
from Hayward, California, commonly prescribes homeopathic medicines for people who injure themselves. He has found consistently that
a single remedy is rarely as effective as a mixture of remedies for the
treatment of injuries. *Arnica 30,* for instance, may be effective in treating the shock that a person experiences from an injury, and it can help
to heal injury to soft tissue, but if nerve tissue is also injured, *Hypericum
30* will be helpful, and if bone tissue is also injured, *Symphytum 30* or
Ruta 30 will be indicated too. Dr. Subotnick commonly prescribes
single remedies in his own formulas as well as formulas made by
homeopathic manufacturers.

Despite the benefits of homeopathic mixtures, they also have their
limitations. There is general agreement in the homeopathic community that these medicines are most effective for providing temporary
relief of symptoms. Ultimately, an individually chosen constitutional
homeopathic medicine is often necessary to enact a deeper cure of
chronic symptoms.

Even though combination medicines do not "cure" a person
deeply, neither do the vast majority of single medicines taken for relief
of acute conditions. For instance, *Euphrasia 30* may ease allergy symptoms, but it will not cure the underlying allergic state. Thus, combination remedies and single remedies for acute conditions have a similar
range of benefit.

The reason why constitutional medicines can act considerably
deeper than remedies for acute symptoms is that constititutional medicines are individually prescribed for a broader range of symptoms and
are generally prescribed in higher potencies. The special benefits of
single homeopathic medicines is evidenced when a constitutional
medicine in a high potency is individually prescribed. In such cases,
these homeopathic remedies have the potential for a real, deep healing, leading to a significant or complete removal of specific symptoms
and an overall improvement in health.

Some homeopaths suggest that homeopathic combination medicines tend to suppress a person's illness, not cure it. However, there is
no evidence of this, and further, it doesn't make sense. Every plant or
animal product is inherently a combination because it is a mixture of
various proteins, carbohydrates, minerals, trace minerals, and other

substances. Virtually all homeopathic medicines, except for a small number of pure mineral products, are made from a combination of ingredients. The only difference between most homeopathic medicines and homeopathic formula products is that homeopaths have done provings on the individual medicines (as noted, provings are experiments in which human subjects take continual doses of a specific substance until symptoms of overdose are created).

It should also be said that classical homeopaths only theorize that combination medicine will suppress symptoms. In my experience and that of the vast majority of homeopaths with whom I've talked, we have never seen a single clear case of suppression from a combination medicine. Even in the rare cases in which some homeopaths theorized that a combination medicine suppressed a person's disease, it is uncertain whether the outcome was the result of any treatment or simply the result of the natural progression of the disease.

Some homeopaths claim that a combination medicine as well as the wrong single remedy both have the potential to change a person's symptoms without curing them, making it difficult to find the single correct homeopathic medicine. This potential problem may be real, but it is still unverified. Some patients are difficult to treat, and whenever a patient has previously self-treated with homeopathic remedies or has been treated by an unknown or unconventional homeopath, there is a tendency for homeopaths to blame previous homeopathic care, often without foundation.

Although homeopaths will probably argue these issues forever, I sincerely hope that we can avoid black-and-white answers postulating that combination remedies are either cure-alls or the devil's doings. Perhaps at this time we will realize that there are numerous ways to heal people with homeopathic medicines, as well as with many other systems of healing.

More Classical Than Thou?

Some classical homeopaths are the most vocal against the use of combination medicines. It must be noted that the term "classical homeopathy" originally referred to the type of homeopathy practiced by its founder, Samuel Hahnemann. In part as a reaction to physicians of his day who commonly prescribed several powerful drugs concurrently, Hahnemann insisted on using extremely small doses of only a single remedy at a time. However, as previously noted, recent evidence from an Oxford-trained scholar, Rima Handley, has confirmed that during the last ten years of Hahnemann's life, he gave most of his patients two different medicines to take daily, one in the morning and one at night.[6]

This prescription of more than one medicine a day to a patient was a common practice not only of Hahnemann's but also of many of the leading twentieth-century British and French homeopaths.

Hahnemann was always experimenting with new and different ways to perfect the science of homeopathy. Before we become dogmatic in practicing one type of homeopathy or another, we too may need to explore and experiment with different prescribing strategies, and we must humbly acknowledge that some people may have different experiences than our own.

Sadly, there has been and still is a harsh dogmatism from a select number of people who call themselves "classical homeopaths." Although they don't practice like Hahnemann, they insist that using only a single medicine, usually in only a single dose, is the only appropriate way to practice homeopathy. They further insist that practitioners who prescribe homeopathic medicines differently should not call themselves homeopaths or their remedies homeopathic medicines.

The dogmatism that some homeopaths express is further evidenced by the fact that many leading homeopaths, past and present, have not openly acknowledged their own diversion from the single-remedy school of thought. They voice a real fear that their colleagues will shun them, and thus they are afraid of "coming out of the homeopathic medicine closet."

The tendency of some homeopaths to be "more classical than thou" hurts dialogue between practitioners who prescribe homeopathic medicines in different ways.

Practical Information about Combination Medicines

Combination medicines are generally mixtures of low-potency remedies because high-potency medicines have to be more strictly individualized for most effective treatment and combination medicines are generally used without this individualized care. Some formulas will have the same potencies, some will have varying potencies, and some will have several potencies of each remedy. As yet, there has not been any formal research comparing the efficacy of these varying ways to make combination medicines.

When using self-prescribed homeopathic combination medicines, take doses similar to doses of single remedies. Take them more frequently when experiencing intense pain or discomfort—usually every other hour, though possibly every hour at the most intense times. During mild pain or discomfort, take them every four hours or simply three or four times a day. These remedies should be taken only as long as pain or discomfort persists, not longer. You will usually notice relief of symptoms after a night's rest or within twenty-four hours. If improvement isn't noticed within two or three days, stop taking the remedy. You have several options if this first remedy isn't working adequately. Consider taking another company's combination remedy (sometimes one company's formula will be more effective for your unique symptoms than another's), try figuring out which single remedy you may need, or consider seeking professional homeopathic care.

Discussion of homeopathic combination medicines would not be complete without recognition that some combination remedies may be more effective than others. Because some homeopathic medicines are known to antidote others, and some medicines are even known to work against the action of other remedies, formulas that do not rely on the experience of previous homeopaths may not be as effective as those that do (an appendix in Kent's *Repertory* provides a detailed table listing those remedies which antidote others). Further, some homeopathic combinations include so many substances that some people wonder if this makes them more effective or less. Research on this subject would certainly be worthwhile. A final concern is that some homeopathic formulas contain deep-acting homeopathic medicines in the 30th or higher potency which are best prescribed by professional homeopaths.

Using Single and Combination Medicines

While combination remedies may have a place in one's medicine chest, the power of the individually chosen single homeopathic medicine should never be underestimated. The correctly chosen homeopathic medicine can effectively heal a person's chronic or even hereditary condition. The correct medicine can also raise the individual's overall level of health so that he or she is more resistant to physical and psychological ailments, acute and chronic.

There is a place in healing for both single-ingredient medicines and combination-formula products. Combination formulas provide a convenient and dependable source of homeopathic care which complements the use of single-ingredient homeopathic medicines.

ELEVEN

Your Homeopathic Medicine Kit

Every home should have a first-aid kit, and homeopathic medicines should be an integral part of it. Just as important as bandages is *Calendula* gel, ointment, or spray to help heal a wound or burn. And just as important as aspirin is *Arnica* for injuries, as well as many common homeopathic remedies for fever, infections, headache, indigestion, and allergy. One never knows when illness or injury will occur, and if you do not have homeopathic medicines readily available, you are more likely to have to rely upon less safe conventional medicines. Illness often begins late at night, at a time when you may not be able to purchase homeopathic medicines.

It is also useful to have on hand some homeopathic formula products for the common ailments that are experienced in your household. As mentioned previously, these combination formulas are valuable in treating acute ailments, especially when one cannot determine which single remedy is needed or when that single remedy isn't immediately available.

Homeopathic medicine kits are available through numerous homeopathic companies (see page 368 for a list) and in selected health food stores and pharmacies. There are good homeopathic medicine kits containing from twenty-eight to forty-eight remedies, as well as some minikits with six to eight remedies. Homeopathic manufacturers provide very impressive discounts on these kits, which are often one-half or even one-third the cost of purchasing the individual medicines. They provide this special discount as a way to encourage you to place future orders of individual medicines with their company. It's a win-win situation that's hard to beat.

You may want to purchase more than one kit. One should remain at home. You may want a kit at your place of work, and you may also want one of the travel kits for your car's glove compartment or trunk (travel kits that carry thirty-eight remedies and are the size of a paperback book are now available; these kits are perfect for cars, large purses, and/or luggage). Not only will having a kit at work and one in your car be helpful to you at those times when illness or injury befall you, but you can be extremely helpful to your friends and colleagues at work and on the road when you are able to pull out a needed and useful homeopathic remedy for what ails them.

Homeopathic medicine kits are not just for people who are seriously into homeopathy. They are for anyone who wants to nip common infections in the bud, anyone who wishes to avoid the side effects of conventional drugs, and anyone who wants to self-treat him- or herself and the whole family as a first method of healing.

The following list of remedies is recommended for assembling your own kits, but it is not meant to be exhaustive. Most kits assembled by homeopathic manufacturers have a good selection of remedies, though depending on the common ailments that you, family members, and close friends experience, you may want to add to these recommendations.

It is generally recommended that you have a kit of medicines in the 6th potency and another kit in the 30th potency. If you must choose one, note that people who are extremely new to homeopathy and who feel less confident in their homeopathic skills should obtain a kit in the 6th potency, while those who have some experience in homeopathy and feel more confident should obtain a kit in the 30th potency. You might even consider having a travel kit of 30th-potency remedies for your car and a 6th-potency kit for your home. This way you can often have two different-potency kits readily available to you.

The Home Medicine Kit

The medicines recommended here are the most frequently used remedies for common ailments and injuries. Homeopathic companies usually sell kits that include most of these remedies. You will generally need to supplement whatever kit you obtain with only a couple more medicines

Aconitum	Ignatia
Allium cepa	Ipecacuanha
Apis	Kali bichromicum
Arnica	Lachesis
Arnica gel, ointment, or spray	Ledum
Arsenicum	Lycopodium
Belladonna	Magnesia phosphorica
Bryonia	Mercurius
Calendula gel, ointment, or spray	Nux vomica
Cantharis	Phosphorus
Chamomilla	Podophyllum
Cocculus	Pulsatilla
Colocynthus	Rhus toxicodendron
Euphrasia	Ruta
Ferrum phosphoricum	Spongia
Gelsemium	Staphysagria
Hepar sulphuricum	Sulphur
Hypericum	Symphytum
Hypericum gel, ointment, or spray	(37 remedies)

The "Second String"

You may want to supplement your home medicine kit with these remedies. By reading this book, other self-care books, or possibly a homeopathic *materia medica,* you will learn about the many applications of the following remedies. If you think that you, a family member, or a close friend may possibly need one of them, consider adding it to your kit. (As noted, individual homeopathic medicines are quite inexpensive, usually costing between $4 and $6.)

Antimonium tartaricum

Borax

Calcarea phosphorica

Carbo vegetabilis

Cinchona

Coffea

Cuprum

Eupatorium perfoliatum

Hamamelis

Kali phosphoricum

Natrum muriaticum

Natrum phosphoricum

Phytolacca

Sabadilla

Silicea

Veratrum album

(16 remedies)

The Child Kit

The following remedies are the most common remedies for treating infants and children. All of these remedies are a part of the Home Medicine Kit. These remedies are listed because some families may want to obtain multiple bottles of them.

Aconitum

Arnica

Arnica gel, ointment, or spray

Belladonna

Bryonia

Calendula gel, ointment, or spray

Chamomilla

Cocculus

Colocynthis

Gelsemium

Hepar sulphuricum

Hypericum

Hypericum gel, ointment, or spray

Ipecacuanha

Ledum

Magnesia phosphorica

Mercurius

Ferrum phosphoricum
Podophyllum
Pulsatilla
Rhus toxicodendron

Nux vomica
Spongia
Symphytum
(24 remedies)

THE ATHLETE'S KIT

Most of these medicines are already in the Home Medicine Kit (the starred remedies are not); however, serious exercise enthusiasts may want to have additional bottles of all these remedies. Some people may even want to carry them in their gym or aerobics bag, bicycle pouch, or whatever carrying case they bring to their workouts. Not only might you benefit from being prepared, you might also be extremely helpful to others.

Apis
Arnica
Arnica gel, ointment, or spray
*Bellis perennis
Bryonia
Calendula gel, ointment, or spray
*Cuprum metallicum
Hypericum
Hypericum tincture or spray

*Lacticum acidum
Ledum
Rhus toxicodendron
Ruta
Symphytum
*Sport Injury gel or ointment (there are numerous formula products available for sports injuries)
(15 remedies)

THE BIRTH BAG

The following remedies are commonly indicated during labor and childbirth. The starred remedies are *not* included in the Home Medicine Kit. These remedies can all be invaluable in helping women to maintain their strength and health during labor and to have healthy babies.

Aconitum

Arnica

Arnica gel, ointment, or spray

Belladonna

Bryonia

Calendula gel, ointment, or spray

*Caulophyllum

*Cimicifuga

Gelsemium

Ignatia

Ledum

Hypericum

Pulsatilla

Rhus toxicodendron

*Sabina

*Sepia

Staphysagria

(17 remedies)

Practical Issues in Using Homeopathic Medicines

Homeopathic medicines, like any type of medicine, are safer and more effective when taken with some basic knowledge about their use. This chapter provides specific, practical information so that users of homeopathic medicine can get the best results and the safest treatment possible.

WHAT TO AVOID WHEN TAKING A HOMEOPATHIC MEDICINE

Homeopathic medicines are not like vitamins, herbs, or conventional drugs. Homeopathic microdoses are sensitive to various environmental factors, and without some basic information about what to avoid, people can accidentally antidote the beneficial effects of a remedy or even neutralize an entire bottle of homeopathic medicine. Antidoting can prevent the healing process from beginning, or it can stop or reverse the healing process once it has begun.

Some homeopaths claim that antidoting happens relatively often, while most believe it is a rare event. This discrepancy may be the result of practitioners who believe that their remedy initially acted, when the patient may actually have responded to a placebo effect, not the medicine. In such cases, the practitioner and the patient may theorize that a substance antidoted and stopped the early healing effects of the medicine, when in fact the remedy was not the correct one, and the therapeutic benefits were primarily the result of the placebo effect.

Many homeopaths assert that a truly correct remedy cannot be antidoted and only those remedies which are partially correct create a potential problem. This subject is controversial and unresolved among homeopaths.

Whether antidoting is a common or infrequent event, it is generally recognized that what may antidote one person's remedy may not necessarily antidote another's. Also, high-potency medicines seem more susceptible to being antidoted than low-potency remedies, and single doses of a remedy tend to be more easily antidoted than multiple doses.

One theory about why homeopathic medicines are vulnerable to being neutralized is that the microdoses may consist of some type of electromagnetic or energetic imprint which can be demagnetized or erased by certain substances or stresses. Just as a tape recording or a piece of film can be erased or damaged by magnetic fields or heat, homeopathic medicines can be similarly affected.

Because the issue of antidoting remains unresolved, homeopaths prefer to be conservative and tend to recommend that their patients avoid whatever may *possibly* antidote a homeopathic medicine, especially after they have just spent twenty to ninety minutes in an initial or follow-up interview with a patient trying to find his or her individualized remedy. They therefore do not want the patient to do anything that may possibly interfere with the effects of the remedy.

Thus, if you have sought professional homeopathic care, it makes sense to avoid those things that may antidote the remedy for at least a couple of weeks after taking the medicine, and in some instances for a longer time. If you are self-treating for an acute condition, you should avoid these substances until the acute ailment has subsided:

Coffee: Coffee is one of the more common substances considered to antidote homeopathic medicines. However, because 40 percent of the French population uses homeopathic medicines and French homeopaths rarely notice an appreciable response to coffee, the problem that coffee may cause remains unresolved. It should be noted, however, that French law allows the use of homeopathic medicines only at or under 30c. The apparent lack of antidotal effects of coffee on homeopathic remedies among the French may be due to the fact that they do not use high-potency medicines.

Decaffeinated coffee rarely antidotes homeopathic remedies, though some clinicians claim that they have seen it happen in rare instances. Caffeine itself is not thought to be the antidoting agent, since sodas and aspirin, which both contain caffeine, are not known to cause any problem. The antidotal effects of coffee are probably due to neither caffeine nor any single ingredient but rather to all the chemical constituents of the coffee bean.

Camphor and camphorated products: This aromatic herb tends to be in certain lip balms and muscle-relaxing creams such as Ben-Gay, Heet, Campho-Phenique, Tiger Balm, and Noxzema.

Mint and mentholated products: Mouthwashes, cough drops, and toothpastes sometimes contain these ingredients.

Electric blankets: These blankets are thought to disturb the bio-electrical processes of the body and may interfere with the action of a homeopathic medicine.

Dental drilling and teeth cleaning: Dental work, for some unknown reason, sometimes antidotes a homeopathic medicine. It is conjectured that it may have this action because there are many acupuncture points under the teeth, and dental work may "short-circuit" the effects of the homeopathic remedy.

Some conventional drugs: It is presently not firmly established which conventional drugs antidote which homeopathic medicines, though the corticosteroidal drugs such as cortisone and prednisone have been found to antidote more than others.

In addition to the above-listed substances which can sometimes antidote a medicine, homeopaths recommend that one avoid ingesting any food or drink (except water) fifteen minutes before and after taking a homeopathic remedy. While this avoidance may be useful when taking a single dose of a constitutional remedy, it is less important when taking lower potencies in repeated dosage.

Touching Homeopathic Medicines

Some homeopaths claim that it is important to avoid touching homeopathic medicines with one's fingers. Instead, when taking a homeopathic remedy, one should either place the medicine from the bottle or box directly into the mouth—preferably under the tongue, letting it dissolve there—or pour the medicine into the cap of the bottle and then into the mouth.

Homeopaths have concerns about touching the remedies for two reasons. 1) Of greater importance, they think that the person's hand may have strong odors on it which may antidote the remedy; and 2) of lesser importance, they are concerned that someone other than the person for whom the remedy is prescribed will touch the medicine and will experience its effects merely from skin contact. Although there is no danger in this, some classical homeopaths prefer that the patient avoid exposure to any homeopathic remedies except the single remedy prescribed for that person.

Confusion about touching homeopathic medicines is predictable because both of the above concerns are real but a bit overblown. For instance, it is possible that a person will have a strong odor on his or her hands, but nothing in the homeopathic literature has ever demonstrated a problem from this. Still, homeopaths have preferred to err on the side of caution.

As for being affected by a homeopathic medicine simply by touching it, there are some cases of this happening, though it is rarely a problem because the person touching the remedy is most often the person taking it. In instances when a parent is giving a remedy to an infant or child, it is extremely unlikely that any effect will be observed, because of the short time the person holds the remedy.

Some controlled studies on tadpoles (see Chapter 4) have shown that homeopathic medicines can affect them even when the medicine is in a bottle partially submerged in their water. This research and homeopaths' clinical experience suggests that a homeopathic medicine and its container emanate some type of energy which influences people who merely touch it, though this influence stops as soon as the touching stops.

This research is quite fascinating, and more studies are vital to learn about the phenomenon. In the meantime, if you are *taking* the medicine, don't worry. If you are *giving* the medicine to another, try to avoid touching it directly to your skin for long periods of time (touching a medicine for prolonged periods is very difficult to do!). And don't worry if you are carrying someone else's medicine, just as long as it is not directly touching your skin for prolonged periods (once again, rarely a problem).

How to Take Care of Homeopathic Medicines

If homeopathic medicines are given proper care and storage, they will remain potent for many decades—often longer. Some homeopaths today utilize remedies made in the nineteenth century.

It is, however, important to know that too much heat and/or light, and certain odors can diminish their potency. Here are some basic guidelines for keeping and storing the remedies to ensure that they maintain their healing benefits:

- Avoid exposure to temperatures higher than 100 degrees.

- Prevent exposure to long-term direct sunlight or other intense light.

- Keep separate from strong-smelling odors, especially camphor, perfumes, and mothballs (it is generally recommended that you avoid placing remedies in medicine cabinets because of the presence of such odors, either past or present.

- Avoid potential contamination by quickly replacing the cap on the homeopathic bottle.

- Keep the medicine in the original container, though you can place several doses in folded-up sheets of clean paper so that a child can take them when away from home.

- If any medicine falls to the floor, it is best to throw it away rather than place it back in the bottle.

- Keep homeopathic medicines out of the reach of children, not because they are dangerous but because they are sweet, and children can easily decimate your supply.

Some people have expressed concern that microwaves and airport X-ray security detectors may have an antidoting effect on homeopathic medicines. Although there has been no research on the effects of X-rays, there has been recent research on the effects of microwaves. A study in Austria tested the effects of microwaves on homeopathic potencies.[1] *Argentum nitricum* in the 24x, 25x, and 26x were placed on top of and in front of a microwave oven, which was turned on for up to two hours. This experiment showed that all three potencies still showed biological activity, as evidenced by marked increase in the germination pattern of seeds, suggesting that the remedies were still active and that exposure to microwaves did not have any noticeable effects on them. Despite this single study, more formal research is essential in order for homeopaths and consumers to know with greater certainty what factors may antidote the remedies.

FACTORS THAT AFFECT THE SPEED OF ACTION OF HOMEOPATHIC MEDICINES

The correct homeopathic medicine acts immediately, though its effects may not be felt immediately. What is meant by this perplexing statement is that while the correct remedy will immediately initiate a healing response, the sick person may not manifest noticeable physiological and psychological changes until a later time.

One rule of thumb that homeopaths use to estimate the speed of improvement is that a patient's complaint will tend to disappear at a speed similar to the speed at which it manifested. For instance, someone with a rapid-onset fever, headache, abdominal cramp, or allergy will generally experience an equally rapid diminution in symptoms after taking a homeopathic medicine. Generally, people with acute ailments will notice considerable improvement within twenty-four hours after taking a homeopathic medicine. If they are in considerable pain, there is usually noticeable relief within several hours.

On the other hand, someone who has a heart condition, chronic skin rash, deep-seated respiratory problem, or other chronic ailment will tend to heal in a considerably slower manner. Homeopaths find that such a patient usually notices some degree of improvement within the first week or two, though they estimate that it takes at least one month for every year that a person has had a condition to experience significant improvement or cure.

These estimates, however, are simply gross approximations, and there are numerous factors that can either speed up or slow down the healing process, though even these factors will have variable effects:

The older the person, the slower the healing process.

The more conventional drugs a person has used, the longer they have been used, and the more powerful and suppressive those drugs are (especially the corticosteroids), the slower the healing process will be.

Genetic weaknesses tend to slow down the healing process.

More information on the prognosis for specific ailments treated homeopathically is provided in Part III.

THE MYTH OF THE DANGERS OF HOMEOPATHIC MEDICINES

Some physicians and consumers incorrectly believe that certain homeopathic medicines are dangerous because they are made from poisonous substances. Just because some homeopathic medicines are made from known poisons, including arsenic, mercury, and snake venoms, does not mean that these medicines are poisonous. As every toxicologist knows, the actual dose of the substance determines whether it is dangerous.

Despite this widely acknowledged principle of toxicology, the Canadian government does not presently allow certain known poisons to be included in homeopathic combination medicines, even in a homeopathic microdose. Strangely enough, the Canadian government allows these same known poisons to be sold in single ingredient homeopathic microdoses. Hopefully, government regulators will soon acknowledge their biases against homeopathy and create more enlightened regulation of homeopathic medicines.

It is widely acknowledged that homeopathic medicines are so small in dose that they are generally recognized as safe. The U.S. Food and Drug Administration (FDA) recognizes that the vast majority of homeopathic medicines are safe enough to warrant their classification as over-the-counter (OTC) drugs. This means that they are legally considered drugs, but one does not have to be a medical doctor to prescribe or obtain them. Most countries throughout the world regulate homeopathic medicines in a similar way.

The only homeopathic medicines that are not considered OTC drugs are those same remedies in less dilute form. For instance, *Ar-*

senicum album 6x (arsenic) is an OTC drug, but *Arsenicum album 1x* is a prescription drug because in this undiluted, concentrated dose it is a potentially dangerous substance which only medical doctors can obtain and prescribe.

The FDA receives advice from homeopathic pharmacists and physicians to determine what doses are safe for the general public. The Homeopathic Pharmacopoeia Convention of the United States (HPCUS) is a nonprofit organization recognized by Congress in the Federal Drug and Cosmetic Act with a board consisting of homeopathic pharmacists and homeopathic physicians. Drawing from research in conventional toxicology and clinical medicine, the HPCUS makes its determinations as to what doses are appropriate for consumer use (OTC), what doses should be available via a doctor's prescription, and what doses should not be made available at all.*

Some people worry about taking homeopathic medicines for certain conditions, such as fevers. They are concerned that the homeopathic medicine may increase their fever and potentially create a greater problem than if they were left untreated. Although a homeopathic medicine is chosen for its capacity to cause symptoms similar to those a person is experiencing, homeopaths commonly discover that symptoms which are potentially dangerous to a person generally decrease, while the symptoms which may increase are those that are superficial to the individual's health and which will generally benefit the person (see Chapter 2 for more detailed discussion on the healing process).

Some women worry about using any drugs during pregnancy, labor, or lactation, though this is generally an excellent time to take homeopathic medicines. These medicines are considerably safer than conventional drugs, and taking them during this time is thought to be beneficial to the infant as well as the mother. One of the few potential problems that homeopathic medicines can create for pregnant women

---

*The manual for the manufacture of homeopathic medicines is the *Homeopathic Pharmacopoeia of the United States (HPUS)*. This book is valuable primarily for companies that want to learn how to make homeopathic medicines, and is not practical for practitioners or the general public. It provides a listing of official homeopathic medicines, the precise dose in which a medicine is either an OTC or Rx drug, the criteria for inclusion in the *HPUS*, the guidelines for homeopathic combination medicines, and the legal requirements for labeling homeopathic medicines. To obtain a booklet that abstracts this information, write to: *Homeopathic Pharmacopoeia of the United States*, P.O. Box 174, Norwood, PA 19074.

is that some remedies, such as *Caulophyllum,* are known to strengthen uterine muscles and speed up labor. Women who take this remedy late in pregnancy may deliver earlier than expected. (For further discussion on the benefits of homeopathic medicines for pregnant, laboring, and lactating women, see Part III, pages 199–208.)

Even though homeopathic medicines are considerably safer than conventional medicines, present laws require all drugs to carry warnings stating that pregnant or nursing women should seek the advice of a health professional before using them.

Parents will be pleased to know that even if an infant ingests an entire bottle of homeopathic medicine, there has never been a reported case of any problem resulting.

THE MYTH OF THE SAFETY OF HOMEOPATHIC MEDICINES

While some people overexaggerate the dangers of homeopathic medicine, others overexaggerate their safety. Before discussing this important issue, we must realize that the word "safe," like the word "pure," means so much and yet so little. In their "purest" forms, very few things are totally pure or safe, and yet we can safely say that certain things are at least relatively "pure" or "safe."

If we were to use these words only when their precise and absolute definitions were followed, we would rarely, if ever, use them. Instead, we generally use them in a relative context. For instance, "pure" chocolate is not always pure because there are often various contaminants which creep into chocolate vats (and I do literally mean "creep," for cockroaches like this sweet stuff so much that it is impossible to keep them out of it; because of this, the FDA allows a certain number of cockroach parts in chocolate, without requiring that it be mentioned on the ingredient label). This is but one of the many times when the FDA occasionally fudges on its own definitions of "pure" as well.

Like the concept of purity, the concept of safety must be understood in a relative, not absolute, context. This introductory information is important because homeopathic medicines are commonly described as safe, and although they are considerably safer than conventional medicines, it would be incorrect to say that they are perfectly or completely safe.

Can homeopathic medicines cause symptoms?

The basic tenet of homeopathy, the principle of similars, asserts that a medicine is good for treating the specific pattern of symptoms that it is known to cause if given in large dose. For example, an experimenter may give *Belladonna 30x* to a group of subjects. When doing a proving of *Belladonna 30x,* the provers will take the medicine several times a day for several weeks. Not every prover will develop symptoms, for unknown reasons, though it is suspected that only certain people are hypersensitive to the microdoses of *Belladonna* or of any substance. The prover is instructed to write down whatever symptoms are experienced in as much detail as possible.

These symptoms can and will dissipate and disappear when:

- the person stops taking this medicine,

- a single dose of a higher potency of this medicine is given to him,

- he is prescribed a potentized remedy that causes similar symptoms to those he is experiencing,

- he is prescribed a potentized remedy that is known to antidote the action of the first remedy, or

- he takes crude doses of a substance, such as coffee or camphor, which is known to sometimes antidote the effects of the remedy.

Whether you are part of an experimental proving or simply taking a homeopathic medicine for self-care, you *can* on rare occasions develop symptoms from taking a homeopathic remedy, though these symptoms do not usually last very long, and tend to go away shortly after you stop taking the remedy. It is helpful to know that people who are already ill rarely experience symptoms of a proving from taking an incorrect remedy, because their bodies are presently consumed with a more formidable challenge of disease.

Just as one can drink too much carrot juice and develop orangy skin, one can take homeopathic medicines too frequently and develop the symptoms that substance is known to cause. And just as carrot juice should not be considered dangerous in ordinary amounts, neither should homeopathic medicines. Wheat and soy products are generally considered healthy sources of nutrients, but some people who are allergic to these foods can develop mild or sometimes serious symptoms if they are ingested. One should therefore not drink carrot juice in utter abandon, nor eat foods to which one is allergic. Likewise, one should not take homeopathic medicines continuously. If you think you are having a hypersensitive reaction to a homeopathic remedy, simply stop taking it. If the reaction is caused by the remedy, its effects will be brief.

It is important for homeopathic manufacturers to educate both consumers and retailers that homeopathic medicines are medicines; they are not supplements to be taken every day. People should take a homeopathic medicine for a limited time and only when they are experiencing a specific set of symptoms for which the medicine is indicated. If these symptoms disappear, it is not necessary to take the medicine any longer. If the symptoms change, it may be necessary to take a different remedy or formula which most accurately fits the new set of symptoms. (Further information about self-prescribing is provided in Chapter 7.)

Are certain potencies more dangerous than others?

Homeopaths commonly use substances that are known poisons. However, the *HPUS* provides strict definitions of doses that are known to be dangerous. After consultation with homeopathic pharmacists and physicians, as noted, the FDA develops guidelines that define the lowest potencies that can be made available to the public (the lowest potencies are those which are the least diluted and therefore the most concentrated crude doses of the medicine). These more dangerous dosages either require a physician's prescription or are simply not available.

At the other extreme, most homeopathic pharmacies do not encourage the retail sale of high-potency (highly diluted) homeopathic medicines—such as 200, 1M, 10M, 50M, or CM (M stands for 1,000; CM stands for 100,000)—unless the consumer has some knowledge of homeopathic medicines. Homeopathic manufacturers may sell these medicines to natural food stores or pharmacies, but they encourage retailers to keep them behind the counter and to sell them only when a customer is knowledgeable or when a physician has prescribed those particular potencies.

These high potency medicines are not dangerous in the traditional sense of toxicology. They are simply deeper-acting medicines which have the potential to create a healing crisis—that is, an increase in certain superficial symptoms (often skin symptoms) as the homeo-pathic medicine stimulates the person's deeper internal health.

If a homeopathically uneducated person experiences a healing crisis, he may not realize that these new symptoms are actually bene-fiting his health and may become anxious or even seek conventional medical treatment for the new symptoms. Such a medical intervention may significantly reduce the healing benefit of the homeopathic med-icine, which may not be easily reestablished.

GUIDELINES AND WARNINGS FOR CONSUMERS PURCHASING MEDICINES

As a result of homeopathy's growing popularity and increased respect in the medical community, it isn't hard to predict that more companies will begin to market homeopathic medicines. Some of these compa-nies will market high-quality products and will have accurate and legal labeling on them, while others may market low-quality products with labeling that is either obviously or possibly illegal. This section will try to educate you to tell the difference.

As noted, all homeopathic medicines are made according to spe-cific pharmacological procedures detailed in the *Homeopathic Pharma-copoeia of the United States* (*HPUS*). There is a right way to make these medicines and a wrong way. However, it is difficult for the average consumer on her own to know if a homeopathic manufacturer is complying with the rules set down by the *HPUS*. While the large homeopathic companies are often inspected by the FDA, smaller com-panies sometimes slip through the regulatory cracks. This doesn't necessarily mean that the smaller homeopathic companies are doing something illegal, but they are not as carefully regulated.

Because the doses of medicinal substance cannot always be verified in a finished product due to the exceedingly small dose, consumers and physicians have to rely upon the integrity of a homeopathic man-ufacturer and the vigilance of the FDA for quality assurance. Although homeopathic practitioners have been harassed by conventional med-ical organizations since homeopathy's inception, the homeopathic manufacturers have had a good relationship with the FDA. This good relationship benefits everyone interested in the field.

Now that the homeopathic market is becoming considerably larger, new companies, some ethical and some not, are emerging and beginning to sell their products. Some of these products may not be legal according to FDA and *HPUS* standards. Keep in mind that just because a specific homeopathic medicine is illegal doesn't mean that it is ineffective. However, if a company chooses to fudge on legal issues, one must ask if they are also fudging on the way they are making the homeopathic medicines. The following guidelines will help you to determine when a homeopathic product is illegal.

The homeopathic medicine is marketed to treat a serious or chronic disease. If a label or any literature on a homeopathic medicine says that it can cure or benefit people suffering from cancer, heart disease, diabetes, AIDS, or any serious or chronic disease that requires medical diagnosis or medical monitoring, it is not considered a legal product.

The homeopathic product does not list the strength of each ingredient (i.e., 6x, 6c, 6LM). There have been instances when manufacturers have incorrectly confused herbalism with homeopathic medicine and have simply placed herbs in pill form and called them homeopathic medicines on the label. Such labeling errors are illegal. The way you can tell is if the strength of each ingredient is not listed. Because homeopathic medicines are legally considered drugs, manufacturers must have a drug manufacturing license to make them.

The labeling on homeopathic medicine lists the substances only in English, not in Latin. Manufacturers can choose to list the ingredients only in Latin, but they are not allowed to list them only in English.

The product contains potentized doses of a food substance. Some companies have sought to market homeopathic doses of foods to which some people are allergic, such as milk, cheese, wheat, grains, soy, etc. Because these products are not listed in the *HPUS,* they are not legal homeopathic medicines. There are a small number of food substances that have become legal homeopathic medicines, such as onions (*Allium cepa*), oats (*Avena sativa*), and asparagus (*Asparagus officinalis*), but these are exceptions to the rule.

The product contains liver, spleen, cartilage, ligament, muscle, or other bodily parts. While there are a small number of homeopathic medicines made from glands, including *Adrenlin, Pituitarum posterium,* and *Thyroidium,* there are no legal homeopathic medicines made from organs, connective tissue, or muscle.

The homeopathic product contains vitamins. Vitamins may be helpful in crude doses, but they are not legally recognized as homeopathic medicines.

The homeopathic medicines are put in Band-Aid-type bandages that are to be placed on acupuncture points. Although placing homeopathic medicines on acupuncture points seems clever and may be helpful, there have never been any published studies on this form of homeopathy. The FDA does not consider it a legal form of dispensing homeopathic remedies. Until solid evidence shows it to be effective, the homeopathic community has supported the FDA on this issue.

In addition to the above-listed caveats on the potential illegality of homeopathic products, there are a couple of other warning signs that consumers should watch for in the marketing of homeopathic medicines:

Be wary of homeopathic products that are marketed to help you lose weight. Although homeopathic medicines can be effective in helping people lose weight, there are no single or combination homeopathic remedies that will help everyone do so. Homeopathic medicines can be helpful in improving digestion, elimination, and metabolism, but such medicines need to be individually prescribed to a person's unique pattern of symptoms.

The above warning also applies to medicines marketed for sexual dysfunction.

Be wary of homeopathic medicines being marketed primarily to "stimulate the immune system." Although homeopathic medicines can certainly have this benefit, there is no homeopathic single or combination formula that will augment everybody's immune system. Such treatment requires individualized care.

Homeopathic medicines will not be effective for treating baldness, except in the rare instances that hair loss is associated with a physical illness. Treating hair loss in such cases requires professional homeopathic care.

Topical applications of homeopathic medicines for skin diseases such as eczema or psoriasis are usually ineffective. Because skin diseases represent internal diseases that manifest on the skin, they require internal and individualized homeopathic treatment. (See the section on skin conditions, beginning on page 251.)

The labeling on homeopathic medicines is required to inform consumers how often remedies should be taken, but it should also state for how long they should be taken. Homeopathic medicines should not be taken continuously, unless they are prescribed in such a way by a professional homeopath. Proper labeling on homeopathic medicines should inform consumers when they should stop taking the remedy if symptoms persist or worsen.

Some common questions asked by consumers about homeopathic products are:

Is there any difference between products from different homeopathic companies?

Homeopathic medicines are generally considered generic drugs because they are supposed to be made in the same way. However, some companies may begin with fresher ingredients, they may have more sophisticated technologies to ensure that there is no contamination in their products, and they may have higher standards of quality in manufacture. Presently, because there have not been any surveys that compared such manufacturing standards, homeopaths tend to purchase homeopathic medicines from the companies that have been in business a long time.

Is there any difference between the different homeopathic combination formulas for a specific ailment?

Most homeopathic formula products contain slightly different combinations of medicines. While one formula may be effective for you, it may not be effective for your friend with the same ailment because she may have symptoms requiring a medicine that is in a different formula. One of the benefits of combination medicines is that they contain several ingredients, creating a broader spectrum remedy for a larger number of people. Despite this benefit, a formula may not work for you if you do not have the symptoms that match any of its ingredients. This is when using an individualized remedy can be useful.

One other way to know that a homeopathic formula may be more likely to be effective than another is if the formula does not contain any remedy that antidotes another remedy. Nutritionists note that certain nutrients help each other's assimilation into the body when consumed together, while other nutrients can disrupt this assimilative process. Likewise, homeopaths have found that certain remedies antidote or even disrupt the action of other remedies.

Some homeopathic companies make their formulas using the common remedies for a specific ailment, but they place remedies that antidote each other in the same formula. While this will not necessarily make the medicine useless, it may decrease its power. To find out which remedies antidote others, read the appendix on the relationship of remedies in Kent's *Repertory*. The edition of Boericke's *Pocket Manual of Materia Medica with Repertory* that was published in India (not the one published in the United States) also has this index.

Single homeopathic medicines commonly list a specific ailment on their label, but not necessarily the ailment for which I was intending to take it. Will this remedy be helpful to me?

Because homeopathic medicines are usually considered over-the-counter drugs, they must list at least one condition they are effective in treating. For instance, the labeling on *Nux vomica* may say it is effective for "indigestion," even though this remedy is used to treat headaches, insomnia, and many other conditions unrelated to indigestion. The listing of a condition on the label does not mean that it is the only condition the medicine treats; it generally means that it is just one of the more common ailments for which it is helpful.

The Limitations of Homeopathy

Homeopathic medicines are miracle workers to many people, though homeopathy, like every system of medicine, has its limitations. There are situations in which homeopathic medicines will not be effective or are simply not appropriate. These natural remedies are not cure-alls and cannot do the impossible, though people are frequently surprised at their ability to do the improbable.

The most serious limitation to the use of homeopathy is that it is sometimes difficult to find the correct individualized homeopathic remedy. This problem is more apt to occur when a person does not have many unique or individualizing symptoms on which to base a remedy. It is also sometimes difficult to find the correct remedy If someone is presently taking conventional drugs (the primary reason for this is that normal symptoms are masked behind the effects of the drug).

The seriousness of a person's complaint does not determine its curability by homeopathic medicines. A homeopath may commonly prescribe remedies that heal people of serious and chronic ailments, but may not be able to find the correct remedy to heal someone with a recurring mild headache or a nonextensive case of psoriasis. Homeopaths theorize that the vitality of a person's overall immune and defense system determines his or her curability. There is no list of specific diseases that homeopaths find incurable, because of the wide differences in people's experience with a disease, as well as their own immune and defense system's response to it.

There are also other instances when homeopathy may not be effective:

The patient truly needs surgical intervention. As noted in the chapter on pre- and postsurgical treatment in Part III, homeopaths are not "against" surgery. Like most health professionals, homeopaths recognize that there is an appropriate place for surgery and realize that homeopathic medicines cannot cure certain extreme conditions.

A patient is not telling the truth to the homeopath. Because the homeopath relies upon a unique pattern of symptoms to find an individualized remedy, a serious problem occurs when the patient doesn't truthfully describe his or her symptoms. Despite this limitation, homeopaths can, in some instances, observe enough objective and subjective characteristics of the patient to prescribe an effective remedy.

Emergency medical treatment is required. In emergency situations, a patient needs immediate medical treatment that can provide certain life-saving effects. Although homeopathic medicines can be helpful in many emergency situations, they do require individualization and one cannot always assume that the correct remedy has been prescribed. In such situations, it makes sense to utilize conventional medical therapies concurrent with homeopathic medicines.

Lifestyle factors are the primary cause of a person's ailment. There are numerous personal lifestyle choices that commonly lead people to illness, including poor nutritional habits, cigarette or cigar smoking, overconsumption of alcohol, coffee, or drugs (recreational or therapeutic), and a sedentary lifestyle. While homeopathic medicines may strengthen a person so that these unhealthful actions will have reduced negative effects, repeated or excessive unhealthy behaviors will still likely lead to chronic illness.

There is an obstacle to cure. Homeopaths acknowledge that there are sometimes environmental factors that are so physically and/or psychologically stressful that they create an obstacle to cure. For instance, exposure to certain doses of toxic substances will create symptoms of an acute or chronic nature. Similarly, the physical or psychological stresses experienced in certain activities or jobs can be significant enough to create an obstacle to being cured by a homeopathic medicine.

Despite these limiting influences, the potential benefit that homeopathic medicines provide considerably outweighs the few risks and limitations associated with them. And the guidelines provided in this chapter on how to handle, store, and dispense homeopathic medicines and what to avoid when taking a remedy should increase the chances of homeopathic medicines working for you and your family in the safest and most effective way possible.

Can Homeopathy Help Me?
Specific Conditions

The purpose of this section is not simply to teach readers how to treat themselves or their families, but also to help them better understand the homeopathic approach to dealing with common health problems.

The logic of using homeopathic medicines will be discussed, as will the potential and limitations of using them for self-care and under professional homeopathic care.

This section will inform readers of the key remedies to consider for common complaints. There is not space in this kind of book to provide detailed information about every possible remedy for every condition. Rather than write many volumes, I have chosen to refer readers to other books or articles which will provide more detailed information about treating the specific condition discussed.

Although specific homeopathic medicines will be discussed in this section, self-care and family care are encouraged only for the acute non-life-threatening conditions. Information is provided on the homeopathic treatment of many chronic ailments, such as cancer, heart disease, drug addiction, and AIDS, which are not covered in most other homeopathic books. This information is meant not to encourage self-treatment but to provide insight into how homeopaths treat these conditions and what experiences they have had. Professional homeopathic and/or conventional medical care is always recommended for all serious and life-threatening ailments.

When applicable, discussion of controlled clinical and laboratory studies and clinical experience is provided to elucidate the possibilities of using homeopathic remedies to treat specific ailments. However, even when research has shown that homeopathic medicines have been effective in treating people suffering from a specific condition, this does not necessarily mean that homeopathy will help everyone with that ailment. The emphasis *in homeopathy on individualization of treatment pervades this book, and I apologize if this statement is not repeated in every chapter.*

Also, it is not the intent of the book to cover all the possible lifestyle, environmental, and genetic factors that may lead to or affect one disease or another. Although they are important, the focus here is on the homeopathic treatment of common ailments.

This section is a good place to begin your experiential inquiry into the question: Can homeopathy help me?

Conditions of Infants

The fact that millions of parents have successfully used homeopathic medicines to treat the common conditions of infants belies the notion that these natural remedies are simply placebos. Such infants are indeed fortunate, for they are given not only effective medicines but safe ones to start off their lives in a healthy way.

There are real concerns about the unknown short- and long-term effects of conventional medications in treating infants. Few controlled studies have been done on the effects of drugs on infants, which suggests that doctors may not know with certainty the safety or efficacy of their medicines on these tender and vulnerable human beings.

Of particular concern is the fact that so little is known about the safety of the doses used in many drugs for treating infants. Dosage is often determined by the body weight of the infant, but pediatricians readily acknowledge that this is a crude way to make that determination.

Dr. Joe Graedon, pharmacologist and author of *The People's Pharmacy,* warns parents and doctors about giving drugs to infants: "Their immature organ systems often deal with drugs much differently than their grown-up version will a few years later, and the differences can lead to anything from uncomfortable reactions to deadly ones."[1]

Homeopathic medicines are obviously safer than conventional drugs, and they are particularly effective in treating a wide variety of acute and chronic ailments of infants. Homeopaths, in fact, have commonly observed that infants respond extremely rapidly to homeopathic medicine. Although it is not known why infants generally respond faster than adults, it is believed that their body's defenses are stronger and less encumbered.

The easiest way to give a homeopathic medicine to an infant is by crushing the pellets between two spoons and pouring the powder directly into the mouth. Because the medicines are sweet-tasting, infants have no problem taking these medicines and usually even like them.

CIRCUMCISION

A large percentage of baby boys are being circumcised these days. Whether a parent has this procedure done for religious, medical, or cosmetic reasons, there are two homeopathic medicines that are invaluable for treating the pain and shock the infant experiences. **Arnica 6** or **30** is indicated immediately before and after the circumcision, while **Staphysagria 12** or **30,** a remedy known for treating stab wounds, is indicated about fifteen minutes later (**Arnica** and **Staphysagria** can be alternated every fifteen minutes for the first hour). Although the infant may not seem to experience pain at this time, it is still a good idea to give these medicines to relieve the pain and shock of the surgery.

It is also recommended to apply **Calendula** gel or ointment to the penile incision several times daily until healed.

TEETHING AND COLIC

It is incredibly frustrating to have to endure the crying, kicking, and screaming of infants as they suffer through teething and colic, and it is incredibly gratifying to give a homeopathic remedy to a teething or colicky infant and watch the often rapid soothing effects that it has. It is no wonder that so many parents have fallen in love with homeopathy.

Homeopathic medicines are effective in treating many common conditions for which there are no effective conventional medications. Teething and colic are two such conditions. The correct homeopathic medicine generally will stop a teething or colicky infant from crying within seconds.

Parents can either find an individually chosen medicine or use one of the combination homeopathic formulas for each of these conditions.

The following remedies are commonly given for either teething *or* colic.

Chamomilla is indicated when the infant is hyperirritable, especially when he demands something but then refuses it, and when nothing consoles except rocking. **Belladonna** is useful when the infant has a flushed face, reddened and often dry mucous membranes (especially the lips), dilated pupils, frightful dreams, and a tendency to kick, scream, or bite. **Calcarea carbonica** is helpful for pudgy, fair-skinned infants whose heads perspire and who have a sour smell and sour discharges.

The following remedies are primarily useful in treating teething infants. Because some crying in infants may be the result of colic rather than teething, it is recommended to review the possible remedies for colic, too.

Calcarea phosphorica is indicated in infants who experience teething later than normal (after twelve months), especially thin infants. **Coffea** treats many teething symptoms similar to those treated by **Belladonna** (flushed face, dilated pupils, shiny redness of the cheeks), but rather than the delirium and frightening delusions that **Belladonna** infants experience, **Coffea** infants are restless, excitable, and hyperactive. **Plantago** is valuable when the infant has ear pain concurrent with teething. In such cases, rub the tincture of this remedy directly on the gums and place a couple of drops, which have been diluted in half with water from a sterile dropper, into the ear.

Colic is generally recognized as unexplained crying by an infant, though it is usually assumed to be related to abdominal pain. Since such crying may also be result of teething, it is recommended to review the possible remedies for teething. The following remedies are primarily useful in treating colicky infants.

Pulsatilla is helpful when colic is aggravated by heat or warm rooms and is relieved by open air, cool air, and parental attention. **Pulsatilla** infants are known to strongly desire sympathy and attention. Distinct from **Chamomilla** infants, who tend to yell and scream when they are in pain, **Pulsatilla** infants weep in a sweet way that beckons the parent or anyone to comfort them. **Aethusa** is indicated for colicky infants who cannot tolerate any milk. They vomit, experience diarrhea, and have stomach pains. **Lycopodium** is an effective remedy for colicky babies who experience their symptoms between four and eight P.M. or after midnight. These babies cannot stand the pressure of tight-fitting diapers or clothing and are aggravated by heat.

Colocynthis is the indicated remedy when the baby pulls its thighs up against its abdomen while lying on the back crying, commonly with arms flailing. While adults who need **Colocynthis** tend to have abdominal cramps that are relieved by digging a fist into the stomach area, infants who need this remedy experience relief when they are draped over the shoulder of a parent or when the parent massages or presses on the abdominal area. Babies who need **Magnesia phosphorica** have similar symptoms as those who need **Colocynthis,** though they tend to be considerably less irritable during their episodes of colic.

Most parents find that these remedies relieve at least the acute teething or colic episode, though sometimes the remedy for the acute situation is also the infant's constitutional remedy. In such instances, this remedy tends to prevent future acute problems or at least reduce the intensity of the acute episodes that are experienced.

Dose: The 6, 12, or 30th potencies are the most commonly indicated. The correct remedy usually acts within seconds, so a second dose is only sometimes necessary. However, additional doses may be needed during the next bout of teething or colic, though it may occur in as little as thirty minutes.

DIAPER RASH

Diaper rash can be treated effectively with homeopathic medicines. Topically, **Calendula** is an excellent remedy for diaper rash, and there are numerous forms of external application in which it can be used, including gel, ointment, spray, and even soap. The gel and spray are preferred over the ointment because they allow the skin to breathe more easily, though the benefit of the ointment is that it is not as easily wiped or washed off and is thus able to have longer exposure on the skin.

A select number of homeopathic gel formulas for diaper rash are available that include **Calendula** as well as other useful ingredients, including some that include homeopathic doses of **Candida albicans,** a yeast that is known to cause some cases of diaper rash.

Calendula soap can be used in place of normal soap, and it is one of the richest and most soothing soaps you will ever use. It is so wonderful for a baby's skin that you will probably want to begin using it yourself.

Resources

Note: In addition to the following books for treating infants and children, many of the general self-care homeopathic books listed in Part IV have information to help you treat the ailments of infants.

Miranda Castro, *Homeopathy for Pregnancy, Birth, and Your Baby's First Year*. New York: St. Martin's, 1989.

Paul Herscu, *The Homeopathic Treatment of Children: Pediatric Constitutional Types*. Berkeley: North Atlantic, 1991.

Randall Neustaedter, *The Immunization Decision*. Berkeley: North Atlantic, 1990.

Dana Ullman, *Homeopathic Medicine for Children and Infants*. Los Angeles: Tarcher, 1992.

Janet Zand, Rachel Walton, and Bob Rountree, *Smart Medicine for a Healthier Child*. New York: Avery, 1994.

Children's Conditions

Most parents feel that they are at the mercy of their doctor and the health care system for the treatment of their children's illnesses. Parents usually feel they are not adequately knowledgeable about their child's health or about possible treatments, and worst of all, they tend to be fearful that the simplest complaint may represent a serious disease. While it is certainly true that it is not always easy to know when medical care is indicated and when it isn't, there are many simple homeopathic medicines that parents can learn to use to significantly reduce the need for doctor visits. And while this natural treatment may or may not reduce the possibility of the child becoming seriously ill, parents who become empowered by treating their own children with safe and effective remedies are less apt to be overwhelmed with anxiety and fear of that possibility.

Pediatricians commonly acknowledge that the majority of visits to them are not medically necessary. There are numerous simple home care treatments that parents can learn to use to safely and effectively treat their children. By so doing, they can reduce unnecessary trips to the doctor, decrease their health care bills, and avoid unnecessary medical testing and treatment.

Medical care for children, like that for pregnant women and infants, needs to be conservative. When asked about drugs prescribed for children, Ralph E. Kauffman, chairman of the American Academy of Pediatrics committee on drugs, told the *Los Angeles Times*, "Safety and effectiveness in children have not been established." And Dr.

Edwin N. Forman, professor of pediatrics at Brown University, reminds us, "Children are not little adults, when it comes to calculating doses or anticipating side effects." Homeopathic medicines provide a considerably safer alternative and should often be considered as a first method of treating sick children.

MUMPS, MEASLES, CHICKEN POX, AND GERMAN MEASLES

Homeopathic medicines are commonly used to treat childhood diseases such as mumps, measles, chicken pox, and German measles. Although many children are now given immunizations to prevent these diseases during childhood, some evidence suggests that people who were immunized as children may have to get reimmunized throughout their lives or they will get the disease later, when it can be considerably more dangerous. Also, mothers who were immunized against these diseases do not appear to confer to their infants the antibodies that normally provide temporary prevention; thus there are increased chances of infants getting these diseases, which is more dangerous than getting it a few years later.

One remedy recommended for a child at the *very beginning* of any of these childhood ailments is **Aconitum.** It is particularly indicated when the child develops a fever with a sudden onset of symptoms. It is often effective in helping a child get over these ailments swiftly and without complications.

For mumps, consider **Belladonna, Phytolacca,** or **Pulsatilla.** **Belladonna** is valuable when the child has a flushed face, a throbbing headache, much drowsiness but difficulty falling asleep, and swollen glands that are hot to the touch (the child will radiate so much heat you may even feel warmth without touching the body). **Phytolacca** is effective when a child has stone-hard throat glands, commonly on the right side. The child may also have throat pain that extends to the ear. One symptom particularly characteristic of children who need this remedy is throat pain when sticking out the tongue. **Pulsatilla** should be considered when children who are approaching puberty get the mumps. It is also indicated when the child has little or no thirst, is sensitive to warm rooms, and has a strong desire for cool open air (or an open window).

Some common remedies for measles are **Belladonna, Gelse-**

mium, Kali bic, and **Pulsatilla. Belladonna** is indicated when there is a sudden onset of fever, a reddened face, and a high fever. The child tends to be drowsy, perhaps delirious, and has difficulty falling and staying asleep. **Gelsemium** is useful when the onset is slow and when the child experiences general fatigue with a great sense of heaviness of the limbs along with the fever and rash and sometimes dizziness or wooziness. Despite the fever, children who need this remedy have little or no thirst. **Kali bic** should be prescribed when the child has a ropy, stringy yellow or greenish nasal discharge and burning tears. The child's salivary glands are noticeably swollen, and stitching pains may be felt extending from the ear into the head or neck. When a child has a relatively mild case of measles, **Pulsatilla** is commonly the medicine, especially when the child is whiny (though not sobbing) and has a great need for consolation. Rarely useful when there is a high fever or a great deal of pain, this remedy is indicated if the child has a dry cough when lying down at night which tends to become loose during the day. The child may have some ear pain, some tearing from the eyes, and a profuse creamy yellow or greenish nasal discharge. It is useful to know that research has shown that in addition to homeopathic medicines, vitamin A significantly reduces complications from measles (in the study 200,000 IU for two days was used).

Other than **Aconitum,** an extremely common remedy for chicken pox is **Rhus tox.** Derived from poison ivy, this remedy can almost be considered a routine prescription for the itching eruptions created by chicken pox. This itching is worse at night, aggravated by scratching, and better when taking a hot bath.

Common remedies for German measles include **Belladonna** and **Pulsatilla. Belladonna** should be used when the child experiences a sudden onset of high fever with a flushed face and reddened lips. Again, the child radiates enough heat that warmth can be felt without even touching the skin. The fever is usually higher at night, during which time the child tends to be agitated, sometimes delirious, and has wild dreams during sleep. A child who needs **Pulsatilla** has less intense symptoms. A chill may accompany the fever, even though the child is averse to warm rooms and has a strong preference for open windows and open air.

Dose: Give the 6, 12, or 30th potency every two hours during intense stages of the ailments and every six hours in more mild stages. Consider another medicine if no changes occur after forty-eight hours.

CHILDHOOD DIARRHEA

Childhood diarrhea is considered the most serious public health problem in many developing countries because of the dehydration that can kill a child. In severe cases, conventional medicine offers oral rehydration therapy (ORT), and although this treatment prevents dehydration, it does not reduce the symptoms of diarrhea. A recent study published in *Pediatrics* has shown that children given individually selected homeopathic medicines get over the diarrhea 20 percent faster than children treated with a placebo.[1]

Childhood diarrhea is not a serious problem in developed countries, but it is a common and irritating problem that can often be quickly cured with homeopathic remedies. (For information about the common remedies for diarrhea, see "Digestive Disorders," page 240.)

EAR INFECTIONS

Ear infections are another common condition of children, and in fact, American parents take their children to doctors more often for ear pain than for any other ailment. Although physicians commonly prescribe antibiotics for ear infections, there is great debate about their efficacy. A considerable number of ear infections result from viral infections or from allergies, and antibiotics are ineffective for these conditions. While some studies have shown that antibiotics are helpful for ear infections, a similar number have suggested that placebos are equally effective. A review of twenty-seven studies published in the *Journal of the American Medical Association* concluded that only one of every nine children with acute ear infection experiences improvement as a result of taking antibiotics, and only one of every six children who have an ear infection with effusion (fluid against the eardrum) improve with antibiotics.[2]

Presently, doctors tend to prescribe antibiotics because they don't know what else to do. However, the newest research recommends that these potentially harmful drugs not be prescribed for children with ear infections unless the infection persists for three months or the child experiences much pain or shows loss of hearing before this time.[3] It makes sense for physicians and parents to consider safer methods, such as homeopathic medicines, during these first three months.

Recurrent ear infections are often treated with ear tubes, but research is equally inconclusive about the efficacy of this surgical intervention.

Homeopaths and parents commonly observe extremely positive results without any side effects when using homeopathic medicines. Besides effectively treating acute ear infections, homeopathic medicines often prevent them from recurring.

There are a limited number of homeopathic formula products specifically for ear pain, though this condition can be more effectively treated with individualized medicines. The most effective way to prevent recurring infections is through professional constitutional care.

The following remedies should be considered for ear infection or ear pain: **Aconitum** is useful primarily during the first 24 hours after onset of an ear infection. The condition tends to start after exposure to cold wind and results in a fever, possibly a runny nose or dry cough, and a hot and painful external ear. These children are restless, appear anxious and fearful, and usually are worse after midnight. Children who need **Belladonna** have a noticeably reddened ear (usually but not always the right ear), often a flushed face and dilated pupils and shiny eyes, with throbbing pain that causes great agitation, and they get some relief by sitting semierect or being treated with warm applications. These children may be delirious with a high fever; when they are able to sleep, they have wild, fitful dreams; and during sleeping or waking states they tend to cry out in pain, bite, kick, or strike people nearby. **Chamomilla** is beneficial for the hyperirritable child who is inconsolable, except for the temporary relief he gets from being rocked. He is hypersensitive to touch, cold, and drafts, and will fly into a rage from them. **Pulsatilla** is effective for children whose condition is aggravated at night and by the warmth of the bed or heat of any kind, who feel some relief with cool applications, and who may experience a yellow or greenish discharge from their ears or nose. These children tend to be thirstless. Distinct from **Chamomilla** children, who will throw a tantrum from the pain they experience, **Pulsatilla** children have a persistent sweet cry that commands sympathy. They tend to be clingy, do not want their parents to leave them, and benefit greatly from comforting. **Mercurius** is effective in treating advanced stages of ear infection. Typically, there is an offensive ear discharge, swollen neck glands, profuse sweating, bad breath, and much saliva from the mouth, which tends to wet the pillow. **Mercurius** children are aggravated by both heat and cold and have their worst symptoms at night.

Other remedies to consider for ear problems are the following: **Ferrum phos** is useful during the early stages of ear infection when the child doesn't have strong or clear symptoms other than redness in the ear and mild irritability. **Kali mur** is valuable for treating ear infections when the child has nasal congestion with a greenish-yellow ear discharge or a white, opaque mucous discharge. There is also a stuffy sensation in the ear with some hearing loss. **Hepar sulphur** is indicated for hyperirritable children who wake shrieking with pain at night, like that for which **Chamomilla** treats. These children are extremely sensitive to cold, touch, and pain. **Hepar sulphur** is useful primarily when the ear has an offensive discharge and the child may experience pain extending from ear to ear. He or she may also have concurrent nasal congestion with an offensive discharge. **Graphites** tend to be indicated for left-sided ear infections, especially when there has been repeated ear discharge with the infection. **Verbascum** (oil of mullein) is useful primarily in treating external ear infections, and is usually given in tincture form directly into the affected ear(s).

Dose: Give a dose of the 6, 12, or 30th potency every two to six hours depending on the severity. Stop when there is definite improvement. If there is no improvement after twelve hours or at least three doses, consider another remedy.

HYPERACTIVITY AND ATTENTION DEFICIT DISORDER

The most commonly prescribed conventional drug for this condition is Ritalin. However, because Ritalin is an amphetamine-like drug, if it is given to a nonhyperactive child or to an adult, it will highly stimulate them. And yet, if given to hyperactive children, it will slow them down. Caffeine has the same effect.

Ritalin and caffeine have a classic homeopathic effect on hyperactive children. Homeopaths sometimes use homeopathic microdoses of caffeine, coffee, and other stimulants when treating such children. The difference between the conventional and homeopathic treatment is that the homeopathic medicine is in considerably smaller dose and is prescribed individually to the unique symptoms of each child's hyperactivity.

While parents may use homeopathic medicines to treat an acutely overactive child, it is recommended that children who are chronically hyperactive or who have been diagnosed with attention deficit disorder (or a similar diagnostic name) seek the care of a professional homeopath. Such care provides the individualized remedy that has the greatest chance of deeply improving the health of the child. The correct remedy is not based just on a child's hyperactive state but on the totality of physical, emotional, and mental symptoms that the child experiences. In some instances, the correct remedy may even be based on the mother's symptoms during pregnancy or breastfeeding or on some idiosyncratic factor that only experienced professionals are trained to find.

Because many potential medicines are used to treat hyperactive children, and because the condition is best treated by a professional homeopath, no short list of recommended remedies for healing this chronic condition will be provided. The following remedies, however, are useful for treating acute episodes of hyperactivity.

Chamomilla is more commonly given to hyperactive infants or young children. These children are restless, fitful, quarrelsome, snappish, hyperirritable, and defiant. They are capricious, demanding something at one moment and then refusing it when offered. They cry loudly and scream and are inconsolable, except for the temporary relief achieved by being held, rocked, or carried. They may experience concurrent stomach pains or digestive problems. Children who need **Arsenicum** experience greater anxiety than anger during these hyperrestless fits. They worry about anything and everything, and are particularly anxious and fearful of being alone or being abandoned. They are conscientious about trifles and can be obsessed with order and tidiness. They tend to be selfish and very possessive with their belongings. Their restlessness can be aggravated at night, especially after midnight. **Argentum nitricum** should be considered when children are extremely impulsive, acting first and thinking about things later. Their hyperactivity can be set off by feelings of anticipation about going somewhere and about participating in a special event, and also after eating sweets. They are impressionable, frighten easily, and suffer from various fears. Like **Arsenicum** children, they are fearful of being alone or being abandoned. They feel hurried internally and act in a hurried fashion. **Rhus tox** is a great remedy for restlessness, not just physical but also mental. **Rhus tox** children have difficulty staying in one place for any length of time. Typically, their minds move from one subject to another at inordinate speed. These children are easily frustrated, and very impatient, and can even be malicious. They can be particularly restless at night. **Coffea** is good for children who are nervous and restless, and are oversensitive and overexcited by stimuli. These children become easily excitable and easily startled, and it is difficult to calm them down. Good news, in particular, can make them uncontrollably energetic.

The nature of each of these substances gives us some insight into why they can be effective in treating hyperactive children. **Chamomilla** is made from the herb camomile, which is known to have powerful tranquilizing effects, especially on children. The reason why it is an effective homeopathic medicine for hyperactivity is that overdoses of camomile create the hyperactivity and hyperirritability that smaller doses are known to relieve. **Arsenicum** is made from a toxic mineral which has been used (illegally) in horse racing because it causes horses to be so restless that they tend to run the track extremely fast. **Argentum nitricum** is made from silver nitrate. Silver is considered one of the most highly conductive metals known, and similarly, children who need it tend to conduct a lot of energy through their bodies. **Rhus tox** is made from poison ivy, which not only creates a highly irritating skin rash, but is known to cause a concurrent hyperrestless state. **Coffea** is made from coffee beans, a known stimulant, and typical of homeopathy, homeopaths use potentized doses of stimulants to help calm hyperactive states.

Dose: Give the 6, 12, or 30th potency every two to four hours during acute hyperactive episodes. Results will generally be observed after one or two doses, but don't consider changing medicines until the child has not experienced any benefits in two consecutive episodes. If you feel a need to change medicines after these two episodes, don't discount the potential of this remedy in the future if the symptoms of the new episodes seem to match those of the remedy.

Growing Pains

Growing pains are a relatively common condition in which children, usually between six and twelve years of age, experience pains in the middle part of the upper and lower legs (distinct from arthritis, where pains are felt in the joints). **Calcarea phos** is the most common remedy for this condition and should be given when no other remedy is obviously indicated. It is particularly indicated in anemic or lethargic children who have bone pains at night, cold extremities, and feeble digestion. **Guaiacum** should be considered when the bone pains are localized to the thighs and hurt even when the child is sitting, the lower limbs feel warm or hot, and pain is relieved by external pressure. **Phosphoricum acid** is used for rapidly growing, tall, and slender children who experience bone pains with great fatigue, especially mental fatigue.

Dose: Use the 6 or 30th potency every two hours in intense pain and every four hours for mild pain. If relief is not observed after three doses, try another remedy or seek professional care.

THE RISE OF CHRONIC DISEASE IN CHILDREN

An almost totally ignored subject today is the significant increase in chronic disease among children. According to a recent comparative survey of American children by the U.S. Department of Health and Human Services, the proportion of children with limitation of activity due to chronic disease has *doubled* since 1960.[4]

Homeopaths theorize that one of the reasons for this significant increase in chronic disease in American children is the increased usage of conventional drugs. The problem is not simply with prescription drugs but also with over-the-counter medications. Parents and physicians commonly give these drugs indiscriminately to children, without realizing that some children may react badly to them.

A U.S. government report on 198 drugs approved by the FDA discovered that more than half of these drugs caused serious reactions that were undetected until after several years of widespread use. Sadly, the drugs reviewed by the FDA for use by children were *twice* as likely to lead to serious reactions as were drugs approved for use by adults.[5] Some of the symptoms that these drugs caused included heart failure, anaphylactic shock, convulsions, kidney and liver failure, severe blood disorders, and even death.

To add to parents' concern, surveys have shown that 20 percent of visits to doctors by children result in the prescription of two or more drugs per visit.[6] Considering the dangers of exposing an infant or child to certain single prescription drugs, the danger increases substantially when two or more drugs are taken concurrently.

While there is certainly an important, even vital place for the appropriate use of conventional medications, most physicians and parents do not presently know about viable and safer alternatives such as homeopathic medicines in the treatment of ailments in children.

Perhaps the fear that many infants and children have of doctors is well placed, even intuitive. Perhaps it is time that we offered them safer natural medicines before resorting to more potentially harmful ones.

RESOURCES

Note: See "Conditions of Infants," page 169, and the self-care books in Part IV.

Randall Neustaedter, "Management of Otitis Media with Effusion in Homeopathic Practice," *Journal of the American Institute of Homeopathy,* 1986, 3–4, 87–99, 133–40.

Michael Schmidt, *Healing Childhood Ear Infections.* Berkeley: North Atlantic, 1996.

Adolescent Complaints

Some parents think that adolescence itself is a disease, but adolescents know they will grow out of it, and they consider adulthood a chronic, lifelong ailment.

Adolescence is traditionally considered the time in a person's life with the greatest turmoil. The maturation of a child into preadulthood is inevitably full of emotional trials and tribulations. It is no wonder that adolescents tend to have more psychological problems than physical health ailments.

Some parents think that rebellion and defiance, insecurity and moodiness, shyness and withdrawal, and self-absorption and selfishness are all typical, expected, and untreatable aspects of adolescence. While varying degrees of these characteristics are certainly typical, extreme cases represent a teenager's discomfort in the world. In the same way that homeopaths commonly treat infants, children, and adults experiencing various disruptive personality traits which cause physical ailments, homeopathic medicines can be used to improve some of the more severe emotional states and behavioral problems of adolescence and prevent their effects on the body.

This certainly does not mean that professional psychological care, family attention, and social support don't have a role. Homeopathic medicines should generally be considered as adjunctive to other sound therapeutic measures.

Emotional Problems

As will be discussed in the section on psychological conditions, homeopathy is wonderfully effective in helping to heal emotional problems, although the majority of these problems require professional constitutional care. Self-care with homeopathic medicines for emotional problems is generally limited to simple and acute conditions treatable by well-known homeopathic medicines. The following remedies are useful for treating emotional states common to adolescents. **Gelsemium** or **Argentum nitricum** are effective for the fear often experienced prior to an exam or a performance. **Gelsemium** is indicated when the person is feeling cowardly and unable to face any challenge. Physically, he or she feels weak and may tremble. **Argentum nitricum** is useful when people feel very anxious and nervous, with great anticipation about what will happen. Physically, they tend to experience diarrhea or flatulence.

Ignatia is a common remedy for children of divorced parents. It is the leading medicine for someone experiencing physical and/or emotional symptoms as a result of not fully expressing grief, a condition often seen in teenagers. As one may thus expect, **Ignatia** is also a common remedy after the death of a loved one or the breakup of a relationship, or from homesickness. Chronic symptoms that emerge from grief, however, require more individualized care.

Dose: **Gelsemium** or **Argentum nitricum** should be given in the 6, 12, or 30th potency one or two times prior to and after the examination or performance (in rare instances, a person may need to take the remedy several times after the event if he is still feeling anxious about it). **Ignatia** should be given in the 30th potency three times a day for one or two days.

Acne

Besides the inevitable emotional turmoil of adolescence, there are certain physical ailments which add to the drama of youth. Acne is one such condition. According to homeopaths, acne, like all skin problems, is not a skin disease but rather a skin symptom of an underlying disease. Because of this, homeopaths do not consider external ointments or gels to be effective or appropriate treatment. Internal remedies are necessary. (See "Skin Conditions," page 251, for more detailed information on the homeopathic perspective and treatment of skin ailments.)

Acne is sometimes difficult to self-treat and is best treated by a professional homeopath based on the totality of a person's symptoms. Still, some benefit is possible from acute remedies for acne.

Kali bromatum is particularly indicated for people with acne on the forehead and/or for sensitive, nervous girls who sigh frequently. **Kali mur** is useful for treating acne with vesicles containing thick, white pus. **Hepar sulphur** is useful for pus-filled acne that is painful and sensitive to touch. **Graphites** are helpful when acne blisters exude a yellow or honeylike pus. **Silicea** provides benefit when every cut becomes infected and tends to create small pits in the face. It is also good for acne with many pustules ("whiteheads"). **Sulphur** is indicated when the person has rough, dirty-looking skin which water and washing tend to aggravate.

For remedies to treat scars that result from acne, see under scarring in "Skin Conditions."

Dose: The recommended dosage of these medicines is the 6th potency three times a day for two to five days.

INFECTIOUS MONONUCLEOSIS

Another condition of adolescence is infectious mononucleosis. Thought to be caused by the Epstein-Barr virus, this disease usually includes sore throat, swollen glands, fatigue, general aching, and loss of appetite. Professional homeopathic care can help reestablish health and should be sought. Because symptoms can vary so much from individual to individual, it is not possible to create a short list of the most common remedies for this condition.

DIGESTIVE PROBLEMS

Adolescents commonly get digestive problems, including stomach cramps, nausea, and gas. When one considers the average teenager's diet of snack foods with high fat, high sugar, and low nutritional content, digestive problems are not surprising. The correct constitutional medicine can dramatically improve a person's health in a significant enough way that the craving for unhealthy foods diminishes greatly; parents commonly express their surprise at the ability of homeopathic medicines to do this. However, many teenagers eat junk foods whether they crave them or not, and no type of medicine will influence this behavior. Still, no matter what food they eat, homeopathic medicines may help teenagers' bodies better assimilate their food and may even reduce some of the pain and discomfort that are felt, though no medicine can deeply heal a person with a significantly nutrition-poor diet. (For common remedies for digestive complaints, see "Digestive Disorders," page 240.)

EATING DISORDERS

Anorexia and bulimia are all too common today, especially among teenage girls. Eating disorders are not simply the result of our society's obsession with food and thinness; they are also related to issues of self-esteem. A growing body of research suggests that physical and sexual abuse is more common than previously thought, and the psychological trauma that is experienced sometimes manifests in disturbed self-esteem which then affects body image and eating patterns.

Homeopathic medicine can be effective in helping a teenager get out of the physical and psychological cycle and rut that led to the eating disorder. It is often more effective when combined with other therapeutic and social-support measures.

Because of the seriousness and intensity of symptoms with eating disorders, professional homeopathic care is required, while self-care is generally inadequate.

(For information on menstruation, see the section on "Women's Conditions," which follows.)

Resources

Trevor Smith, *Homeopathic Medicine: A Doctor's Guide to Remedies for Common Ailments*. Rochester, VT: Healing Arts, 1989.

See also the homeopathic self-care books listed in Part IV, especially Cummings and Ullman's *Everybody's Guide to Homeopathic Medicines*, Ullman's *Homeopathic Medicine for Children and Infants*, Kruzel's *Homeopathic Emergency Guide*, and Lockie's *The Family Guide to Homeopathy*.

Women's Conditions

Eliza Flagg Young, M.D., a nineteenth-century physician, once said, "Every woman is born a doctor. Men have to study to become one." Although this may be a controversial statement, what isn't controversial is that women tend to be the primary health care providers in most families. In the vast majority of homes women are responsible for watching over the health needs of the children, and by their shopping and cooking, they are responsible for fulfilling the nutritional needs of the family.

Because homeopathic medicines are considerably more amenable to home care than are conventional drugs, it is predictable that American women have had a history of interest in homeopathy.

It was not simply a coincidence that a large number of leading suffragettes in America during the nineteenth century were advocates of homeopathic medicine. Susan B. Anthony, Elizabeth Cady Stanton, Julia Ward Howe, Louisa May Alcott, Elizabeth Stuart Phelps, Lucretia Mott, and Clemence Sophia Lozier were but some of the nineteenth century feminists who considered both women's rights and homeopathic medicine to be important ways to create a healthier society.

The famous Ladies Physiological Societies of the nineteenth century were early versions of contemporary women's support groups in which women taught each other about their bodies and how to heal themselves. Because of the significant role that homeopathy played at that time, information about homeopathic medicines was integral in many of these meetings of women.

Even many wives of conventional physicians in the nineteenth century sought the care of homeopaths. At an 1883 meeting of the American Medical Association, one doctor complained, "Too many wives of conventional physicians are going to homeopathic physicians. And to make matters worse, they are taking their children to homeopaths too!"[1]

Likewise today, the vast majority, approximately two-thirds, of homeopathic patients and purchasers of homeopathic products are women. And today, there are approximately three hundred homeopathic study groups, the significant majority of which are led by women and participated in by women.

There is one simple reason why so many women, past and present, have sought out homeopathic medicine: it is a safer and more effective method of healing themselves and their families. Because women tend to seek professional medical care more than men do, they also tend to experience more of its dangers as well as its benefits. When women reach the limits of modern medical expertise and experience some of the harsh side effects of modern medical practices, it is certainly understandable that they seek out alternative health methods such as homeopathic medicine.

PREMENSTRUAL SYNDROME (PMS)

Homeopathic medicines can effectively treat the cramps, bloating, and various psychological symptoms that women commonly experience around their menstrual flow. While serious PMS should receive professional homeopathic attention, occasional or mild PMS symptoms can benefit from self-treatment, with either an individually prescribed remedy or one of the combination formula products.

When cramps are the predominating symptom of PMS, consider **Pulsatilla** (for cramps experienced by women who are gentle, yielding, and easily weepy, and who experience a changeable menstrual flow from month to month, are without thirst, are occasionally nauseous, prefer open air, and tend to feel worse when exposed to heat, which usually aggravates their water retention), **Belladonna** (for intense bearing-down pains or cramps that come on and go away suddenly, and aggravation from motion or any type of jarring or draft, sometimes with a headache), **Magnesia phos** (cramps that are relieved by bending over, by firm abdominal massage while bending forward, or by warmth and warm application, and that are aggravated by cold, cold air, or uncovering), and **Colocynthis** (cramps like those of **Magnesia phos** but the woman is considerably more irritable and restless).

When bloating is the primary symptom, consider **Pulsatilla** (see above), **Sepia** (constipation, lethargy, general weakness felt in internal organs, irritable personality, snappishness, sadness), **Lycopodium** (aggravation of symptoms between four and eight P.M., in warm weather, and with flatulence and backache), and **Lachesis** (aggravation of symptoms during sleep and upon waking; symptoms worse on the left side, pains relieved by the flow).

When moodiness, irritability, and heightened emotions are the main symptoms, consider **Pulsatilla** (see above), **Sepia** (see above), **Ignatia** (emotional vulnerability, especially grief, contradictory feelings, and hysteria), **Cimicifuga** (sharp laborlike pains that dart from one side of the body to the other, possible back pain or sciatica, intolerance of pain, loquaciousness, hysteria, feelings of being overwhelmed, and "I can't take it anymore"), **Lachesis** (loquacious, sharp-tongued, sarcastic, irritable, suspicious, and jealous, with flushes of heat; symptoms worse upon waking and exposure to heat; headaches), and **Nux vomica** (irritable, faultfinding, quarrelsome, competitive; Type-A personality; nausea).

Dose: Take the 6, 12, or 30th potency every two hours during intense symptoms and every four hours for less intense symptoms. Stop taking the remedy if symptoms are gone or quite mild. If there isn't some type of obvious improvement in twelve hours, try another remedy.

CYSTITIS (BLADDER INFECTION)

Another extremely common condition for which homeopathic medicines seem to work wonders is cystitis (bladder infection). While professional homeopathic care and/or medical attention should be sought to treat recurring bladder symptoms and for severe symptoms, an individually chosen homeopathic medicine can alleviate the pain and discomfort of most acute conditions before the woman reaches the doctor's office.

The two most common remedies for acute cystitis are **Cantharis** (burning, cutting pain before, during, and after urination, each drop passing as though it were scalding water, frequent urges to urinate) and **Sarsaparilla** (severe pain at end of urination, burning pain and constant urging; a characteristic but not common symptom is that urine can be passed only while standing). Other remedies to consider are **Berberis** (pain in the thighs and loins during urination, pain extending from the bladder and/or over the abdomen to the urethra), **Pulsatilla** (pain during and after urination as well as when lying down, dry mouth but no thirst), **Apis** (stinging pains with an aggravation of symptoms by warmth of any sort), **Belladonna** (acute pain aggravated by any motion or simple jarring, a sensation of something moving inside the bladder, restlessness at night with wild dreams), **Nux vomica** (constant urge to urinate, short relief when passing small quantities and from warm applications or warm bathing), and **Causticum** (cystitis after surgery, involuntary urination when coughing or sneezing).

Dose: Take the 6, 12, or 30th potency every two hours during intense symptoms and every four hours for less intense symptoms. Stop taking the remedy if symptoms are gone or become mild. If there isn't some type of obvious improvement in twenty-four hours, try another remedy. The correct remedy may need to be taken for up to three days for an acute urinary tract infection.

VAGINITIS

Vaginitis refers to an inflammatory condition in the vagina that is primarily the result of infection (i.e., from *Candida albicans, Trichomonas vaginalis, Gardnerella vaginalis,* or *Chlamydia trachomatis*) or exposure to an irritant (chemical or allergic). The symptoms of vaginitis generally include an abnormal vaginal discharge and itching or burning pains. To understand how and why homeopathic medicines are effective, it is useful to learn something about the nature of vaginitis.

One of the most common types of vaginitis is a yeast infection, usually caused by the yeast *Candida albicans.* The vagina normally is populated by a variety of microorganisms that help to prevent infection. The "good" microorganisms create a chemical environment that inhibits the "bad" microorganisms. They also compete for food with the "bad" infective organisms. If a woman takes antibiotics to treat an infection, whether it is for vaginitis or not, the antibiotics kill both the bad and the good microorganisms, ultimately creating various imbalances in the body, including yeast infections.

The vagina can normally live comfortably with small amounts of yeast, but the killing of good microorganisms by antibiotics allows yeast to grow in significant numbers, creating a yeast infection.

Conventional treatment for yeast conditions is usually antifungal medications or suppositories. While these medications may temporarily decrease the number of yeast cells, they do not increase the body's good microorganisms, nor do they protect the body from future yeast infections.

Other factors that can disrupt the ecological balance in the vagina are a high-sugar diet, birth control pills, and certain hormonal changes, including those caused by pregnancy. Simply getting rid of the yeast, bacteria, or other pathogens growing as a result of the ecological imbalance and leading to vaginitis does not resolve the fundamental stress to the woman's health.

Homeopathic medicines are not antifungal or antibacterial in the conventional sense. Rather, they strengthen a woman's own defenses, which then help her body fight off the fungal infection itself. By this process they do not create the same type of internal ecological disruption that antibiotics cause. Some of the common remedies for vaginitis are **Pulsatilla** (white, yellow, or greenish bland vaginal discharge with vaginal soreness, a weepy, moody, emotionally laden state, thirstlessness; aggravated by heat and relieved in the open air; a common remedy for vaginitis in pregnant women), **Kreosotum** (itching with burning pains, a yellow, putrid vaginal discharge which is acrid and irritates the vaginal lips and surrounding skin; the discharge may stain bedsheets, and is worse in the morning and upon standing), **Borax** (a burning vaginal discharge the color of egg whites; **Borax** tends to be useful for vaginitis that occurs midway between menstrual periods), **Hydrastis** (profuse stringy yellow vaginal discharge with great itching, worse after menstruation), **Sepia** (white, milky, offensive, itchy, and burning discharge which tends to be more profuse in the morning and while walking, sensations of uncomfortable pressure and heaviness in the vaginal area, general fatigue, constipation, irritability, depression), **Graphites** (premenstrual yeast infection, often in overweight women with thin, white, acrid discharge and who may experience a concurrent backache, increased discharge in the morning and while walking), and **Calcarea carb** (thick yellow or milky discharge which tends to cause intense itching, usually in overweight, fair-skinned women, worse before menses and on becoming warm, though they tend to be very chilly; a headache and spasmodic cramps may be concurrent). These remedies are effective not only for yeast infections but also for other types of vaginal infection. In addition, there are numerous homeopathic formula products in pill or suppository form that can be used to treat the acute vaginal infection effectively.

Chronic or recurrent vaginitis should receive professional homeopathic care for an appropriate constitutional medicine.

Dose: Take the 6, 12, or 30th potency every two hours during intense symptoms and every four hours for less intense symptoms. Stop taking the remedy if symptoms are gone or have become mild. If there isn't some type of obvious improvement in 48 hours, try another remedy.

Cysts and Fibroids

A cyst is a usually harmless fluid-filled sac of tissue that may be found in the breast, ovaries, or vagina, or simply under the skin. Small cysts are often imperceptible, and even large ones can sometimes be symptomless unless they are large enough to press on certain organs or nerves. Fibroids are noncancerous growths in or on the walls of the uterus which can lead to abnormal uterine bleeding, painful intercourse, and bladder and bowel pressure.

Cysts and fibroids are relatively common symptoms experienced by women. Conventional medical care ranges from the conservative ("Let's leave it alone and let it go away") to the radical ("We need to remove it before it gets worse or causes any other problem"). Homeopathic treatment for these conditions generally requires professional constitutional care. Some homeopaths have observed that cysts often respond rapidly to the correct homeopathic medicine, while fibroids tend to take longer. Homeopathic remedies for fibroids will not always completely get rid of them, but they do often at least reduce bleeding or other complications. Homeopathic treatment of fibroids tends to be more effective when they are not too extensive.

In reference to the treatment of cysts, a gynecologist from Barcelona recently reported on a study she performed evaluating forty cases of ovarian cysts. After nine months of treatment using individually chosen homeopathic medicines, thirty-six of the forty women had no evidence of a cyst, three had only a right-sided cyst, and one had a cyst on both sides.[2]

ENDOMETRIOSIS

Endometriosis is a condition in which the lining of the uterus gets displaced and appears in various sites in the body, including the ovaries, the bladder, or the bowel. Although the cause of this condition is unknown, it is sustained by ovarian hormones.

Endometriosis can lead to varying symptoms, including heavy, painful periods, breast swelling, backache before periods, infertility, painful intercourse, dizziness, and depression. Conventional treatments for it are diverse and problematic. The conventional pharmacological treatment is with drugs that inhibit ovarian or pituitary hormones. These drugs produce various masculinizing effects, including increased body hair and irreversible changes in the voice. Some physicians recommend surgical treatment in which the displaced cells are burned out with a laser, or removal of the uterus, Fallopian tubes, and/or ovaries.

Because some women experience great pain with this condition, they are desperate for any relief. These conventional medical treatments sometimes provide relief, but at the cost of new problematic symptoms and sometimes at the cost of the recurrence of the original condition.

Michael Carlston, M.D., a homeopath and assistant clinical professor at the University of California at San Francisco School of Medicine, asserts that homeopathic medicines can be very helpful at the early and middle stages of endometriosis, though because of severe scarring during advanced stages of the disease, they are not very effective later on. Endometriosis is not an ailment amenable to self-care; professional homeopathic care is required.

FERTILITY AND CONTRACEPTION

Because homeopathic medicines can be effective in reestablishing health in women's reproductive organs, it follows that they can be helpful in reestablishing fertility. Homeopathic constitutional care, rather than self-care, is necessary for treating problems of fertility.

Some women ask if homeopathic medicines can be used for contraception. The answer to this question is a definitive "No." Homeopathic medicines create healthy people, and in the process of doing so tend to make people more rather than less fertile.

Any pharmacological agent that is strong enough to block conception is also strong enough to cause other physiological disruptions. Birth control pills have been linked to heart disease and to breast cancer, though while some studies have found this latter link, others have not. Various less drastic but still problematic symptoms have also been associated with the use of birth control pills, including increased vaginal bleeding, migraine headaches, bladder infections, depression, and various nutritional deficiencies. Dr. Ronald W. Davey, physician to Queen Elizabeth II, notes that he sometimes uses homeopathic doses of the Pill to treat women who have suffered from side effects of this drug. To get the best results, however, a woman has to have stopped taking the Pill.

Many women have experienced symptoms from the IUD as well. Chellis Glendenning, in her book *When Technology Wounds,* describes her traumatic experiences with the ill-famed Dalkon shield IUD.[3] Ultimately, professional care from a homeopathic physician helped restore her health when no other treatment was effective.

Side effects from conventional drugs and from medical devices generally require the attention of a professional homeopath, unless the symptoms are extremely minor.

MENOPAUSE

Menopause is a natural life phase which some doctors seem to have made into a disease. The fact that women secrete less estrogen in their fifth or sixth decade of life does not signify an ailment but is part of normal body evolution. While it is true that many women experience various symptoms during this change of life, there are many natural ways to deal with them which are safer than the lifelong estrogen replacement therapy that physicians commonly recommend (see resources section on page 197 for details).

Homeopathic medicines are effective for relieving the common symptoms experienced during menopause (hot flashes, vaginal dryness, cramping, bloating, constipation, and emotional swings). Self-care with homeopathic medicines can be provided for these symptoms, though because the symptoms can be so diverse in their effects on women's bodies and minds, it is not possible to summarize the key remedies in this book (also see resources section).

OSTEOPOROSIS

Osteoporosis is one of the serious conditions that some women experience late in life. Because there are several homeopathic medicines, notably **Calcarea phos** (calcium phosphate), which are known to help build stronger bones, it makes sense that homeopathic remedies be considered as part of a woman's health program. However, because osteoporosis can be an insidious condition which develops without obvious symptoms prior to a fracture, women are encouraged to become familiar with the various nutritional and lifestyle factors that decrease the chances of developing osteoporosis. When such efforts are combined with homeopathic medicines, women will inevitably be significantly stronger and healthier.

Dose: Although classical homeopaths prefer to prescribe constitutionally to women just prior to, during, or after menopause, women who have increased risk factors for osteoporosis and are not under professional homeopathic care might consider taking the 6th potency of **Calcarea phos** once a day for three to five days, every month. If, however, the woman is undergoing professional homeopathic constitutional care, this remedy will generally not be necessary.

RESOURCES

Lonnie Barbach, *The Pause: Positive Approaches to Menopause.* New York: Dutton, 1993.

Susan Curtis and Romy Fraser, *Natural Healing for Women.* London: Pandora, 1991.

Chellis Glendenning, *When Technology Wounds.* New York: Morrow, 1990.

Liz Grist, *A Woman's Guide to Alternative Medicine.* Chicago: Contemporary, 1988.

Rima Handley, *A Homeopathic Love Story.* Berkeley: North Atlantic, 1990.

Andrew Lockie and Nicola Geddes, *The Women's Guide to Homeopathy.* New York: St. Martin's, 1994.

Robin Murphy, *Women's Health* (set of seven tapes). Available from Homeopathic Educational Services (page 366). This set of tapes is not for the beginner. It provides useful, practical information for people who already have introductory-level information and books and want to expand their knowledge.

Christine Northrup, *Women's Bodies, Women's Wisdom.* New York: Bantam, 1994.

Dana Ullman, *The One-Minute (or So) Healer.* Los Angeles: Tarcher, 1991.

See also the resources listed under "Pregnant and Laboring Women," page 204, "Breastfeeding and Postnatal Conditions," page 208, as well as the self-care texts listed in Part IV, many of which have good sections on women's health. Of greatest benefit are Cummings and Ullman's *Everybody's Guide to Homeopathic Medicines* and Kruzel's *Homeopathic Emergency Guide.*

Pregnant and Laboring Women

Women inevitably experience a variety of discomforting symptoms during pregnancy, including nausea, indigestion, hemorrhoids, bladder infection, vaginitis, herpes, swelling, headaches, fatigue, and emotional swings. Although some of these conditions are minor enough not to warrant any type of treatment, many symptoms during pregnancy are discomforting enough to merit something to alleviate them. It is understandable that pregnant women often seek treatment from their doctors to provide relief from their nagging symptoms.

Modern obstetricians now realize that whatever therapeutic drugs a pregnant mother takes go through the placenta to the fetus. Because of the many unanswered questions about drug safety, obstetricians generally discourage drug use unless there is medical necessity. Because no one knows what short- or long-term effects these drugs have on physical or psychological development, it is prudent to avoid therapeutic drugs during pregnancy, childbirth, and lactation unless they are truly necessary. This statement is not meant to lay a guilt trip on any woman who feels compelled to reduce the pain of childbirth with a medication or a surgical procedure, for serious distress during labor can have its own complications. Despite the concerns that physicians have about drug use during pregnancy, one survey found that 80 percent of women had taken three or more drugs during pregnancy and an additional three or more drugs during labor.[1]

Part of the reason for this significant drug use is that women and their obstetricians do not know about reasonable alternatives such as homeopathic medicines. Judy Norsigian and Jane Pincus, coauthors of *The New Our Bodies, Our Selves,* note, "Homeopathic remedies can be effective in both major and minor ailments during pregnancy, birth, and the postpartum period. Sometimes homeopathy can help prevent problems and complications in ways that conventional medicine cannot match."[2] Besides the benefits that homeopathic medicines offer in the prevention and treatment of many common ailments during pregnancy, the fact that they are so much safer for pregnant and laboring mothers than conventional drugs makes it all the more convincing that these natural medicines should be considered first, before resorting to the more risky conventional medications.

It should be noted that pregnancy is an excellent time to seek out professional homeopathic care so that a constitutional medicine can be given. A constitutional medicine has the capacity to provide an overall strengthening to the woman, both physically and psychologically, enabling her to experience a healthier and happier pregnancy and labor. Further, constitutional care during pregnancy is thought to provide benefit to the baby, potentially reducing some of the genetic weaknesses that may be passed down.

Most of this chapter will focus on homeopathic medicines recommended for use during pregnancy and childbirth. Readers are encouraged to review other chapters for information on treating conditions common to pregnancy that are not discussed here. For instance, information on treating morning sickness is provided in the chapter on digestive disorders, and vaginitis and bladder infections are covered in the chapter on women's conditions.

USING HOMEOPATHIC MEDICINES WITH MODERN DIAGNOSTIC PROCEDURES

There are times when conventional procedures and homeopathic medicines can be used together. For instance, a significant number of women today have genetic-screening tests performed on their fetuses through modern diagnostic procedures such as amniocentesis and chorionic villus sampling (a newer and slightly more dangerous procedure). Because these diagnostic procedures are invasive by their use of needles to take out fetal tissue, they can shock the fetus and in a small percentage of cases can lead to miscarriage. To reduce the shock and the potential for miscarriage, the homeopathic medicines **Arnica** and **Ledum** are both invaluable. **Arnica** helps the fetus and the mother deal with the shock of these surgical procedures, while **Ledum** is a remedy par excellence for puncture wounds.

Dose: **Arnica 6, 12,** or **30** is best taken just prior to and immediately after the procedure. **Ledum 6, 12,** or **30** should be taken within thirty minutes afterward. Alternate taking these two remedies every hour for two doses of each medicine.

HOMEOPATHY PRIOR TO AND DURING LABOR

In addition to the value of homeopathic medicines for alleviating common symptoms of pregnancy, they are also invaluable during labor. Research has shown that homeopathic medicines can both reduce the time of labor and decrease birth complications. French researchers showed that fifty-three pregnant women who were given a combination of five homeopathic medicines completed labor an average of 40 percent faster than women given a placebo. The researchers also found that only 11.3 percent of those given the homeopathic medicines experienced some type of complication during childbirth, while 40 percent of those given a placebo experienced complications.[3]

The five homeopathic medicines used were **Caulophyllum, Cimicifuga, Arnica, Pulsatilla**, and **Gelsemium.** Each of these medicines was in the 5th potency (5c). This combination of five homeopathic medicines was taken twice a day, morning and night, during the ninth month of pregnancy. It was taken every fifteen minutes after the first contractions, though one should stop taking it after two hours of treatment or if excessive pains have ceased.

This specific combination of five homeopathic medicines is not available in the United States, but each medicine is available individually from homeopathic companies. (Because American and British companies tend to make 6c, rather than 5c, and because there is a negligible difference between the two, it is acceptable to take the 6c of these remedies.)

Most homeopaths do not know about this French study, so there is little experience outside of France with this formula. Whether homeopaths are familiar with it or not, some prefer to avoid any treatment, homeopathic or otherwise, unless the woman is experiencing the symptoms necessary to warrant it. Others feel that certain homeopathic medicines, especially **Caulophyllum** and **Arnica,** are useful to the vast majority of laboring women, and thus these homeopaths suggest that most women will benefit from them. (See dosage instructions.)

Caulophyllum is valuable because it is thought to strengthen uterine muscles, while **Arnica** is valuable for treating the shock and trauma that both mother and infant experience during labor. **Caulophyllum** is particularly indicated when labor does not progress or progresses slowly or when contractions are excessively painful but ineffectual. It is also very useful in helping to expel the placenta after birth.

An Italian study has recently confirmed the benefits of **Caulophyllum**. When one dose of **Caulophyllum 7c** was taken during labor every hour for four hours, labor time was reduced by 30 percent, from 5¼ hours to 3¾ hours.[4] The use of **Caulophyllum 7c** began when the women were at least three centimeters dilated and had at least two contractions every ten minutes lasting at least forty-five seconds.

Women should know that homeopathic medicines do not completely get rid of the pain of labor as painkilling drugs do. However, the correctly chosen homeopathic medicines strengthen the woman so that she can complete labor more easily, faster, and with fewer complications: They ease the birthing process so that she does not seem to need painkilling drugs as often. They also reduce the rate of complications during labor so that a cesarean section or episiotomy is less likely to be necessary.

The laboring woman who uses homeopathic medicines is more likely to go through the childbirth process without conventional drugs of any kind. When one realizes that whatever conventional drugs she takes are being fed directly to the fetus and to the newborn during lactation, there are additional benefits to mother and infant who experience a drug-free delivery.

Dose: Some women take **Caulophyllum 6** or **30** once daily during the last one to four weeks of pregnancy. During labor, it can be taken every hour for up to four doses. **Arnica 6** or **30** is commonly taken once labor has begun every one to four hours, and it is usually taken for a day after delivery, every two to six hours.

BACKACHE DURING OR AFTER LABOR

Homeopathic medicines can also be useful in treating backache during and after labor. It is recommended to alternate **Arnica 6** or **30** and **Rhus tox 6** or **30** every thirty minutes during labor and every three hours after labor until the pain resolves (though not longer than forty-eight to seventy-two hours). External applications of **Arnica** (gel, ointment, spray, or tincture) or of external formula gels that include **Arnica** and other remedies for injury and backache, such as **Rhus tox** and **Hypericum,** should be applied to aching parts of the back.

Sulphur 6 or 30 is useful if the woman experiences burning pains in her back and feels increased general body warmth which is aggravated by exposure to heat and relieved by cold air. **Kali carb 12** or **30** is indicated if she experiences radiating pains from her back and feels chillier than normal. **Sulphur** or **Kali carb** should be taken every three or four hours, though it should not be necessary to take either for longer than two consecutive days.

WHEN CESAREAN SECTION OR EPISIOTOMY IS NECESSARY

Presently, almost 30 percent of American births are by cesarean section, even though the World Health Organization has conservatively estimated that "there is no justification for any region [of the world] to have a rate higher than 10–15 percent."[5] For those women who experience a cesarean section, there are a couple of very useful homeopathic medicines which may help them rebound faster from this surgery. **Arnica 12** or **30** is an important remedy for surgical shock and should be taken every other hour for the first day, and three to six times a day for the next day, depending upon the intensity of pain. **Staphysagria 12** or **30** is a primary remedy for healing surgical incisions. It can be taken concurrently and with a similar frequency, though ideally it should be taken approximately one hour apart from **Arnica**.

If sharp or shooting pains are present after a cesarean, **Hypericum 12** or **30** should be taken also, though at different times than the other medicines.

To help heal the scar of surgery, external applications of **Calendula** in an ointment, gel, spray, or tincture are useful. **Calendula** tincture can be added to a sitz bath (approximately one part of remedy to five parts water). Homeopathic-formula external gels for wounds which contain **Calendula** plus other ingredients can also be extremely helpful.

These same remedies are also useful for women who experience an episiotomy.

RESOURCES

Miranda Castro, *Homeopathy for Pregnancy, Birth and the First Year*. New York: St. Martin's, 1993.

Hans Willem Jansen, *Synthetic Bedside Repertory for Gestation, Childbirth, and Childbed*. Haarlem, the Netherlands: Merlijn, 1992.

Thomas Kruzel, *Homeopathic Emergency Guide*. Berkeley: North Atlantic, 1992.

Richard Moskowitz, *Homeopathic Medicines for Pregnancy and Childbirth*. Berkeley: North Atlantic, 1992.

W. A. Yingling, *Accoucher's Emergency Manual*. New Delhi: B. Jain (reprint).

Breastfeeding and Postnatal Conditions

Breastfeeding is a valuable but not always utilized gift that a mother can give to her newborn. Of greatest importance are the first couple of days after birth, when the breasts secrete colostrum, a milky fluid rich in important antibodies which boost an infant's immunity.

Women commonly experience a variety of complaints during the postnatal period, including exhaustion, insomnia, constipation, sore or cracked nipples, engorged breasts, inverted nipples, breast infection, urinary difficulties, and emotional problems. Readers are encouraged to review other chapters for the treatment of ailments not discussed in this chapter.

Self-care with homeopathic medicine for many of these complaints is quite effective, and the books listed in the previous section provide much useful information. Professional homeopathic care should be sought if self-care is not effective or if symptoms are severe. Also, professional homeopathic care during pregnancy and lactation is invaluable for strengthening a woman's overall health.

AFTER-PAINS

As a result of the great exertion and trauma of labor and the various hormonal changes that occur after the termination of pregnancy, women commonly experience various physical and psychological symptoms. The following remedies should be considered at this time.

Arnica is the primary remedy to help relieve the bruised and sore feelings. Because soreness is experienced by virtually every woman after labor, **Arnica** can almost routinely be given to them. **Cinchona** should be considered if the woman lost a considerable amount of blood and as a result is feeling faint and extremely chilly, and is hypersensitive to touch, noise, and any stimulation. **Pulsatilla** is an excellent remedy for a woman who experiences great emotional instability and moodiness along with her after-pains. This remedy is confirmed if the woman is intolerant of warm rooms and is noticeably relieved by cool or fresh air. **Sepia** is indicated if she has great heaviness in her pelvic region and bearing-down pains as though her uterus may fall out. Along with this sagging feeling, women who need this remedy are exhausted and may have a nagging backache. Emotionally, rather than being weepy like the women who need **Pulsatilla**, women who need **Sepia** are irritable and impatient, especially with loved ones. **Sabina** is useful when the woman experiences a discharge of blood with every pain. It is also indicated when excessive blood was lost during labor and when many blood clots are released. Symptoms that further confirm this remedy is when the woman is overheated and intolerant of any type of warmth.

Dose: Take 6, 12, or 30th potencies every two to four hours during the first couple of days after birth and up to four times a day during the next week. If there is no improvement after forty-eight hours, consider another remedy.

MASTITIS (BREAST INFECTION)

Mastitis is a common condition in breastfeeding women and is usually caused by the blockage of one or more milk ducts, creating increased susceptibility to the colonization and growth of infective organisms. The most common remedies for mastitis (in order of frequency of use, with the first two remedies used the vast majority of the time) are **Belladonna**, **Bryonia**, **Phytolacca**, and **Silicea**. **Belladonna** is indicated primarily when the breast becomes very hot and sore and she experiences throbbing pains. The breast is swollen, bright red or perhaps even shiny red in appearance, and extremely sensitive to touch and even slight motion. The mother may have a fever, and in the worst cases, she may show red streaks from the areola. **Bryonia** is useful when the condition develops more slowly, when the mother is extremely sensitive to any type of motion, and when, despite breast soreness, she feels some relief when lying on her painful breast. Cold applications provide some relief, and she craves cold drinks. **Phytolacca** is helpful in treating mastitis when the breast is hard and lumpy and when the pain wanders to other areas of the chest or other parts of the body. **Silicea** is indicated to heal old lumps or abscesses in the breast.

Dose: Take 6, 12, or 30th potencies every two to six hours up to four times. If there is no change after twenty-four hours, consider another remedy.

CRACKED OR SORE NIPPLES

Cracked or sore nipples are another common condition of breastfeeding women and are best treated externally with **Calendula** gel or tincture, though it should be washed off just prior to breastfeeding. If this external application isn't effective, the following internal remedies should be considered: **Castor equi** is considered a specific for this condition. In other words, unless another medicine is clearly indicated, use this remedy. **Hepar sulphur** is useful when the woman experiences splinterlike pains in the nipple that are extremely sensitive to touch or cold. There may also be some bleeding from the nipple. **Phytolacca** is indicated when the pain radiates over the woman's entire body and/or when the nipple is also hard and lumpy. **Graphites** are generally indicated for chilly, overweight women who develop swollen and hard breasts. **Silicea** is helpful for thin, delicate women who have recurring sore nipples and recurring uterine pains when nursing.

Dose: Take the 6, 12, or 30th potency after every nursing for one or two days. If relief is provided but is not complete, continue taking the remedy every other nursing for up to seven days and then stop for several days before taking it again. If there is no relief after twenty-four hours, consider another remedy.

Having too much or too little milk can also be treated with homeopathic medicines, though these conditions are best treated by a professional homeopath.

It is increasingly common for women to use homeopathic medicine for the treatment of many physical ailments, but too many women do not recognize their value in treating emotional problems. Many women experience postnatal blues, and homeopathic medicines are wonderfully effective in treating it. **Sepia** is one of the most frequently prescribed remedies for it, though individualized care, preferably with a practitioner, is recommended.

RESOURCES

Note: See "Pregnant and Laboring Women" for resources. Moskowitz's *Homeopathic Medicines for Pregnancy and Childbirth* and Castro's *Homeopathy for Pregnancy, Birth and the First Year* have good information for the layperson on homeopathic and general health care for lactating women, while Jansen's *Synthetic Bedside Repertory for Gestation, Childbirth, and Childbed* has the most information for the practitioner.

Men's Ailments

There are presently numerous women's magazines that keep women informed about their health and how to maintain it, and yet there are very few magazines focused on men's health. This isn't the fault of publishers. Men do not seem as interested in their health as do women. In fact, men often ignore their health until the discomfort of an ailment is so intense that it can no longer be denied.

BENIGN PROSTATIC HYPERPLASIA

Recent studies have suggested that 50 to 60 percent of men between the ages of forty and sixty experience a common disorder of the prostate gland called benign prostatic hyperplasia (BPH). Despite these high statistics, it is amazing how few men know about this condition until they actually get it. The prostate tends to enlarge as a man gets older, and this swelling can constrict the urinary passage. This condition is characterized by increased urinary frequency, nighttime awakening to urinate, delayed onset of the urinary stream, and reduced force upon urination.

If left untreated, BPH can lead to bladder obstruction, resulting in a more serious condition of urine retention in the blood called uremia, which may require surgical intervention and/or dialysis.

The acute symptoms of BPH can be self-treated with homeopathic remedies, though it is generally recommended to seek professional care for this chronic condition. Self-care can be considered as long as there is no significant pain or discomfort and only minor symptoms are experienced, such as increased frequency of urination. The most common remedy for BPH is **Chimaphilla umbellata** (characterized by retention of urine with an enlarged prostate, frequent urging, soreness in the prostate, worse with pressure, especially when sitting; a sensation of a ball or simply a painful swelling in the perineum, which is between the anus and the genitals). Other remedies to consider are **Pulsatilla** (pain after urination, pains in the prostate which extend into the bladder or pelvis; pains worse when lying on the back, a thick, bland, sometimes yellow or greenish discharge from the penis, thirstlessness, desire for open air; in a man who feels and tends to show his emotions), **Clematis** (urine passed drop by drop, dribbling after urination, urethral stricture with BPH), **Apis** (last drop of urine causes burning pain; sharp stinging, aggravation of symptoms by heat and warm rooms, sensitivity to touch), **Staphysagria** (burning in urethra even when not urinating, retained urine, impotence), **Selenium** (dribbling of semen during stool or when sitting, premature ejaculation; worse on hot days), **Baryta carb** (chilly, physically slow and mentally dull; bed-wetting), **Kali bic** (prostate pain worse on walking, relief from standing still, pain extending from the prostate to the penis, burning in the urethra after urination, thick, sticky discharge at the tip of the penis), and **Causticum** (pressure and pulsations in the prostate extending into the urethra and bladder after a few drops of urine have passed, incontinence during a cough or sneeze, loss of pleasure from orgasm).

Benign prostatic hyperplasia appears when a mass of glandular tissue, known as an adenoma, forms at the base of normal prostatic tissue. One study using homeopathic medicine to treat 37 men with an adenoma (19 of whom also had chronic prostatitis) showed that 80 percent of the patients experienced significant improvement in their symptoms, mostly within the first two months of the six-to-nine-month experiment.[1] Of the 27 patients with frequent nightly urination, 23 improved. The same number of patients also noticed improved urinary stream. Of the 19 patients with groin, perineal, and loin pain, 18 experienced improvement. In addition to this reduction in symptoms, 14 out of 16 patients who previously had lower than normal urinary testosterone levels experienced increased levels after homeopathic treatment. Although the size of the prostate itself did not decrease, the patients self-reported improvement in their symptoms as well as in their overall state of health. These men were individually prescribed homeopathic medicine in the 30c to 10m potencies.

Dose: Take the 6, 12, or 30th potency three times a day for one to four days. Stop as soon as symptoms improve. If there is no improvement after waiting at least two weeks after the last dose, consider another remedy.

PROSTATITIS

Men can also experience an infection in the prostate gland called prostatitis, most commonly between the ages of twenty and fifty. The prostate gland is susceptible to both acute and chronic infection. The acute infection is usually characterized by severe pain in the prostate area and possibly extending to the genitals, pelvis, or back, along with an increased desire to urinate, burning upon urination, difficulty starting urination, penile discharge, fever, and generalized weakness.

The symptoms of chronic infection of the prostate tend to be milder, including dull aching in the prostate region, dribbling of urine, and difficulty starting or maintaining a full stream. Even after the prostate rids itself of bacteria, the problem may persist for unknown reasons.

The remedies for prostatitis are similar as those for benign prostatic hyperplasia.

CANCER OF THE PROSTATE

Prostate cancer is one of the slowest-growing cancers; it is so slow-moving that most men diagnosed with it die of other diseases before it kills them. Although modern medical diagnostic measures can now diagnose prostate cancer in its early stages, clinical research has shown that surgical and drug treatments for this condition do not improve health or longevity and may in fact, due to their side effects, worsen health. Several leading physicians have now gone so far as to discourage men from even getting tested for prostate cancer, especially if they are not having any urinary symptoms.[2] The majority of men with prostate cancer are symptomless, though some men experience similar symptoms as those with benign prostatic hyperplasia.

Although prostate cancer is slow-growing, it is still a relatively common cause of death in men. While aggressive medical treatment in the early stages is not recommended, it does make sense for men with prostate cancer to consider safer natural therapies such as homeopathic medicine. Although there have not yet been any controlled trials on the homeopathic treatment for this condition, this safer natural therapy is more prudent than conventional measures.

TESTICLE AND SCROTUM PROBLEMS

Testicle and scrotum problems definitely require professional medical attention, though for severe pain, self-care using homeopathic medicines can be a godsend. For enlarged or painful testicles, consider **Clematis** (the first choice, especially when the right testis is affected and there is burning pain in the penis during ejaculation and tingling in the spermatic cord and urethra), **Aurum** (swelling of the lower part of the testis, with aching pain worse at night and from touching or rubbing), **Staphysagria** (strong sexual urgings, especially for masturbation, despite pain), **Apis** (swelling worsened by heat or warm applications), **Pulsatilla** (pressing and drawing pain from the penis extending to the abdomen or thighs), and **Argentum metallicum** (pain as though the testicles were bruised).

Ideally, professional homeopathic care should be sought, even if conventional painkilling drugs need to be taken concurrently.

RESOURCES

Stephen Cummings and Dana Ullman, *Everybody's Guide to Homeopathic Medicines*. Los Angeles: Tarcher, 1991.

Thomas Kruzel, *Homeopathic Emergency Guide*. Berkeley: North Atlantic, 1992.

Andrew Lockie, *The Family Guide to Homeopathy*. New York: Fireside, 1993.

Note: It is recommended that you complement the rather limited information on self-care of men's ailments in these books with the more detailed information provided in Boericke's *Pocket Manual of Materia Medica with Repertory*.

Conditions of the Elderly

"May you die young . . . as late in life as possible."

Some of the world's leading thinkers and artists have done their greatest work after sixty years of age. The abilities of Sophocles, Goethe, Chagall, Kant, Picasso, and numerous others became increasingly sophisticated with age.

While some people age like a good bottle of wine, others age less gracefully. And sadly, the vast majority of physicians and other health professionals are inadequately trained in the proper care of our elders.

MEDICAL ELDER ABUSE

Despite the graying of the world's population, there are few physicians who specialize in geriatric medicine. While one might hope and expect that this deficiency of knowledge would lead to a conservative practice of medicine, just the opposite occurs today. On the dispensing of medications, for example, Dr. Warren Davidson, a representative of the Canadian Medical Association's coalition on the medication of the elderly, asserts, "Seniors are being drugged silly. We have a serious problem and it's getting worse."[1]

A Harvard study found that approximately 25 percent of Americans over sixty-five were prescribed drugs that they should almost never take.[2] A Canadian survey by researchers at McGill University uncovered the shocking fact that during a one-year period nearly 50 percent of elderly people were prescribed a questionable, high-risk drug.[3] Another survey revealed that 70 percent of physicians who treat Medicare patients failed an examination on prescribing for elderly patients.[4]

Many older people take an inordinate number of pills, sometimes as the result of errors by physicians and sometimes as the result of their forgetting or not telling the doctor what other medications other physicians have already prescribed for them.

The problem is not only the kinds and numbers of drugs being prescribed to the elderly but also the doses. Physicians commonly prescribe the same doses of drugs to older people as they prescribe to younger people, not knowing that older people are more sensitive to certain drugs. Diazepam (Valium), for example, is metabolized differently by older people and tends to remain in their bodies longer.

The author of the above-mentioned Harvard study, Dr. Steffi Woolhandler, noted, "A lot of the problem is that doctors frequently ascribe side effects of drugs to old age. If a patient loses memory or loses balance, they say it's old age."[5]

Although people over sixty years of age make up only 17 percent of the American population, they account for 51 percent of deaths due to drug reactions, according to a U.S. General Accounting Office report.[6] Drug-related health problems are responsible for one third of hospital and one half of nursing home admissions.[7]

The elderly have a problem not only with many prescription drugs but with common over-the-counter medications as well. Even short-term use of ibuprofen, for instance, has been shown to cause serious kidney and gastrointestinal problems in people over seventy.

The treatment of the elderly requires judicious use of medication. Due to the sometimes frail tendencies of the elderly, it makes sense to use safer therapeutic measures such as homeopathic medicine before resorting to more risky conventional therapies.

HOMEOPATHIC MEDICINES FOR THE ELDERLY

Because the elderly often suffer from multiple concurrent complaints, it is appropriate to consider utilizing a holistic approach such as homeopathy which provides an integrated method of treating the whole person and the variety of symptoms and syndromes that are experienced. Also, the elderly sometimes experience idiosyncratic symptoms that do not fit any of the disease categories common to conventional medicine, and homeopathy is a therapeutic modality that particularly thrives on such individualizing characteristics.

In addition to treating specific symptoms, homeopathic medicines have the capacity to strengthen overall resistance to disease. Because the elderly often suffer from reduced resilience when ill, homeopathic medicines should be an integral part of their health care.

Some people ask if any specific homeopathic medicines help to promote longevity, and the best answer is that they all seem to do so, because any therapy that is truly effective in improving health tends to promote longevity. This may explain why homeopaths have a reputation of living and practicing into very old age. Homeopaths theorize that homeopathic constitutional medicines, as discussed in Chapter 2, have the greatest impact on longevity because they seem to have the most profound effect on a person's overall quality of life.

While the elderly may experience a certain number of conditions that are somewhat unique to them, the vast majority of their complaints are the same problems experienced by others, no matter what their age. Because of this, readers should review the sections that relate to the specific complaints an elderly person might experience. Following is a list of these common complaints and their respective places in this book:

- osteoporosis: see "Women's Conditions," page 189

- increased urinary frequency and prostate problems: see "Men's Ailments," under "Benign Prostatic Hyperplasia," page 209 or "Women's Conditions," under "Cystitis," page 191

- constipation: see "Digestive Disorders," page 240

- insomnia: see the chapter on this subject, page 268

- arthritis: see the chapter on this subject, page 264

- cancer: see the chapter on this subject, page 295

- heart disease: see the chapter on this subject, page 289

- emotional problems: see "Psychological Conditions," page 303

- dizziness: see "Conditions of Travel and Recreation," under "Motion sickness," page 323, for common dizziness remedies

- when surgery is necessary: see "Pre- and Postsurgical Treatment," page 342

- injuries: see the chapter on this subject, page 329

Some of the most common symptoms that accompany increasing age are vision and hearing difficulties. These symptoms, from a homeopathic perspective, should not be understood or treated as local problems but as constitutional issues that require treatment of the totality of the person. This perspective is not uniquely homeopathic, for even Hippocrates once stated, "To heal even an eye, one must heal the head and even the whole body."

It is also important to note that some "symptoms" that elderly people commonly experience should not be considered symptoms. For instance, elderly people generally do not have as much energy as they did when they were younger. It is inappropriate to diagnose fatigue in the elderly, unless a significant level of fatigue is experienced. Likewise, elderly people tend to eat less and therefore have fewer bowel movements. Just because an elderly person does not have a daily movement does not necessarily mean that he or she is constipated.

INCONTINENCE OF URINE

As a result of decreasing tone in the bladder muscles as people age, urinary incontinence becomes increasingly common. Urinary incontinence is a symptom, not a disease. As such, it is best treated as part of a constitutional treatment by a professional homeopath. If such care is not readily available, some of the following acute remedies may be helpful.

Causticum is useful if dribbling or loss of urine is experienced when coughing, sneezing, or laughing, if there is weakness in the bladder sphincter as evidenced by delayed starting and stopping of urination, or if there is a tendency to be more incontinent during cold weather than warm weather. **Belladonna** is indicated when incontinence is experienced in people whose sleep is so deep that they do not wake to urinate. They also tend to be restless during sleep and sometimes delirious upon waking. **Gelsemium** is useful for incontinence that results from anticipation of a special occasion. **Sabal serrata** is effective for elderly men who suffer from incontinence associated with an enlarged prostate (best used in the tincture or up to the 3rd potency). **Baryta carbonica** should be considered when incontinence is associated with senility. **Equisetum** is thought to be a generic remedy for involuntary urination when used in low potencies (best used in tincture or up to the 6th potency) and should be considered when no other remedy is obviously indicated.

Dose: If incontinence is primarily experienced during sleep, take the 3 or 6th potency (unless otherwise indicated) one or two hours before bedtime and another dose at bedtime. If incontinence is experienced at any time, take the 3 or 6th potency three times a day for a week, unless improvement is noticed earlier. If there is no improvement, wait a week, and repeat doses of the same remedy for another week. If no improvement occurs after this, try another remedy in a similar fashion.

Leg cramps

Decreased exercise and reduced muscle tone lead to many complaints, including leg cramps. The following remedies are often helpful in providing relief of leg cramps. **Nux vomica** is helpful for people who experience cramps that are worse at three to four A.M., when they are chilled, or after drinking alcohol, taking drugs, or overeating. These people get some relief from the warmth of a bed. They may also experience cramps in the foot, with irritability, constipation, indigestion, headache, and nausea. **Rhus tox** is indicated when there is great restlessness along with the leg cramps, which are worse when the person is chilled, especially during damp weather, upon initial motion, when lying in bed or sitting still. Symptoms tend to be relieved by continued motion. **Sulphur** is indicated when cramps are worsened by the warmth of a bed, when the person wakes around five A.M. in pain, and when cramps in the foot are experienced. **Ambra grisea** is known to be useful in the elderly who are suffering from senility and/or when there are cramps in the thighs. **Calcarea carb** is most commonly given to pale-skinned, overweight people who are easily chilled. People who need this remedy experience cramps in the thighs, calves, and feet at night. **Kali carb** is indicated when a person gets cramps in the thighs which are worse from two to four A.M. **Calcarea phos** is valuable when symptoms are worse in the late winter/early spring while the snow is melting, or when symptoms tend to develop after a prolonged or severe acute illness. This remedy is also useful when the cramps are worse from exposure to cold or drafts.

Dose: To cure or significantly reduce the frequency and intensity of leg cramps, it is best to seek a constitutional remedy from a professional homeopath. To treat the acute leg cramps, take one of the above remedies in the 6, 12, or 30th potency; another dose can be taken thirty to sixty minutes later if necessary.

BEDSORES

While people with bedsores generally need to be under the care of a physician, the following remedies can provide complementary care. **Arnica** is the most frequently used remedy for bedsores because one of the symptoms it is known to treat is a bruised sense that leads people to feel that everything is too hard against their bodies, even a pillow or a bed. **Arnica** is a primary remedy for shock and trauma of injury or of overexertion. Sometimes it helps to heal the initial problem that caused the person to be bedridden. **Calendula** is best applied externally (in a slightly diluted tincture, spray, or gel), and helps to heal relatively shallow bedsores. An external application that contains both **Calendula** and **Hypericum** is even more preferable. **Hypericum** can be used both internally and externally. It is used internally when the person feels sharp and/or shooting pains from sores (in a slightly diluted tincture, spray, or gel or in a combination external application with **Calendula**). Externally, it is useful for deep bedsores. **Graphites** should be used when the bedsores exude a thick yellow or honeylike fluid that dries into golden crystals on the skin. **Lachesis** is known to treat advanced stages of bedsores and is useful when the ulcers have a purplish edge around them, bleed easily, and are extremely sensitive to the touch. Typically, the symptoms are particularly bad in the early morning upon waking. **Petroleum** is indicated when a person with very dry skin develops bedsores that itch intensely, especially at night and in bed. This remedy tends to be more useful during the winter than the summer. **Silicea** is helpful when any cut or sore ulcerates, when the ulcers develop much pus, and when they are extremely sensitive to the touch.

Dose: Use the 6 or 12th potency three times a day for up to a week. If no obvious changes have occurred after a week, try another remedy. External applications can be applied concurrent with internal remedies.

ALZHEIMER'S DISEASE (AD)

It should first be noted that many elderly people suffer from varying degrees of confusion and senility but do not necessarily have Alzheimer's. As mentioned earlier in this chapter, some of them have been prescribed conventional medications which cause forgetfulness and confusion. In fact, these side effects are so common that good physicians must do what they can to systematically take their elderly patients off select medicines to determine if mental symptoms are drug-related.

Alzheimer's disease is a serious condition that is inappropriate for self-care with homeopathic medicines. While little can be done to help people in advanced stages of Alzheimer's, professional treatment with homeopathic medicines may play a useful role in preventing it and in treating its early stages.

Several autopsy studies have found higher concentrations of aluminum in the brains of people with AD than others. The most common sources of this exposure include the use of aluminum cookware, antiperspirants, and antacids. While it is not yet certain to what degree these various substances lead directly to increased concentrations of aluminum in the brain, it makes sense to avoid possible exposure to this metal.

There is a tendency to believe that because some people with the disease do not have traces of aluminum in their brain, aluminum does not lead to Alzheimer's. This same logic would assert that tobacco does not cause lung cancer because not everyone with lung cancer smokes. Indeed, aluminum is not the cause of *every* case of Alzheimer's, but it seems prudent to suggest that repeated or excessive exposure to aluminum can increase the chances of getting this serious ailment.

Further evidence of the link between Alzheimer's and aluminum can be observed by reviewing homeopathic materia medica which list the symptoms that aluminum is known to cause and cure. Dr. Andrew Lockie, a British homeopathic physician, has compared the known symptoms of Alzheimer's with known toxicology of aluminum and has uncovered a significant match.[8]

This finding does not mean to imply that homeopathic **Aluminum** is the only remedy for this condition, though it does suggest that it is one of several potentially important remedies when given in homeopathic doses.

The one and only remedy that people might consider for self-care treatment of AD is **Gingko biloba.** This remedy is a plant medicine taken from one of the world's oldest and hardiest trees. **Gingko biloba** is known for its effects on improving circulation to the brain and is presently the drug most commonly prescribed for *any* condition by physicians in Germany (although it is considered a "drug" in Germany, it is legally considered an herb in the United States, even though it is usually sold in pill form). Because improving circulation to the brain can be important in preventing and treating various senility states, natural therapies such as **Gingko** that augment circulation will inevitably play an increasing role as our society ages.

Although **Gingko biloba** is also a homeopathic medicine, as noted it is primarily marketed in the United States as an herb, and it is best in treating presenility and senility syndromes in unpotentized doses.

THE LAST STAGES OF LIFE

Death is part of life, just as shadows are part of light. That said, homeopathic medicines can be used during the last stages of life to decrease pain and discomfort and sometimes to snatch the person away from death's door.

There are two homeopathic medicines that are called "grave robbers": **Carbo vegetabilis** and **Arsenicum.** These remedies are known to greatly relieve the profound pain that the late stages in life can bring, and sometimes bring people back from the brink of death. **Carbo veg** is indicated when the person is almost lifeless. The body is cold, pulse imperceptible, lips bluish, and breathing either oppressed or quickened due to the difficulty oxygenating themselves. Typically, despite their listlessness, these people demand that windows be left open and others fan them to help them breathe.

Arsenicum is helpful for those who are extremely weak but are also restless and fearful. Despite their exhaustion, they feel uncomfortable staying in one position. They experience many fears, especially fear of death. Their fears are particularly strong at night and when alone. They experience great anguish and demand that doctors and anyone "do something" to help them. **Arsenicum** is also a leading remedy to help reduce the pain experienced by people with malignant cancers.

One of my own experiences with prescribing **Arsenicum,** which may provide some insight into the value of homeopathic medicine in such instances, was to my mother on her death bed. Dying of pancreatic cancer, she was experiencing great abdominal pain, for which her physician prescribed painkilling drugs which aggravated her constipation and increased her pain as a side effect. I gave her a dose of **Arsenicum 30,** and literally seconds later, she said, "Oooops." When our family looked quizzically at her, she admitted, "I had an accident in the sheets."

Although I have been involved with homeopathic medicine since 1972, I am still always amazed at how fast homeopathic medicines sometimes work. I expressed my appreciation for homeopathic medicine at that moment, to which my physician father responded that no medicine can act that fast, and I retorted, "Yes, they can!" Hearing this banter, my mother looked up at me and jokingly remarked, "If your medicine acted as fast as you say it did, then you take responsibility for cleaning these sheets." She kept her sense of humor and her dignity to her dying day.

RESOURCES

Although there are presently three books that at least briefly discuss using homeopathic medicines to treat conditions of the elderly, none of them provide detailed or comprehensive information on the subject. It is recommended that you supplement these books with other homeopathic self-care guidebooks listed in Part IV. To further improve your use of homeopathic medicine, consider using a *materia medica* and a repertory. The best book to get first is Boericke's *Pocket Manual of Materia Medica with Repertory.*

Andrew Lockie, *The Family Guide to Homeopathy*. New York: Fireside, 1993.

Trevor Smith, *Homeopathic Medicine: A Doctor's Guide to Remedies for Common Ailments*. Rochester, VT: Healing Arts, 1989.

Keith Souter, *Homeopathy for the Third Age*. Saffron Walden, England: C. W. Daniel, 1993.

Common Infections

Homeopathic medicine gained its greatest popularity during the mid- and late 1800s, primarily because of the significant successes it achieved in treating the many serious infectious disease epidemics that raged during that time, including scarlet fever, typhoid fever, yellow fever, and cholera. The death rates in homeopathic hospitals from these diseases were one half to as little as one eighth of the death rates in conventional hospitals.[1]

Besides this history of success in treating the serious infectious diseases of the nineteenth century, homeopathy also has an impressive body of experience in treating the many common acute infectious conditions experienced today. Modern medicine prides itself on its ability to treat infectious diseases with antibiotics, but one should be aware of the fact that homeopathic medicines are also effective in treating various minor and major infections, and without the side effects that antibiotics create. Also, because many contemporary infectious conditions are the result of viral infection and antibiotics are primarily useful in treating bacterial infections, specific alternatives such as homeopathic medicines can be more useful in controlling viral diseases.

While it would be inappropriate to ignore the substantial benefits that antibiotics offer in the treatment of common bacterial infections, it would be equally inappropriate to ignore their limitations as well as the problems their overuse creates. For many years, doctors have had to prescribe stronger and stronger antibiotics, and predictably, we are now witnessing increasing numbers of antibiotic-resistant strains of bacteria. Harvard professor and Nobel Prize–winning chemist Walter Gilbert predicted in *Time* in 1981 that "there may be a time down the road when 80 to 90 percent of infections will be resistant to all known antibiotics."[2]

One factor that is speeding up this resistance to antibiotics is their inappropriate prescription. Numerous studies have shown that 50 to 60 percent of antibiotic use is unnecessary. In addition, we are exposed to a significant amount of antibiotics that are fed to farm animals and ultimately make their way into us through our ingestion of milk, egg, and meat products.

To make matters worse, the overuse of antibiotics also kills off beneficial bacteria and creates ecological disruption in the body, often leading to other types of infections and chronic conditions. *Candida albicans* is but one of the fungal infections that result from overuse of antibiotics, and one can expect new microorganisms and new diseases to emerge unless alternatives to antibiotics are more rigorously sought.

A 1994 *Newsweek* cover story called "Antibiotics: The End of Miracle Drugs?" suggested, "A better strategy might be to abandon antibiotics altogether in favor of different kinds of drugs."[3]

Homeopathic medicines may be this different kind of drug.

Before discussing specific homeopathic remedies for various infectious diseases, it is important to clarify one of the basic misconceptions about infections. Contrary to common belief, bacteria and viruses do not always "cause" disease. It may be more accurate to say that bacteria and viruses are generally the "results" of disease.

Just as bacteria do not begin infecting and decomposing an apple unless the apple has become old or bruised, they do not create an infection in a human being unless there is a weakened condition that is favorable to their growth. Toward the end of Louis Pasteur's life, even he recognized that susceptibility to infection predisposes a person to infection and that this has greater predictive value of the risk of infection than the germ itself.

An exception to this general rule occurs when individuals become infected with a new microorganism to which they have not previously been exposed. The body's response to this infection, whether it be a foreign flu virus or a new cold virus, is usually to create fever and inflammation, which are the defensive strategies it has developed to adapt to and defend against future infections from this microorganism. The very process of fever and inflammation, while serving to fight infection, also results in the body's learning how to fight this same type of infection in the future. If, however, the sick person takes an antibiotic which kills the infective organism before the body develops some type of inflammatory response on its own, the body may not have had the opportunity to learn how to defend itself from this kind of infection in the future.

Antibiotics are commonly prescribed for treating all kinds of infectious diseases, even though they are useless for infections that are not of a bacterial nature. One such infection is the common cold, which is the result of a virus, as are most throat infections and many common respiratory, digestive, and ear infections.

The incentive and logic of this approach, which primarily seeks to attack microbes rather than raise host resistance, were crudely described by an executive from a leading drug company, who said in the *American Druggist*, "We count on bugs adapting to drugs. That's how we keep our jobs."[4]

While it may be convenient for some people or companies that bugs adapt to drugs, the vast majority of people benefit from safe, effective treatments for infectious conditions. Here is where homeopathic medicine has something to offer.

The homeopathic approach to treating people with infectious disease is the same individualized method that is used in treating any condition. However, people suffering from acute infections sometimes do not have many unique or differentiating symptoms, thus making it difficult to find the correct homeopathic remedy. In such cases, one can consider using a homeopathic formula product, especially when the sick person has not had recurrent infections. If he or she has had chronic infections, professional homeopathic attention is generally indicated, either because a constitutional remedy is needed or because a rarer acute remedy is indicated.

Some evidence of the efficacy of homeopathic medicines in treating respiratory infections was provided in a double-blind, placebo-controlled randomized trial performed on 175 Dutch children suffering from recurrent upper-respiratory-tract infections.[5] The children in the treatment group were prescribed a constitutional medicine for their overall health as well as acute medicines for their acute respiratory infections. The study found that the children given homeopathic medicine had an 18 percent better daily symptom score.

This study also found a 54.8 percent reduction in the use of antibiotics in children given homeopathic medicines, while children who received a placebo experienced a 37.7 percent reduction in antibiotic use. (The reason for the significant decline in antibiotic usage in *both* groups was that the parents of both groups received written advice on adequate nutrition.) The number of children given a placebo who had to undergo adenoidectomy was 24 percent higher than the number of children given homeopathic remedies.

The Common Cold

The common cold is precipitated by viral infection. As a result of the infection, the body's immune system attacks and kills cold viruses, and in the fight, some of its own white blood cells are killed. The body then creates a liquid substance called mucus as a way of flushing out these dead viruses and cells. The reason why conventional medicine does not have a "cure" for the common cold is that they misunderstand it. Trying to dry up mucous membranes with over-the-counter drugs as a way to stop a runny nose simply inhibits the body's natural efforts to rid itself of dead cold viruses and dead white blood cells.

Because homeopathic medicines mimic and augment the body's own efforts to responding to cold viruses, they help the body heal itself. Homeopathic remedies can usually cure a cold within twenty-four hours.

There are many homeopathic medicines to consider when treating the common cold. Two of the more frequently used remedies during the first twenty-four hours of a cold are **Aconitum** (after exposure to cold weather or drafts, restlessness with increased thirst, especially for cold drinks) and **Ferrum phos** (tiredness and vague symptoms of the beginning of an illness). After the first twenty-four hours, consider **Allium cepa** (profuse nasal discharge that irritates the nostrils, sneezing, watery eyes; symptoms worse in a warm room), **Euphrasia** (profuse bland nasal discharge with burning tears that irritate the lower lids and cheeks), **Nux vomica** (symptoms after overeating, overdrinking, drug use, overwork, and undersleeping, frequent sneezing upon waking, fluent nasal discharge during the day and congestion at night), **Gelsemium** (fatigue, wooziness, headache in the back part of the head, thirstlessness), **Kali bic** (thick, purulent, stringy, sticky nasal discharge, usually yellow), **Eupatorium perf** (hoarseness and cough worse in cold air, muscle aches and bone pains, fever, morning chill), and **Pulsatilla** (yellow or greenish bland, creamy nasal discharge that is worse in a warm room and at night). In addition to these remedies, various homeopathic formula products for colds are available.

Although aspirin will not cure the common cold, some physicians prescribe it because it tends to reduce fever and relieve some of the aches and pains frequently associated with a cold. Because physiologists recognize fever as an important defense of the body, it is becoming increasingly common for physicians to discourage aspirin use except when fever is particularly high. One interesting study showed that the nonindividualized prescription of a homeopathic medicine, **Eupatorium perf 2x,** was at least as effective as aspirin in providing relief for people with colds, and did so without the side effects for which aspirin is known.[6] One can only wonder how much more effective an individualized remedy or homeopathic formula product would be when compared with aspirin.

Dose: It is recommended to use the 6, 12, or 30th potency every two hours at the beginning of the cold for three or four doses and then one dose every four hours. You should not have to take a remedy for more than two days. In fact, relief from a cold is usually noticed within a couple of hours or at least after a night's sleep. If some degree of improvement is not noticed after twenty-four hours, try another remedy.

COUGH

The body's cough reflex is classically understood as an important defense of the organism. The fact that conventional over-the-counter drugs tout their ability to suppress a cough doesn't necessarily make it something to brag about, except in the case of extremely irritating coughs which have not been amenable to effective treatment with homeopathic or other natural medicines.

Sometimes homeopathic treatment for a cough results in a temporary exacerbation of coughing, most often turning unproductive coughs into productive ones, and thus enabling the person to expectorate mucus which may be impeding respiration. Although this increase in symptoms may make it appear that the person is getting worse, the homeopathic medicine is actually enabling the body to clear its bronchial airways and is thus speeding up the healing process.

The homeopathic remedies for cough are similar to those used for a cold, so readers are encouraged to consider those. Other remedies to consider are **Bryonia** (dry cough that is aggravated by motion of any kind; chest must be held to reduce pain from coughing), **Spongia** (dry, barking cough, usually before midnight, aggravated by talking, lying down, or cold drinks, cough from a tickling in the throat or chest; cough may be relieved after eating or drinking, especially warm drinks), **Phosphorus** (many different types of cough, any of which will be made worse by cold air, talking or any type of exertion, eating, or lying on the left side; craving for cold drinks though they may aggravate the cough), **Drosera** (dry, spasmodic, hoarse, croupy, barking cough, repetitive and sometimes choking cough, with a tickling in the chest, worse when lying down; must apply pressure to chest to reduce pain from coughing; difficulty catching breath), **Rumex** (a cough that is set off by tickling in the neck and chest, especially at the pit of the throat, aggravated by touch or pressure to the throat or larynx, by cold air, and at night, which tends to prevent sleep), **Antimonium tartaricum** (a cough with rattling in the chest, yet inability to cough up mucus, great exhaustion due to shortness of breath; particularly useful in the very young and very old), and **Ipecacuanha** (cough with nausea and vomiting, usually worse in warm humid weather).

French researchers compared a placebo cough syrup with a homeopathic formula of ten homeopathic medicines in the 3c potency in a syrup.[7] The results showed that twenty of the thirty patients given the homeopathic syrup experienced relief of their dry or hacking cough, while only eight of the thirty patients given the placebo syrup experienced a similar degree of relief.

Dose: Take the remedy three to six times a day, depending on the intensity of the symptoms. Stop when symptoms abate or significantly improve. Consider changing remedies if no changes occur after forty-eight hours.

INFLUENZA

People suffering from influenza, like people with any fever, may require medical attention in rare situations when the fever reaches 103.5 degrees or higher and does not respond to treatment after six hours, or when an infant under six months of age experiences any fever. The good news is that homeopathic medicines are extremely effective in helping the body deal with influenza and other fevers.

Treating influenza with homeopathic medicines is usually quick and effective. In fact, the most popular cold and flu remedy sold today in France is a homeopathic medicine, **Anas barbariae 200c** (commonly marketed as *Oscillococcinum,* though also available under different names). This product has a 50 percent market share in France, meaning that sales of this product are so high that it represents 50 percent of *all* cold and flu products sales in the entire country. Research published in conventional medical journals has confirmed it to be effective in almost twice as many people as a placebo is.[8]

Despite this positive research, homeopaths have observed even better results when a more individually chosen medicine was used. Some of the common medicines recommended for flu treatment are **Aconitum** (first stages of the flu, especially when there is a rapid onset of symptoms, and/or symptoms brought on by exposure to cold or drafts), **Belladonna** (sudden onset of symptoms, high fever, wild dreams, flushed face, reddened lips and mucous membranes), **Ferrum phos** (slow onset of vague, nonsevere symptoms of flu with few individualizing characteristics), **Gelsemium** ("dizzy, drowsy, and droopy"; overall fatigue, difficulty raising extremities or even opening the eyes completely, headache in the back part of the head, thirstlessness), **Bryonia** (muscle aches from any type of motion, dry mouth and mucous membranes with great thirst for cold fluids, headache in the front part of the head, aggravation of symptoms in warm rooms, extreme irritability, desire to be left alone and to keep very still), **Arsenicum** (anxiety and fear that symptoms represent a serious illness, desire for company and sympathy, symptoms worse at and after midnight, fever with chills, great thirst but only for sips of water at a time, restless, especially in bed), **Eupatorium perf** (intense aching in the bones, especially in the morning, chills but thirst for cold fluids), and **Rhus tox** (fever with restlessness, especially at night in bed, achiness that is worse on initial motion and better on continued motion; chilly, worse by exposure to cold).

Dose: Take the 6, 12, or 30th potency every two to six hours, depending upon the intensity of the symptoms. The correct remedy will resolve the flu within a night's rest. If you wake up feeling partially better, take at least two or three more doses. Stop if you begin to feel significantly better. If you do not wake up even partially better, consider another remedy.

SORE THROAT

Throat infections are a common complaint for which doctors often scare people into getting antibiotic treatment. Doctors are usually not seriously concerned about the throat symptoms per se, but are fearful that they may be due to strep bacteria and, if left untreated, may possibly lead to rheumatic fever, a potentially dangerous, even life-threatening condition.

Although strep infection may at one time have led to rheumatic fever, this no longer seems to be the case. Rheumatic fever has been extremely rare over the past several decades, both in antibiotically treated and untreated individuals. An outbreak of rheumatic fever among children was reported in the *New England Journal of Medicine,*[9] but two thirds of these children did not even have a sore throat for three months prior to onset of the disease. Of the eleven children who were given a throat culture, eight tested positive for strep. Even though these children were prescribed antibiotics, all developed rheumatic fever.

This research raises serious questions as to whether sore throats are related to rheumatic fever, and, further, whether antibiotics do anything to actually prevent it.

Although antibiotics may not provide the protection against rheumatic fever that doctors hope, these drugs at least partially diminish symptoms of throat discomfort. However, research shows that they reduce symptoms only one day earlier than for those given a placebo. Of additional concern, because many sore throats today are the result of viral infection, antibiotics are not effective for these and may ultimately be more disruptive to a person's health than no treatment at all.

In light of these meager results and the attendant side effects from antibiotic use, it makes sense to investigate the benefits of homeopathic medicines for throat infection. One can without much difficulty find a homeopathic medicine that is known to treat the individualized symptoms of people with sore throats. If one is unable to individualize or if that single medicine is not readily available, a homeopathic formula for sore throat is a reasonable alternative.

The following are some of the common remedies for acute sore throat pain, all of which can be given to children or adults. **Aconitum** is called the "homeopathic vitamin C" because it is most useful at the very beginning of an infection as a way to prevent it from developing. It is good when the sore throat begins after exposure to cold or drafts and the person may also have a cold. **Belladonna** is a very common remedy when a right-sided sore throat pain begins suddenly, there is burning pain, and no pus has yet developed. The throat is scarlet-red, and the person will have a fever, flushed face, and reddened lips. **Arsenicum** is useful for burning throat pains that are particularly aggravating at and after midnight and are relieved by frequent sips of warm water. **Hepar sulphur** is indicated when there is a sense of a stick in the throat, throat pain extends to the ears, and symptoms are aggravated by touch, cold drinks, and cold air. **Rhus tox** treats sore throat pain that is worse on initial swallowing and relieved by frequent swallowing, especially warm fluids. **Lycopodium** is helpful in treating right-sided sore throats or those that start on the right and move to the left, and are aggravated by cold liquids and relieved by warm ones. **Mercurius** is effective for those very painful, deeply red and swollen sore throats which are aggravated by both cold and warm liquids or foods, especially in people with foul breath who are freely perspiring and actively salivating at night on their pillows. **Lachesis** is good for left-sided sore throat pain which is worst upon waking and aggravated by empty swallowing, tight clothing around the neck, or a slight touch to the throat, while being relieved by cool or cold liquids. **Phytolacca** is useful for throat pain that extends to the ears, especially when swallowing saliva and drinking warm fluids. One characteristic symptom that will confirm this remedy is pain at the root of the tongue when sticking it out. There are also usually concurrent swollen glands.

Relief from throat pain is usually observed within a couple of hours or at least after a night's rest. Because some sore throats can be dangerous, consult books such as *Everybody's Guide to Homeopathic Medicines* to learn when medical attention is indicated.

Dose: Take the 6, 12, or 30th potency every two to six hours over a two-day period (stop sooner if there is significant improvement). If there is no obvious relief after twenty-four hours and if symptoms are not just mild, consider another remedy.

Resources

Michael Schmidt, Keith Sehnert, and Lendon Smith, *Beyond Antibiotics*. Berkeley: North Atlantic, 1993. This book provides an excellent overview and critique of modern antibiotic usage, and discusses over fifty specific ways (mostly nutritional) that individuals can strengthen their immune system.

Note: For more detailed information on how to use homeopathic medicines to treat common infections, see the homeopathic self-care texts listed in Part IV. People interested in supplementing knowledge from this and various other books should consider obtaining a set of seven cassette tapes, *Fevers and Infectious Diseases*, by Robin Murphy, N.D. (distributed by Homeopathic Educational Services, Berkeley; see page 366).

Headaches

In Greek mythology, Zeus developed a headache after he discovered that his spouse Hera had conceived without any male help. Zeus' headache was diagnosed by the midwives as pregnancy, and he gave birth to Athena in an early form of cesarean section by having his head split open by an ax.

This mythical diagnosis and treatment certainly sounds strange and barbaric. Yet it was a common treatment until 1800 for physicians to drill into the skulls of headache patients and remove pieces of bone (this procedure was called trephining).

Such treatment is considered inhumane today, and yet we must humbly ask if people in the future will consider our modern medical treatment of headaches to be insensible too. Physicians readily acknowledge that modern medications do not cure headaches. The use of powerful analgesics to kill pain, vasodilators and antihistamines to expand blood vessels, vasocontrictors to narrow blood vessels, muscle relaxants to reduce tension, and diuretics to decrease water retention at best provide only temporary relief. However, each may create various side effects, including headaches.

Two of the most common types of headaches are tension and migraine headaches. Tension or muscle-contraction headaches refer to head, scalp, neck, and upper back pains that arise from the tightening of muscles in these areas. Pain results from these muscles being overworked and from the constriction of blood vessels to the head. Migraine or vascular headaches are generally thought to cause deeper and more throbbing pain than tension headaches. Although physicians previously thought migraines were the result of abnormal dilation and then constriction of the blood flow to the head, new research acknowledges that the condition is considerably more complicated than this and may involve a blood (platelet) disorder or a disorder of the central nervous system.

Conventional drugs may be ineffective because they are prescribed to inhibit the natural defenses that the body is deploying in order to deal with various stresses it is experiencing. While a conventional drug may effectively reduce or increase blood flow to the head, it does not influence the underlying complex syndrome that is creating the headache in the first place. In contrast, a homeopathic medicine is individually prescribed to mimic the person's symptoms which represent the body's wisdom and its effort to heal itself.

It is interesting to note that one of the common doctor-prescribed drugs for migraine headache is called Cafergot, which is a mixture of caffeine and ergot. It is prescribed because these substances are known to contract dilated arteries in the head. Ironically, caffeine and ergot are both known to cause head pain in overdose. Because of this, homeopaths commonly use these substances in homeopathic microdoses, not for everyone with migraine but only for those people with the unique pattern of symptoms that each substance has been found to create. **Coffea,** for instance, is indicated for people with head pain "as though a nail were driven through the head," especially in people who are restless, excitable, oversensitive to noise, touch, and odors, and who may also suffer from insomnia.

Many people with headaches seek homeopathic care because conventional medicine has little to offer most headache sufferers. A British homeopath assessed forty-three patients with chronic headaches during an eighteen-month period of time.[1] The following results of their homeopathic treatment were obtained:

- 65 percent said their head pain was reduced within the first month.

- 16 percent said their head pain was moderately improved during the first month.

- 19 percent noticed no improvement.

- 56 percent said improvement persisted for the eighteen months of the study.

- 32 percent said moderate improvement persisted during this time.

- 12 percent said no improvement persisted during this time.

In addition to this survey, one double-blind study using homeopathic medicines to treat patients with migraines showed a significant difference in those patients given an individually chosen homeopathic medicine as compared to those given a placebo.[2] Sixty patients were involved in this study, of whom thirty were given a placebo and thirty were given a 30c potency every fifteen days for four doses (both groups of patients were formally interviewed by a homeopath, and neither the doctor nor the patients knew which received the real medicine). The homeopath prescribed one or two remedies which he could choose out of a group of twelve medicines. An impressive 93 percent of patients given an individualized homeopathic medicine experienced good results, while only 17 percent of patients given a placebo experienced a similar degree of relief.

The medicines used to treat these patients with migraines (in order of frequency) were: **Belladonna**, **Natrum mur, Silicea**, **Gelsemium**, **Ignatia**, **Sulphur**, **Lachesis**, and **Cyclamen.**

Homeopaths generally list many different medicines when asked which are common remedies for headache. This is because there is such a large number of possible remedies, some of which are good for migraine headaches and some for tension headaches, some for the acute phase of the headache, and some for the chronic underlying condition from which the headache springs.

The following remedies are often helpful in treating the acute headache, and in rare instances they can significantly reduce the frequency and intensity of chronic headaches. However, it is best to seek professional homeopathic care to cure chronic headaches.

One final note about headaches is that it is generally recommended that you avoid coffee and caffeinated products. Caffeine is known to cause headaches, and homeopaths have often found that homeopathic medicines for headache sufferers are antidoted by coffee consumption. It is presently unclear if coffee directly antidotes the action of the remedy or if the coffee simply creates new symptoms in sensitive people.

Tension Headaches

Tension headaches typically manifest in a dull, steady ache either in the forehead, temples, back part of the head, or upper neck. A sense of constriction or tightness is felt.

Nux vomica, **Bryonia**, **Gelsemium**, and **Belladonna** are four of the most common remedies for treating tension headaches. **Nux vomica** is the classic remedy for the modern era. It is indicated for people who experience headaches after overindulging in food or drink (especially rich foods and alcoholic beverages) or after overworking and undersleeping. It is also useful for people who have taken many drugs, either therapeutic or recreational. Typically, **Nux vomica** is given to Type-A people who push themselves to achieve, who use various stimulants to continue to perform, and who become irritable and anxious from the pressures and lack of rest.

The primary characteristic of the headache sufferers who need **Bryonia** is that their pain is aggravated by any type of motion, including walking, bending over, coughing, or even moving their eyes. The pain is positioned anywhere over the forehead, and is usually accompanied by nausea, constipation, and irritability. Firm pressure or lying upon the painful part of the head provides some relief of pain.

Gelsemium is a primary remedy for pain in the back of the head. These pains commonly extend to the rest of the head and may include a sensation that a band is around the head. People who need **Gelsemium** tend to feel weak, heavy, and dizzy, and so wiped out that they can barely open their eyes (their eyelids droop). A unique and characteristic symptom of such people is pain relief after urination.

Belladonna is indicated when the headache comes on very suddenly and may disappear and reappear suddenly as well. Typically, these types of headaches are pulsating and throbbing, and the pain is aggravated when the person lies down flat, by any motion of the head or eyes, from light, sound, jarring, and even drafts. Some relief is obtained by applying firm pressure, standing or sitting, or bending backward.

The following remedies are also useful but are less commonly indicated: **Argentum nitricum** is effective in treating restless, possibly hyperactive children or adults with strong cravings for sweets, and head pain which is relieved by firm pressure or binding of the head. **Coffea**, as noted, is indicated for head pains "as though a nail were driven into the head," hypersensitivity to noise, touch, and odors, and restlessness, usually with insomnia. **Ignatia** is effective when head pain begins after a grieving experience or any powerful emotional state. **Kali phos** is valuable for headaches after excessive mental exertion, with weakness in the stomach.

Dose: Improvement is usually noticed after two or three doses of the 6, 12, or 30th potency, which may be taken every hour for intense pain and every four hours for mild discomfort. Stop taking the medicine whenever some degree of relief is observed.

MIGRAINE HEADACHES

Migraine headaches tend to be more profound and varied than tension headaches. Sufferers may experience various concurrent symptoms with their migraine, including changes in vision, dizziness, slurred speech, weakness or numbness on one side of the body, and various other neurological symptoms.

Some homeopathic medicines are known to treat people who experience greater pain on one side of the body or the other. If a person has pain on the right side, it is less likely that one of the remedies known for treating left-sided symptoms will be indicated. However, if a person has a migraine on both sides, all remedies can be considered, and determination of the correct remedy may be based on other symptoms.

Cluster headaches were previously assumed to be a type of migraine headache, though they presently are in a class of their own. Because people with cluster headaches experience some of the same problems of vasodilation as people with migraines, and because there is some overlap of symptoms, some of the medicines listed below can be used for the acute stages of cluster headaches, though it is recommended that professional homeopathic care be sought for the best results.

General Migraine Pains

Natrum mur is one of the most common migraine remedies. It is particularly indicated when people experience head pain that is worse from sun and light, at ten A.M. (or from ten A.M. to three P.M.), before and after menstruation, from reading, and after a grieving experience.

Typically, the pain feels as if hammers were beating the head. A cold, hay fever, or herpetic eruption may be experienced concurrently.

Ignatia, like **Natrum mur**, is useful in people who get a migraine after an emotional experience. These emotionally sensitive people may have just experienced a romantic disappointment or grief, and as a result of this, they are prone to frequent, deep sighing. Typically, they tend to experience a lump in their throat and/or difficulty swallowing along with their headache.

Right-sided Migraines

Belladonna is indicated for a throbbing headache with pains that come and go rapidly, are aggravated by light, jarring motion, noise, sun, and heat, and are relieved by cold applications, hard pressure, lying in the dark, and sitting semierect. The person may have a bounding pulse and a hot, red face.

Lycopodium is recommended when head pain is worst between four and eight P.M. and in warm rooms or from the heat of a bed, when the pain starts on the right side and then shifts to the left side, and when gastric symptoms are also experienced, especially excessive gas. A characteristic look of the person who needs this remedy is a furrowed brow or jowls and early graying of the hair or beard. These people tend to be irritable and bossy.

Sanguinaria is a remedy for right-sided headaches usually prior to menstruation. It is also good for people who experience headaches from exposure to the sun, or people who get recurring headaches in a consistent pattern, such as every seven or twenty-eight days. When people experience relief of their head pain after vomiting and/or belching, this remedy should be considered.

Chelidonium is indicated for right-sided headaches with concurrent right-sided pains, including facial neuralgia, liver pains, or back pains. This remedy is known to be helpful in people who have liver or gallbladder disease and who crave hot drinks.

Left-sided Migraines

Spigelia is effective in treating head pains over the left eye and frontal region, especially when the head is extremely sensitive to touch. It is also indicated for sinus pains or left-sided facial neuralgias which begin after exposure to cold or to cold, wet weather and yet are relieved by cold applications and by lying on the right side with the head erect.

Lachesis is typically indicated when head pains are aggravated upon rising in the morning and the pain is felt at the root of the nose and on the whole left side of the head. Warmth and sun aggravate the head, while open air and hard pressure provide some relief. Head pains are also worse prior to menstruation and are relieved with the commencement of the flow.

Iris is useful when the head pain is combined with nausea, vomiting, and blurred vision. These symptoms are aggravated by eating sweets and by exposure to heat, while open air and gentle motion provide some relief.

Sepia is effective when the person experiences a migraine concurrent with nausea, especially when relief comes either from being quiet while lying down or from rigorous exercise. The head pain is aggravated by stooping, coughing, light, jarring, and exposure to warm rooms.

Dose: Improvement is usually noticed after two or three doses of the 6, 12, or 30th potency, which may be taken every hour in intense pain and every four hours in mild discomfort. Stop taking the medicine whenever some degree of relief is observed.

RESOURCES

Dale Buegel, Blair Lewis, and Dennis Chernin, *Homeopathic Remedies for Health Professionals and Laypeople.* Honesdale, PA: Himalayan, 1991.

Stephen Cummings and Dana Ullman, *Everybody's Guide to Homeopathic Medicines.* Los Angeles: Tarcher, 1991.

Thomas Kruzel, *Homeopathic Emergency Guide.* Berkeley: North Atlantic, 1992.

Digestive Disorders

"Indigestion" is, figuratively speaking, a "waste can" term for a wide variety of digestive symptoms, including nausea, vomiting, heartburn, flatulence, and stomach pain. This condition, medically termed gastritis, is often the first way that people experience symptoms of stress.

Indigestion can result from the food one eats, the amount and combination of foods ingested, and even from the emotions one experiences during and after eating. Indigestion can also result from unknown factors that affect assimilation of food, for the body does not assimilate all nutrients equally well.

Digestive symptoms can range from simple, temporary conditions to chronic, debilitating disease, and these symptoms can be local, digestive system–centered ailments or systemic conditions that manifest in various places, not just the digestive system.

Most of the common digestive symptoms that people experience can be treated at home without medical supervision. However, persistent digestive complaints or severe symptoms warrant medical attention.

When Hippocrates said, "Let food be thy medicine," he did not mean to say or imply that food should be one's only medicine. He readily acknowledged the value of various substances as medicinal agents. That is why Hippocrates also noted, "Through the like, disease is produced and through the application of the like, it is cured." In so doing, the father of medicine recognized homeopathy's principle of similars. And when homeopathic medicines are combined with sound nutritional practices including nonrushed eating and thorough chewing of food, one significantly decreases the chances of experiencing digestive difficulties.

Nausea and Vomiting

Nausea and vomiting are important inherent defenses of the body. Though these defenses tend to be more active during infancy and childhood, the symptoms are ways that the body seeks to rid itself of irritating and potentially poisonous substances. Homeopathy's principle of similars makes infinite sense in treating such symptoms, since it is wise to aid the body's efforts to get rid of irritating substances, rather than simply suppress the body's response as conventional drug treatments tend to do. In fact, homeopathic remedies can sometimes cause sick people to vomit as an effective way to relieve their indigestion.

Acute nausea and vomiting can be effectively self-treated with homeopathic medicines, though when these symptoms are experienced recurrently, it is best to seek professional homeopathic care.

One of the most common homeopathic medicines for treating acute nausea and vomiting is **Ipecacuahna,** made from an herb known to cause nausea and vomiting if taken in crude doses. It is primarily useful in treating the symptoms it is known to cause: constant nausea which is not relieved by vomiting, vomiting with gagging, lack of thirst, a surprisingly clean tongue despite strong feelings of nausea, aggravation of symptoms from warmth, and some relief of symptoms from being in the open air. A headache, cough, or heavy menstruation may accompany the nausea.

Ironically, one of the classic studies which physicians commonly refer to as showing the power of placebos was a study in which doctors prescribed ipecac to patients suffering from nausea (ipecac is a drug derived from the ipecacuahna plant, which is known to cause nausea and vomiting). The physicians didn't tell the patients what they were being given and simply informed them that it was a new drug that was effective in treating nausea. Much to the physicians' surprise, the ipecac did not aggravate their nausea, and in fact, it actually alleviated it. The experimenters asserted that this study proved "the power of placebo." Sadly, however, they were woefully ignorant of homeopathic principles, for this experiment didn't prove the power of placebo so much as it proved the homeopathic law of similars.

Arsenicum is another common remedy for acute nausea and vomiting, especially when they are the result of food poisoning. Typically, the person who needs **Arsenicum** cannot stand the sight or smell of food and has a strong thirst but can tolerate only sips at a time. The person may experience burning pains in the stomach, burning pains in the throat as a result of irritating vomitus, and burning pains in the anus as a result of excoriating diarrhea. **Arsenicum** is a leading remedy for food poisoning.

Nux vomica is a remedy for acute nausea and vomiting, commonly the result of overeating, drinking alcohol, or food poisoning, and often accompanied by flatulence, bloating, heartburn, and either diarrhea or constipation. People who need **Nux vomica** usually experience the worst symptoms in the morning upon waking. They feel some relief from warmth, warm applications, and warm drinks. These people wake unrefreshed and are highly irritable. This remedy provides relief from hangovers and also helps deal with digestive upsets aggravated by therapeutic or recreational drugs.

Bryonia is known to be effective in treating nausea that is aggravated by motion (just getting up or stooping can lead the person to vomit), and also aggravated in a warm room and by heat. Even though their stomachs are sensitive to touch, people who need this remedy are at least partially relieved by lying on them. Some relief is also experienced in cool or open air and by resting. These people also have a significant thirst, usually for cold drinks though they may experience some relief from drinking warm fluids. A headache in the front part of the head may be concurrent.

Podophyllum should be considered when the person also experiences diarrhea with nausea and vomiting. Typically, the diarrhea is painless, profuse, offensive, and expelled with gushing force. There is much gurgling in the abdomen prior to having a stool and much gas released with the diarrhea.

Pulsatilla is helpful in treating people with indigestion after eating rich foods or pork. They have bloating, abdominal distension, and sometimes a headache. They tend to be thirstless. This remedy is more often given to children and women than to men.

Other useful though less commonly indicated remedies to consider are **Colchicum** (when the person suffers from severe nausea simply at the sight or smell of food), **Phosphorus** (when he or she eats something cold or icy and then vomits it once it is warmed in the stomach), **Sepia** (a major remedy for nausea during pregnancy), and

Veratrum album (when a person has projectile vomiting and diarrhea, and is extremely chilly; it is also a common remedy for nausea prior to menstruation).

Dose: Take the 6, 12, or 30th potency every two to eight hours, depending upon the severity of symptoms (the more intense the symptoms, the more frequent the recommended repetition). If symptoms are strong and no changes have occurred in six hours, consider another remedy. If symptoms are mild, wait for at least twenty-four hours before changing remedies. Stop taking any medicine if some improvement is experienced.

ACUTE DIARRHEA

Acute diarrhea is an important defense the body deploys to hasten the elimination of bacteria or other irritating substances. Conventional drugs which "control" or "manage" diarrhea tend to slow this natural defensive effort. Although these drugs may effectively stop the diarrhea, they tend to create more irritating gastrointestinal symptoms, neurological syndromes, and dependency on the drug as the result of suppressing the body's natural defenses.

A double-blind, placebo-controlled study which showed the efficacy of homeopathic medicines in treating acute diarrhea was recently published in *Pediatrics,* the journal of the American Academy of Pediatrics.[1] This study indicated that Nicaraguan children suffering from acute diarrhea experienced a significant relief of symptoms when prescribed an individually chosen homeopathic medicine, as compared with children prescribed a placebo.

As noted previously, this study is of particular importance because acute diarrhea is the most serious public health problem in many developing countries. Approximately 5 million children die every year as the result of dehydration caused by diarrhea.

Although acute diarrhea is not as serious a public health problem in developed countries, it is still a common and discomforting problem to both children and adults. Fortunately, homeopathic medicines can be very effective in treating people with symptoms of diarrhea.

People with diarrhea who may benefit from **Arsenicum** have stools that are acrid and tend to burn the anus. Most typically, people who need **Arsenicum** develop symptoms as the result of eating spoiled or tainted food or eating too much fruit. They usually feel exhausted, yet are restless in bed, unable to find a comfortable position. They are also very anxious and tend to feel fearful about being alone. Their worst symptoms are at and after midnight, and they are very thirsty but only for sips of fluids at a time. They are extremely chilly, and cold drinks tend to irritate them, while warm drinks provide some relief. They tend to break out in a cold sweat, and feel better when covered.

People who need **Podophyllum** usually experience gurgling in the abdomen with a very sudden urge to have a stool. The stools are profuse and offensive-smelling, and are usually expelled with great force and little pain, followed by great exhaustion after each stool. These people may experience severe weakness in the anal sphincter, causing a sensation that they cannot hold anything inside the rectum. Their diarrhea is aggravated by eating, drinking, and moving around and may alternate with a headache. They may gag and have empty retching, they have a great thirst for cold fluids, and they may experience painful cramps in their feet, calves, and/or thighs. This diarrhea is sometimes experienced in teething infants and in children who have eaten a lot of fruit.

Chamomilla is indicated primarily in infants and children, especially when they are extremely irritable, quarrelsome, fitful, and inconsolable. Typically, they ask for something and then reject it once it is offered. Only rocking and being carried provide temporary relief of their discomfort. They are aggravated by heat, worse in the evening until midnight, and better from cold drinks. Teething or colicky infants who experience diarrhea tend to need this remedy. Their diarrhea tends to be offensive, green, and slimy, like chopped grass, and it smells like rotten eggs.

Mercurius is known to be most effective in treating people with diarrhea who have the "never completely done" sensation—that is, no matter how many times they have diarrhea, they still feel that they have more left. Typically, they experience much retching during release of the stool, and the stool may have some blood in it. This retching tends to exhaust them. They are sensitive to extremes of temperature and may at one time feel chilly and at another time feel feverish. In any case, their symptoms are worse at night. They sweat profusely, have offensive breath, usually salivate onto the pillow, and tend to be quite slow and weak both physically and mentally. They commonly have a strong thirst for cold fluids.

Sulphur is a remedy for people who experience a sudden, involuntary expulsion of their diarrhea, including when they think they are passing gas. The diarrhea is thin, watery, offensive, acrid, and smells of rotten eggs. It tends to be painlessly expelled, and the most frequent problems are at 5 A.M. and at night. Cold sweat on the face and feet are common, and these people are very thirsty for cold drinks and have little appetite. Emotionally, they are irritable and weepy with indifference to their appearance and to their bodily odors.

Veratrum album is indicated when people have diarrhea and vomiting and are very chilly and weak. Despite being chilly, they tend to crave ice cold drinks. They may also have a bloated abdomen and experience stomach cramps.

Dose: Take the 6, 12, or 30th potency after each time you have a stool that is not normally firm. If symptoms are strong and no changes have occurred in twelve hours, consider another remedy. If symptoms are mild, wait for at least twenty-four hours before changing remedies. Stop taking any medicine if obvious improvement is experienced.

ACUTE CONSTIPATION

The frequency of defecation varies from one person to the next. A person is not necessarily constipated just because he or she does not have a stool every day. Constipation refers more to the difficulty one has in expelling stools, and the symptoms one has if unable to, than the actual frequency of stools.

Acute constipation can often be treated through dietary means (fiber-rich foods and adequate liquids), exercise, and/or prudent use of herbal laxatives. Homeopathic medicines can augment the efficacy of lifestyle changes. Some of the most common remedies are **Nux vomica, Bryonia**, and **Calcarea carb.** Homeopathic combination formulas can also be wonderfully effective in treating constipation.

Nux vomica is indicated when the person has constant urges to stool but is unable to pass it. Small amounts can sometimes be expelled, but this provides only temporary relief. It is also useful when the constipation is related to overeating, alcohol consumption, or drug use (therapeutic or recreational).

Bryonia is indicated when the person's mouth and anus feel excessively dry as are their stools. Food tends to sit like a lump in their stomach because their digestive juices have similarly dried up. A headache in the forehead or behind the eyes or nose which is very sensitive to any type of motion is commonly experienced at the same time.

Calcarea carb is typically used in overweight people with flabby skin tone. They have no urge to have a stool. They do not feel any ill-effects of constipation, and children with constipation may even feel better during this condition. They experience heartburn and have sour burping.

Dose: You should need to take only between three and six doses of the 6, 12, or 30th potency in twelve hours. If no changes have occurred, consider another remedy.

Hemorrhoids

Hemorrhoids, which are swollen blood vessels in the anal area and which tend to accompany constipation, can readily be treated with homeopathic medicines. If a person has had hemorrhoids for a long time, homeopathic medicines may relieve the pain and reduce the bleeding, but they will not always be able to reverse the tissue changes that have occurred.

The late British homeopath Richard Hughes claimed consistently good results in treating hemorrhoids using **Nux vomica 3x** before breakfast alternating with **Sulphur 3x** upon retiring. There are, however, other remedies to consider. **Hamamelis** is a remedy for bleeding hemorrhoids and for varicose veins. This remedy is also good when the anus feels raw and sore and when pulsations are felt in the rectum. **Aesculus** is indicated when the hemorrhoids don't bleed, but the person experiences a sense of a lump or fullness and burning pains in the anus, as well as sharp sticking pains up into the rectum. People who need **Aesculus** may also be chilly and feel chills up and down the back, though they tend to feel some relief from exposure to cool, open air.

In addition to various internal remedies, there are also some external applications that are effective. These external applications come in gel or ointment form and usually include **Hamamelis** and **Aesculus**, as well as **Collinsonia** (for habitual constipation with bleeding,

also a sense of small sharp sticks in the rectal area, with a sense of constriction) and **Aloe** (for hemorrhoids "like a bunch of grapes," ameliorated by cold bathing, possibly with diarrhea in which the person is
driven out of bed to run to the toilet and sometimes has to hurry to
the toilet after eating and drinking, or if a stool is accidentally released
after flatus).

Dose: You generally need to consider taking two doses a day of the 6,
12, or 30th potency for up to four days. Stop taking the remedy if
some type of improvement begins. External applications, likewise,
only need to be applied twice a day for up to four days.

FLATULENCE AND BLOATING

Flatulence and bloating are extremely common problems. Almost
everyone at least occasionally experiences gas problems, especially
after overeating, eating certain gas-causing foods such as beans or cab-
bage, or eating too rapidly. Some people experience them frequently,
and the discomfort to themselves and others may vary from minor to
significant. Often such problems are chronic and require professional
constitutional care. It is difficult to prescribe a remedy based only on
the symptoms of gas and bloating, and since these symptoms are usually accompanied by others; homeopathic medicines are more effective when prescribed on the broader symptom complex.

    Carbo veg helps relieve people who suffer from great distension
and offensive gas from almost all types of food. They get some relief
from the release of gas and desire carbonated drinks because they seem
to help in releasing it. **Cinchona** is useful when there is more pain
than distension, frequent rumbling in the abdomen, and no relief from
releasing gas. **Raphanus** is a common remedy for people who have a
distended abdomen but are unable to expel gas. **Colocynthis** is effective when there is more pain than distension, and cramps that are relieved by bending over.

    Nux vomica is indicated when people get gas from overindul-
gence in food and drink, especially if alcohol or drugs (therapeutic or
recreational) are also ingested. Typically, those who need this remedy
experience their worst gas symptoms upon waking. They may want to
vomit but can't, except after much retching, and may feel a need to

defecate but can't, except with much pushing. Besides the various physical symptoms, they are extremely irritable. **Bryonia** is useful in people who have similar symptoms as those listed for **Nux vomica**, though people who need **Bryonia** will be more aggravated by any type of motion, and their abdomens will be extremely sensitive to touch. Also distinct from **Nux vomica**, these people are aggravated by warm rooms and heat and relieved by coolness and open air. **Pulsatilla** is more commonly indicated for women and children, especially after eating rich, fatty foods. They will be averse to warm food or drinks and to warmth in general and will feel some relief by exposure to cool or open air. They may taste previously eaten food when they burp, and they will tend to be thirstless.

Besides the above single remedies, the homeopathic combination formulas for indigestion and gas can be used and are often effective.

Dose: Take the 6, 12, or 30th potency every four to six hours. If improvement is not noticed after twenty-four hours, consider another remedy. Stop taking the medicine if symptoms improve in any way.

ABDOMINAL CRAMPS

When a person experiences abdominal cramps, **Magnesia phos, Colocynthis,** and **Belladonna** are common remedies to consider. **Magnesia phos** should be considered when the cramps are temporarily relieved by warmth, warm drinks, or bending over. **Colocynthis** is helpful when the cramps are relieved by bending over or applying firm and steady pressure to the painful area. People who need **Colocynthis** also tend to be considerably more irritable than those needing **Magnesia phos**. **Belladonna** is effective when the cramps come and go rapidly in waves, when simple motion or jarring aggravates the symptoms, and when the pain is intense enough to cause even a small degree of delirium.

Dose: Take the 6, 12, or 30th potency every one to four hours, depending upon severity of symptoms. If relief isn't experienced within twelve hours, consider another medicine. Stop taking the medicine when any noticeable improvement is observed.

ULCERS

Gastric and duodenal ulcers require the supervision of a physician because a perforated or bleeding ulcer can create a life-threatening condition. Gastric ulcer refers to ulceration occurring in the main body of the stomach, while duodenal ulcers occur in or near the duodenum, which extends from the lower part of the stomach to the first part of the small intestine. Typically, abdominal pain and distress are felt forty-five to sixty minutes after eating, and the use of antacids and ingestion of food provide temporary relief.

It is recommended that one concurrently seek professional homeopathic care for ulcers. Some of the more common remedies that homeopaths use include: **Phosphorus, Kali bichromicum, Hydrastis, Arsenicum, Argentum nitricum, Nux vomica, Lycopodium, Pulsatilla, Mercurius corrosivus, Kali carbonicum,** and **Nitric acid** (see Kruzel's *Homeopathic Emergency Guide* and Boericke's *Pocket Manual of Materia Medica with Repertory* for detailed information on each of these remedies). These remedies can be very effective, though patients are also encouraged to become more conscientious about eating better and reducing their stress.

IRRITABLE BOWEL SYNDROME AND INFLAMMATORY BOWEL DISEASE

Irritable bowel syndrome (IBS), also called colitis, spastic colon, or simply nervous stomach, refers to a functional disorder of the colon or large intestine. People with IBS have abdominal pain and suffer from chronic diarrhea and constipation which alternate and debilitate. Despite these symptoms, medical examination cannot find disease or tissue change. Inflammatory bowel disease (IBD) includes more serious conditions such as Crohn's disease and ulcerative colitis in which there is disease and cellular damage in the large intestine that can be confirmed through medical examination by X-ray or sigmoidoscopy (internal examination of the large intestine).

IBS and IBD both require professional homeopathic care. Self-treatment with remedies for the acute diarrhea or constipation that is experienced can be effective in providing temporary relief, though more significant improvement in health requires constitutional care. Still, one study showed that ninety-one patients with IBS who were given **Asafoetida 3x** experienced noticeable improvement in symptoms compared to people with IBS who were given a placebo.[2]

RESOURCES

Stephen Cummings and Dana Ullman, *Everybody's Guide to Homeopathic Medicines*. Los Angeles: Tarcher, 1991.

Thomas Kruzel, *Homeopathic Emergency Guide*. Berkeley: North Atlantic, 1992.

Andrew Lockie, *The Family Guide to Homeopathy*. New York: Fireside, 1993.

Skin Conditions

The human skin is a masterpiece of evolution. It regulates bodily temperature, waterproofs the body, and defends against and even destroys invading pathogens. It is considered the largest human organ, and every square inch of skin is a highly sophisticated feat of engineering with 19 million cells, 625 sweat glands, 90 oil glands, 65 hairs, 19 feet of blood vessels, 19,000 sensory cells, and over 20 million microscopic animals.

Homeopaths do not consider skin diseases to be actually diseases of the skin; they are internal conditions which create symptoms that manifest on the skin. From this point of view, it doesn't make sense to treat skin symptoms primarily with external applications, nor does it make sense to use steroidal drugs, as is extremely common today in dermatology, because they are specifically prescribed to suppress the immune system's natural response to an irritating or allergenic substance. Although these treatments "work," they do not heal the underlying disease and tend to cause various side effects that can be worse than the original symptoms.

The homeopathic approach to treating people with skin conditions is to find a medicine that is known to cause and cure the totality of symptoms they are experiencing, not just their skin symptoms. This comprehensive assessment leads to an individualized homeopathic remedy that will help to initiate a healing response. Professional homeopathic care is generally necessary for skin conditions, and thus information on homeopathic self-treatment is not provided in this chapter, except for a limited number of acute skin problems.

The good news for people with chronic skin problems is that homeopaths have observed that people who suffer from such conditions *tend* to be healthier and live longer than those who do not. Homeopaths believe that these people are strong enough to push their internal ailments onto the skin. Despite the fact that these people may not look healthy, they often are healthier than the rest of us.

While these observations by homeopaths may provide some consolation to people with chronic skin ailments, the vanity that lurks within most of us may make it difficult to fully accept this good news. Once again, we are lucky that homeopathic medicines exist, because they are so effective for skin complaints. We can have the luxury of being both vain and healthy.

ECZEMA

Eczema is also called atopic dermatitis, which is simply a technical way of saying that it is an allergic inflammation of the skin. The derivation of the word "eczema" provides insight into how this condition should and should not be treated. "Eczema" derives from Greek and means "result of boiling over." If, in fact, eczema is a condition in which something under the skin is boiling over, putting a lid on it will not be very effective, since the steam will simply seek to escape along the sides of the lid. And if the lid is held on firmly, an internal explosion becomes imminent. But putting a lid on it is what people do when they take steroidal medications or other drugs that merely suppress their eczema symptoms, driving the disease deeper into their bodies and creating the potential for more serious health problems in the future.

Eczema is best treated internally, usually by a professional homeopath. The exception is that one can apply external applications of **Calendula** when a rash becomes inflamed or infected. Such treatment often provides some nourishment and relief to the skin, though it is not expected to heal the condition.

A British physician surveyed 130 consecutive cases of patients with eczema.[1] He treated 87 children who had eczema of an average duration of 4.33 years. Almost 90 percent of these children were either better or much better during the average period of treatment of 2.5 years. He also observed that the sooner the child began homeopathic care, the better the result.

Because self-treatment for eczema is not recommended, discussion of the individual symptoms for these remedies is not provided.

PSORIASIS

People with psoriasis are commonly treated with many of the same remedies as people with eczema. And like the latter, they are best treated by a professional homeopath.

WARTS

Warts are an extremely common skin condition. Some homeopaths brag that treating warts is very easy, and they generally mention **Thuja** as the most common remedy for them. While **Thuja** is a relatively common remedy for warts, it is not the only one, and it is not frequently useful for all types of warts, such as plantar warts (warts on the soles of the feet). The *Canadian Medical Association Journal* published research on the homeopathic treatment of plantar warts.[2] The double-blind study included 162 patients who were given daily, over a six-week period, a combination of three homeopathic medicines: **Thuja 30c, Antimonium crudum 7c,** and **Nitric acid 7c.** Patients given this combination of homeopathic medicines did not experience any better relief from their plantar warts than those given a placebo.

However, although these three homeopathic remedies are very frequently given to people with warts, they are not generally indicated in the treatment of plantar warts. One year before this study was published, another study showed that over 90 percent of patients who were prescribed individually chosen homeopathic medicines had their warts disappear.[3]

Effective treatment of warts generally requires the professional treatment of the entire person, not just the wart symptoms.

ABSCESSES, BOILS, AND CARBUNCLES

Other common skin conditions are abscesses, boils, and carbuncles (carbuncles are boils that extend into deeper layers of the skin). The first remedy to consider for the first stage of an abscess or boil is **Bel-**

ladonna 6 or **30** (sudden onset of very red, tender eruptions). **Hepar sulphur 30** is a common remedy for later stages of an abscess, boil, or carbuncle, (when the eruption is very sensitive to touch and it holds or has exuded much pus). **Silicea 30** is good when the eruption has persisted and is slow to heal.

Dose: Take a 6 or 30th potency every one or four hours for only one to five doses. This is all that will generally be needed to obtain some relief of symptoms. Don't consider changing medicines for at least twelve hours or after a night's rest, whichever is longer.

SCARRING

Scarring from an injury, surgical procedure, or acne can be significantly reduced and sometimes entirely eliminated with homeopathic medicines. The first remedies to use for scars are external gels that include **Thiosinaminum** and **Calendula**. If they are not available, topical applications of **Calendula** are great for superficial scars; **Thiosinaminum 6** helps to dissolve scars and adhesions; **Silicea 30** helps reduce old scars that become inflamed; **Graphites 6** or **30** is effective when a scar becomes thick.

Dose: Take one of the above remedies three times a day for up to a week. The medicine will usually begin a healing process not immediately observable. Wait one month before trying another remedy.

BURNS

Homeopathic medicine offers much for the treatment of all types of burns, though basic first-aid treatment for burns should be followed. Also, medical attention is recommended for second and third degree burns.

First degree burns, including sunburn, are very effectively treated with homeopathic medicines. It is common to experience significant reduction or complete elimination of pain shortly after using homeopathic medicines, and to find that there is no evidence of a first or second degree burn after twenty-four hours.

The first treatment of choice for burns is external burn gels (such gels should include at least **Calendula** and **Urtica dioica** or **Urtica**

urens). If a formula gel composed of these two remedies is not available, use a **Calendula** gel or spray. Internally, **Urtica urens 6** or **30** or **Hypericum 6** or **30** should be taken. If the pain of a second or third degree burn is significant, **Cantharis 30** is the indicated remedy. Another common remedy for second or third degree burns is **Causticum 30**.

Dose: Take 6, 12, or 30th potencies every one to six hours, depending upon the severity (the more severe the pain, the more frequent the dosage). External applications should be reapplied whenever the injured part is washed or a new dressing is applied.

BLISTERS

Blisters are easily treated and quickly cured with **Calendula** gel, ointment, or spray. If the blister is broken, one should first clean the wound and then apply the **Calendula**. Consider re-applying the remedy once a day or whenever the dressing is changed. If the blister is unbroken, **Calendula** can be apply directly over the swelling. There is controversy in the medical community about whether blisters should or shouldn't be broken, though it is agreed that one should not pull the skin off the blister because it provides a useful shield against secondary infection.

POISON OAK/POISON IVY

Although many of us have cursed the very existence of poison oak and poison ivy, both of these substances have become extremely important homeopathic medicines when potentized. Knowledge of their value as homeopathic medicines, however, does not diminish the itching and irritation that is experienced from the contact dermatitis these plants cause.

Rhus tox (poison ivy) is not the only remedy to consider for poison oak or ivy rashes, though it and **Croton tiglium** are the two most commonly effective remedies. The primary indications for using **Rhus tox** are aggravation of itching at night, from the warmth of a bed and from scratching, reduced itching from warm applications and hot water, and vesicles (pus-filled blisters) in a line of the scratch. People who need **Rhus tox** are extremely restless and may obtain some relief from constantly moving.

Croton tiglium is indicated when the skin feels tight and "hidebound," and there is some difficulty moving the affected part in a way that causes any creasing of the skin. Typically, these symptoms are not as bad after sleeping. The person has intense itching worse at night and by touch or washing and may be relieved by gentle rubbing; however, scratching leads to burning pains. People who need this remedy may have pustules that dry into yellow scabs.

Other remedies to consider are **Ledum** (when relief is experienced from cold applications), **Anacardium** (when there are large blisters filled with yellow liquid, and sufferers become so irritable that they have irresistible urges to swear and curse, and they experience some relief from eating and from immersion in hot water), **Graphites** (when the eruptions exude a glutinous, sticky, honeylike fluid, especially after scratching), and **Sulphur** (when the symptoms are aggravated by the warmth of a bed, by scratching, and by washing; consider this remedy if **Rhus tox,** which fits similar symptoms, doesn't work).

In addition to these individual medicines, there are a number of homeopathic combination formulas available which have a reputation of efficacy.

Dose: Take the 6, 12, or 30th potency every two to six hours, depending upon the severity of symptoms. Stop as soon as obvious improvement is observed.

RESOURCES

The best resources for treating skin complaints are homeopathic repertories and *materia medica*. The best book that combines both is William Boericke's *Pocket Manual of Materia Medica with Repertory*. New Delhi: B. Jain.

See also:

Dale Buegel, Blair Lewis, and Dennis Chernin, *Homeopathic Remedies for Health Professionals and Laypeople*. Honesdale, PA: Himalayan, 1991.

Stephen Cummings and Dana Ullman, *Everybody's Guide to Homeopathic Medicines*. Los Angeles: Tarcher, 1991.

Thomas Kruzel, *Homeopathic Emergency Guide*. Berkeley: North Atlantic, 1992.

Allergies

Contrary to popular opinion, allergies are not caused by an allergen; they are caused by the hypersensitive state of the person to the allergen. It is as though the person is a loaded gun and the allergen is the trigger. The allergen itself does not load the gun; it just sets it off.

Although avoidance of the allergen can provide relief for allergy sufferers, it does not provide a cure but just keeps the sleeping giant of hypersensitivity undisturbed, providing only a temporary reprieve from symptoms. Homeopathic medicines offer the real potential of decreasing this hypersensitivity, sometimes temporarily and sometimes permanently.

Homeopaths have a long history of successful allergy treatment, and they have made some important contributions to our present understanding of allergies. In fact, it was a British homeopath, C. H. Blackley, who in 1871 first noted that seasonal sneezing and nasal discharge were the result of exposure to pollen.[1] An American homeopath, Dr. Grant L. Selfridge, was one of three physicians to start the organization that became the present American Academy of Allergy.[2]

Conventional treatment for many types of allergies includes desensitization shots, which are a homeopathiclike treatment in which small doses of an allergen are injected. However, this use of the "law of sames" in treatment (called isopathy), as distinct from the homeopathic law of similars, is only somewhat effective. Because the allergen is only the trigger to the problem and not the underlying cause, using small doses of the allergen does not always work to desensitize a person.

There are numerous types of allergies and innumerable symptoms that are experienced from them. The most common allergies are respiratory allergies (especially hay fever and asthma), food allergies, and skin allergies, each of which can be successfully treated with homeopathic medicines.

RESPIRATORY ALLERGIES

Respiratory allergies include hay fever and asthma as well as allergies to animal fur, mold, tobacco smoke, and house dust mites. Less common but still sometimes serious are allergies to cosmetics, perfumes, gas, fumes, and household cleaning products. Surprisingly, the most allergenic substance in the world is the house dust mite. The symptoms of respiratory allergy generally include nasal discharge, sneezing, and watery eyes.

Homeopathic medicines are usually prescribed based on the person's unique pattern of symptoms, no matter what he or she is allergic to. To homeopaths, it is important to know the color and consistency of the person's nasal discharge, what factors aggravate or alleviate the symptoms, and what unusual and characteristic symptoms are experienced.

Conventional allergy testing thus is not necessary for homeopathic care, though in some treatment-resistant cases, using potentized doses of the specific allergen can occasionally provide relief when other homeopathic treatments aren't working.

Using single or combination remedies based on the acute symptoms of the allergy can provide valuable relief, but professional constitutional care is necessary to achieve a deeper cure.

HAY FEVER

One of the important studies showing the efficacy of homeopathic medicines was an investigation of the treatment of hay fever noted in Chapter 4. This study tested the result of giving the 30c potency of the pollen of twelve common flowers to patients with hay fever.[3] Those who were given this potentized pollen mixture experienced significant improvement compared with those given a placebo.

The study showed that patients who took the placebo had six times more symptoms than those to whom the homeopathic medicine was given. Further, all subjects in this study were also given a second medicine, an antihistamine, which they were told they could use if the first medicine was not adequately effective. The study showed that those given the homeopathic medicine needed to take the antihistamine one half as often as those given the placebo.

This potentized dose of mixed pollen did not "cure" the subjects' allergy, though it did provide valuable relief for them.

Some of the common individual remedies that are used for the acute phase of a respiratory allergy are **Allium cepa** (profuse watering from the eyes and dripping nose; nasal discharge is acrid and irritates the nostrils and upper lip; sneezing; worse in warm rooms, better in cool air), **Euphrasia** (profuse watering from the eyes, with acrid tears that irritate the lower lids and cheeks), **Sabadilla** (primarily paroxysms of sneezing, usually worse from cold or exposure to odors or perfumes, better from warmth and warm drinks), **Arsenicum** (watery, acrid nasal discharge, complete nasal obstruction, chilliness; better from warmth and heat), **Kali bichromicum** (copious, thick, acrid, stringy nasal discharge, usually yellow), **Nux vomica** (fluent nasal discharge during the day and congested at night, fluent discharge in the open air, aggravation of symptoms after overindulgence in food or drink or after overworking and undersleeping), **Natrum mur** (clear, watery nasal discharge and tearing from the eyes, frontal headache or migraine, possible herpetic eruption), **Pulsatilla** (thick nasal discharge, usually yellow or green; worse in warm rooms, open air, or evening, better from cold applications; thirstlessness; commonly used for children or women), **Arum triphyllum** (profuse acrid nasal discharge, usually on the left side, marked itching of the nose and lips causing the person to scratch and pick at the itching parts, hoarseness), **Wyethia** (significant itching in the nose, throat, and palate of the mouth, compulsion to rub the palate with the tongue), and **Histaminium** (use this remedy when you don't know what else to use).

Homeopathic combination formulas should also be considered for acute allergy symptoms. These remedies provide quick relief for great numbers of allergy sufferers.

Dose: Take the 6, 12, or 30th potency every four hours or during intense symptoms every two hours. Improvement commonly begins after one or two doses. Continue to take doses as long as symptoms remain, unless they are very mild. Consider changing medicines if no improvement is observed after four doses.

ASTHMA

Asthma is generally, though not always, considered the result of an allergic response. Besides being triggered by pollens, fur, feathers, smoke, house dust mites, and inhaled irritants, it can also be triggered by emotional upsets, drugs, caffeine, exercise, and changes in the weather.

A recent study published in the prestigious journal *Lancet* showed the efficacy of homeopathic medicines in the treatment of asthma.[4] This unique study integrated conventional allergy testing to determine which substance asthma sufferers reacted to the most, and then half of the subjects were given the 30c potency of this substance, while the other half were given a placebo. The researchers observed a very significant difference starting the first week and continuing through the end of the two-month experiment. At the end of the study, those who got the homeopathic remedy boosted breathing capacity by 30 to 40 percent, while those given the placebo experienced an improvement of only 12 percent.

It should be noted that homeopaths observe that using potentized doses of the substance to which a person is allergic does not cure the asthma but does provide nontoxic temporary relief. A true cure of this ailment requires professional homeopathic care, and is commonly experienced from good practitioners. Asthma is a serious enough condition that individuals should not simply rely upon self-care but should seek the care of a professional homeopath and/or other medical professional. If necessary, homeopathic medicines can be taken on the way to the doctor or hospital, for the correct remedy often reduces the chances of asthma becoming a medical emergency.

Whether one is under the care of a professional homeopath or not, it is beneficial for asthma sufferers and their families to know how to treat acute asthma attacks. Some of the most common remedies are **Aconitum** (for the initial stages of onset of asthma when the sufferer is frightened and anxious), **Arsenicum** (when symptoms are worse from midnight to two a.m.; soreness and burning in the chest, better sitting upright; anxiousness, fear, restlessness, chilliness, thirst for small quantities frequently), **Ipecacuanha** (for childhood asthma, a rattling cough, nausea and vomiting), **Pulsatilla** (useful in weepy children and women who need sympathy and attention; symptoms usually worse before ten p.m., yellow or green sputum; wants open air; thirstlessness), **Spongia** (dry, croupy cough, difficulty breathing in; cough better after eating or drinking, especially from warm things, worse from dry, cold wind), and **Natrum sulphur** (worse in wet weather, worse at four to five a.m.; chest held when coughing; especially useful in children or in anyone after a grieving experience).

As noted, professional homeopathic constitutional care is quite effective in treating asthma, usually leading to a significant reduction in the frequency and intensity of asthma symptoms.

Dose: Take the 6, 12, or 30th potency every one or two hours, but stop if there is obvious improvement. Repeat the doses if symptoms return. If no changes are observed after four doses, consider another remedy.

FOOD ALLERGIES

Food allergies are a controversial topic in medicine because there are few tests to verify conclusively that people have them. Part of the problem is that many people who think they have food allergies may actually have difficulty digesting certain foods as a result of enzyme deficiencies, but such difficulty does not constitute a formal food allergy. People who do not have the appropriate enzymes to digest foods are thought to have a food intolerance, not an allergy, though distinctions in symptoms between allergies and intolerances are not always clear. Diagnosis of either of these conditions is further complicated by the fact that many people with food allergies or intolerances do not develop symptoms until several hours after eating the trigger food. Additional problems in diagnosis are created by the fact that people sometimes experience digestive problems primarily during certain times of the year, when certain foods are combined with others, or when they are responding to the chemicals or contaminants in the food, not the food itself.

One example of a contaminant in food which can create symptoms is cockroaches. The FDA recognizes that it is often impossible to keep these insects out of food preparation plants, and thus they allow a certain small percentage of cockroach parts in the food. Cockroach parts are known to trigger allergic symptoms, including asthma. In fact, homeopaths use microdoses of it (*Blatta orientalis*) to treat those people whose asthma symptoms match the remedy's. Contaminants in food help explain why sometimes people react to certain foods and sometimes they don't.

It is not necessary for homeopaths to diagnosis with certainty that a person has an allergy or intolerance, and while it is helpful, it isn't always necessary to even know which food or foods are the offending culprits. Instead, the homeopath selects an individualized remedy, based not only on the person's reactions to foods but on the totality of the symptoms.

Homeopaths inevitably ask every patient what foods they crave and are averse to, and what foods cause any type of symptom. Homeopaths ultimately use this important information to find a constitutional remedy which can improve the patient's digestive function so that he or she is less likely to be allergic or intolerant to foods.

People experience so many varied symptoms as a result of food allergies that it is not possible to provide a list of common remedies for this condition.

Skin Allergies

Skin allergies, like any skin symptoms, are not skin diseases but internal diseases that are simply manifesting on the skin. For more details about the treatment of skin allergies, see "Skin Conditions," beginning on page 251.

Resources

Note: Most of the good homeopathic home care books listed in Part IV have chapters on the homeopathic treatment of allergies. The books that have the best and most detailed information are:

Dale Buegel, Blair Lewis, and Dennis Chernin, *Homeopathic Remedies for Health Professionals and Laypeople*. Honesdale, PA: Himalayan, 1991.

Stephen Cummings and Dana Ullman, *Everybody's Guide to Homeopathic Medicines*. Los Angeles: Tarcher, 1991.

Thomas Kruzel, *Homeopathic Emergency Guide*. Berkeley: North Atlantic, 1992.

Barry Rose, *The Family Guide to Homeopathy*. Berkeley: Ten Speed, 1993.

Dana Ullman, *Homeopathic Medicines for Children and Infants*. Los Angeles: Tarcher, 1992.

Arthritis

Sir William Osler, known as the father of modern medicine, once said, "When an arthritis patient walks in the front door, I feel like leaving by the back door." There is one simple reason why Dr. Osler and many other conventional physicians after him have had difficulty facing arthritic patients: conventional medicine offers them little. The lucky ones get temporary relief along with drug side effects; the unlucky ones get only the side effects.

Arthritis is not simply one disease but many. There is osteoarthritis, rheumatoid arthritis, gout, systemic lupus, and bursitis, to name a few. Osteoarthritis and rheumatoid arthritis are the two most common types of arthritis, though they are considerably different. Osteoarthritis is thought to result from the wear and tear on joints with increasing age, while rheumatoid arthritis is an autoimmune disease, in which one's immune system begins attacking the body itself. Gout is a type of arthritis in which only one joint, usually the big toe, is affected; it is caused by a build-up of uric acid in bodily fluids.

Homeopaths believe that all types of arthritis are not just local diseases but the result of a systemic disorder. Even the explanation that osteoarthritis is the result of wear and tear doesn't make sense to homeopaths, because if this were true, people wouldn't tend to get it in only one or two places. As one centenarian said to his doctor when told he had osteoarthritis in his left knee, "Doc, my other knee is a hundred and one years old too, and it doesn't hurt."

Arthritis is one area in which several published studies have shown that homeopathic medicines are efficacious. One previously noted study, published in the *British Journal of Clinical Pharmacology,* showed that 82 percent of patients with rheumatoid arthritis experienced some degree of relief after being prescribed an individually chosen homeopathic medicine.[1] Only 21 percent of patients given a placebo received a similar degree of relief.

Because homeopathic medicines need to be individually prescribed for the unique pattern of symptoms that people experience, controlled studies must be sensitive to this in order to adequately and accurately test the medicines. Another previously noted study on the treatment of osteoarthritis gave half of the subjects a single homeopathic medicine which was not adequately individualized to their symptoms.[2] Because of this faulty research design, this study predictably showed that the homeopathic remedy did not work.

What can a person derive from these studies and from two hundred years of clinical experience by homeopaths? First of all, homeopathic medicines are a safer alternative to conventional drugs in the treatment of arthritis. Second, homeopathic medicines can be efficacious when individually prescribed.

One of the common conventional medicines for gout is the drug colchicine. Colchicine's tendency to create goutlike pains when taken in overdose is predictable from a homeopathic point of view. The herb **Colchicum autumnale,** from which the drug is taken, is commonly used in homeopathy for people with gout, though homeopaths use considerably smaller and safer doses, and individualize it to each person's unique set of symptoms.

Colchicine has such dramatic effects on gout that physicians often prescribe it to people experiencing their first attack of this disease as a way to confirm the diagnosis. However, the optimal dose of this powerful drug causes significant side effects in 80 percent of users.

It is also predictable from a homeopathic perspective that conventional doctors would inject gold salts into people with chronic arthritis. When ingested or injected, gold has a specific affinity for bones and joints, causing symptoms similar to those which conventional medicine is known to treat. In comparison, homeopaths use considerably smaller and safer doses of gold **(Aurum metallicum)** and prescribe it more individually to people with arthritis. Arthritis sufferers who need it tend to experience deep bone pains which are worse at night and from cold. The pains in the joints, especially the hands and feet, are so extreme that people can barely move them. Emotionally, they suffer from great anxiety, profound despair, and deep depression, sometimes with a desire to commit suicide, especially because of the unbearable pain.

Homeopaths have found clinically that homeopathic medicines are particularly effective in treating people with rheumatoid arthritis. Because rheumatoid arthritis is considered a disease of the immune system, the use of homeopathic medicines makes sense because of their affinity to immune response.

Professional homeopathic care for arthritis and arthritis–like conditions is preferred because it can provide great relief of symptoms and even potential cure of these conditions. Self-care with single-ingredient homeopathic medicines or combination formulas can be considered for symptomatic relief, though there are so many possible individual remedies for arthritis that it is not possible to discuss more than a handful of the most common.

Whether a person has one type of arthritis or another, the specific diagnosis does not influence the proper choice of homeopathic medicines. What does matter is the person's unique pattern of symptoms. The following remedies represent some of the common acute syndromes of people with arthritis, especially osteoarthritis, rheumatoid arthritis, bursitis, and gout.

Two of the most common remedies for arthritic pain are **Rhus tox** and **Bryonia. Rhus tox** is indicated when the person has the typical "rusty gate" type of pain—that is, pain that is aggravated on initial motion but ameliorated as motion continues. The pain is also aggravated by rest, during which time the person becomes very stiff. These arthritic pains are worse in cold, wet weather and at night and are relieved by rubbing, heat, and exercise. Sufferers are very restless, constantly wanting to move the affected part.

Bryonia is useful when arthritic pains are aggravated by any type of motion, quite distinct from people who need **Rhus tox** and experience relief from motion. Those who need **Bryonia** are relieved when lying on and placing pressure on their painful areas. They are irritable, anxious about their business or whatever daily affairs they commonly deal with, and become so upset that they prefer and sometimes demand to be alone. A dry mouth, great thirst, and chronic constipation are often experienced.

Two other relatively common remedies for acute arthritis pain are **Apis** and **Ledum. Apis** is derived from crushed bees. Folk medicine has long touted the relief experienced by some people with arthritis after being stung by a bee. Homeopaths have found that bee venom will work only on people who have symptoms similar to those caused by bee venom; swelling with burning or stinging pains which are aggravated by heat and touch and relieved by cold. They prescribe bee venom in homeopathic doses, **Apis.**

Ledum is indicated for joint pain that begins in the foot and eventually moves up the body to affect other joints. Although people who need it are very chilly, their joint pain is relieved by cold applications and aggravated by warm ones or by exposure to heat in general. **Ledum** is also useful for the side effects of steroid injections which people with arthritis sometimes are given.

Dose: Take the 6, 12, or 30th potency of the indicated remedy every four hours in mild pain and every two hours in more significant discomfort. If improvement is not noticed after forty-eight hours, consider another remedy.

RESOURCES

Herbert A. Roberts, *The Rheumatic Remedies.* New Delhi: B. Jain, 1939.

Insomnia

Falling asleep is so easy and yet can be so hard. Actually, it is hard for a lot of people. It is estimated that between 10 and 33 percent of Americans suffer from insomnia.

Scientists previously believed that the body shut down during sleep. We know now this isn't true—the body remains very active. Various physiological processes that are important for physical and psychological health are as dynamically active and complex during sleep as they are during waking consciousness. Whatever interferes with the physiological processes of sleep also interferes with the health processes of the awake person.

Many people use sleeping pills to help them go to sleep. But present research shows that every drug tested for treating insomnia, except one, has been found to lose its efficacy after two weeks, and that one exception maintains its efficacy only for up to four weeks.

Many over-the-counter sleeping pills claim to be "safe, effective, and non-habit-forming," but these claims are not true. Sleeping pills tend to adversely affect people for usually eighteen hours. Some of the common side effects are mental dullness, lethargy, indigestion, circulatory disorders, respiratory problems, blurred vision, skin rashes, high blood pressure, lowered resistance to infection, kidney and liver ailments, central nervous system damage, impaired memory, irritability, anxiety, confusion, and depression.

If these side effects aren't bad enough, experts have noted that many driving accidents are the result of drowsiness caused by sleeping pills. And accidental deaths from unwittingly mixing sleeping pills with alcohol are relatively common.

One way that some people cope with the drowsiness and fatigue caused by sleeping pills is to use stimulants during the day. These stimulants simply aggravate insomnia and the underlying ailment from which the person is suffering.

Not only do people pay the price of using sleeping pills in side effects, they also risk addiction to these drugs. And according to some experts, addiction to sleeping pills is more difficult to break than heroin addiction.

Ultimately, sleeping pills can turn a mild case of situational insomnia into a chronic nightmare.

One of the side effects of antihistamines prescribed for allergy symptoms is drowsiness. Thanks to the creative marketing skills of conventional drug companies, many over-the-counter sleeping pills are primarily antihistamines. But although these drugs make you drowsy, they will not necessarily help you fall asleep.

Scopolamine and bromide drugs were previously recommended by physicians. However, the effective doses of these drugs are not much different from their toxic doses. Some patients taking scopolamine have been committed to psychiatric institutions under the mistaken diagnosis of schizophrenia, when in fact they had simply overreacted to their sleeping pills. As for the bromides, while some physicians encourage the occasional use of sleeping pills, many do not consider bromides to be rational for even limited use.

Not only is conventional drug treatment ineffective for insomnia, sleep experts are now saying that the old device of counting sheep is also ineffective. Counting sheep, they say, requires you to focus mental activity on a specific function, and sleep is a defocusing activity. It is now recommended that you experiment with relaxation exercises.

Although conventional drugs are not safe or effective in treating insomnia, there are numerous homeopathic medicines that are safe, effective, and non-habit-forming. The following remedies are the most commonly indicated homeopathic medicines for insomnia. If you cannot find one that fits your unique symptoms or if the ones you try don't work, you could try one of the many homeopathic combination formulas for insomnia which are commonly available in pharmacies and health food stores. These formulas are actually some of the most popular homeopathic products presently available.

If insomnia continues after you have tried a homeopathic formula or a couple of choices of individual remedies, seek the care of a professional homeopath for constitutional care. People with chronic insomnia should seek professional homeopathic treatment.

In addition to taking a homeopathic medicine, there are a variety of simple home care measures that should be considered (see on page 272 Goldberg and Kaufman's *Everybody's Guide to Natural Sleep* and Ullman's *The One-Minute (or So) Healer)*.

Aconitum is useful primarily for treating insomnia during acute illness. People who need it are excitable, may fear that they are going to die, and usually have wild, fearful nightmares. This remedy is commonly useful for children.

Arsenicum is known to be helpful for those people who have difficulty sleeping after midnight, especially from midnight to two a.m. They suffer from anxiety attacks which drive them out of bed, have despair of life, fear of death, and see the world as threatening and chaotic, are greatly agitated and constantly toss and turn in bed, and desire to have others around, though they tend to feel that they cannot trust anyone (this type of person may respect his or her doctor, but often seeks a second opinion). People who need **Arsenicum** tend to be anxious, restless, chilly, avaricious, and fastidious.

Ignatia is indicated in people who have experienced a recent grief, from the breaking up of a relationship, a fight with a loved one, the loss of someone close, or homesickness. A key sign for determining the need for this remedy is frequent deep sighing or yawning.

Lycopodium was the favorite sleep remedy of Dr. Margery Blackie, the late physician to Queen Elizabeth II. It may be useful for anyone who must take an examination and has difficulty afterward worrying about the outcome of the test. These people suffer from great anxiety and constant thinking about their anxiousness, making it difficult to fall asleep. They tend to wake at three to four a.m. and have difficulty falling back asleep. **Lycopodium** people are known to dream but rarely remember their dreams. People who need this remedy may also tend to wake hungry in the middle of the night. They usually sleep on their right side.

Nux vomica is a key remedy for people suffering from insomnia accompanying drug or alcohol abuse, and should be considered as a primary remedy for those who have abused sleeping pills. It is also a primary remedy for people who are sleepless after mental strain. They may be able to fall asleep, but they wake up very early, commonly between three and four a.m., with a very active mind, especially with worry about their work. They will usually be anxious or angry at other people, rarely at themselves or their own actions. They are light sleepers, and subtle noises will awaken them, usually leading to great anger at the person or thing that is making the noise. During the day, they are usually extremely irritable.

Coffea is indicated when the body and mind are very active and excitable. People who need it either have difficulty falling asleep or wake from the slightest noise. It is especially indicated when the person experiences great anticipation about an upcoming event. **Coffea** should also be considered when a person has insomnia as the result of hearing either good or bad news. It is also useful in people who are heavy coffee drinkers, though it will not be as effective if they continue to drink this stimulating beverage.

Pulsatilla tends to be useful for children and women who are moody and emotional. They tend to be disturbed by a particular song or phrase of a song that runs continually through their head. They may weep because they can't go to sleep and have difficulty sleeping alone. They also have difficulty sleeping in a warm room. They tend to throw off all or most covers and need to have a window open or at least cracked. **Pulsatilla** is also indicated when a person suffers from insomnia after eating much rich food. Typically, these people sleep on their abdomen or back with arms above the head.

Cocculus is indicated in people working the night shift or in lactating mothers, especially those who have been nursing for a long time. These people have lost much sleep due to their difficult schedule, and they feel so exhausted that they have difficulty falling or staying asleep. They tend to be irritable and/or giddy.

Chamomilla is the most common remedy for irritable and fussy infants, especially when they are teething or experiencing colic. They continue crying until they are rocked or held, though they tend to wake up and become irritable again once they are put down.

Magnesia phos or **Calcarea carb** should be considered when insomnia results from leg cramps.

Three homeopathic medicines known to be very effective in treating insomnia when used in either their tincture or low potency are **Passiflora, Humulus lupulus,** and **Avena sativa. Passiflora** is indicated in treating insomnia in infants and the aged, as well as the mentally worried and overworking who have a tendency to convulsions. **Humulus lupulus** is for people who are extremely drowsy but are unable to fall asleep. **Avena sativa** is a common remedy for insomnia in alcoholics and others who have suffered from a chronically debilitating condition. **Humulus lupulus** and **Avena sativa,** when available in tincture form, should include ten to twenty drops per dose, while **Passiflora** requires thirty to sixty drops per dose.

Consider seeking medical care if you have difficulty falling or staying asleep for ten consecutive days or if sleeplessness is the result of a painful condition.

Dose: Take the 6, 12, or 30th potency thirty minutes before bedtime, another dose at bedtime, and, if necessary, every thirty minutes after this for two more doses. If it hasn't worked by then, another remedy should be tried on the next sleepless night.

RESOURCES

Margery Blackie, *Classical Homeopathy.* Beaconsfield: Beaconsfield, 1986.

Philip Goldberg and Daniel Kaufman, *Everybody's Guide to Natural Sleep.* Los Angeles: Tarcher, 1990.

Alonzo Shadman, *Who Is Your Doctor and Why?* New Canaan: Keats, 1958.

Dana Ullman, *The One-Minute (or So) Healer.* Los Angeles: Tarcher, 1991.

Chronic Fatigue Syndrome

Many people believe that chronic fatigue syndrome (CFS) is a new disease. This could not be farther from the truth. Since ancient Greece, physicians have recognized what has been called an asthenic (without strength) condition. At various times in medical history this condition or something quite similar to it has been called nervous exhaustion or enervation. And in more recent times, it has been diagnosed as glandular fever, postviral syndrome, chronic fatigue viral syndrome, chronic fatigue immune dysfunction syndrome (CFIDS), or (in Great Britain) myalgic encephalomyelitis ("myalgic" means pain in the muscles and "encephalomyelitis" refers to inflammation involving the brain and spinal cord).

Despite all the advances in modern medicine, we still do not know much about chronic fatigue syndrome, as evidenced by the simple fact that physicians do not even know what to call it.

Physicians still are not certain if CFS is the result of a single virus or a "cocktail" of several viruses. Several years ago some physicians theorized that it was caused by the Epstein–Barr virus, the same virus that is thought to cause mononucleosis, an ailment in which fatigue is a primary symptom. But too many people with fatigue were not infected with this virus and too many people without fatigue had significant amounts of it for that theory to be accurate.

The reason why CFS is thought to be caused by a virus is that many people experience it shortly after what seems to be a normal viral illness, but then their ailment lingers with increasing stages of debility. It is, however, not yet known with certainty if this syndrome is of viral origin.

Some physicians and sufferers theorize that the disease is the result of exposure to environmental poisons. Others assume that it is an immunological disorder (some think it is an immunodeficient condition, while others think it is due to an overly active immune system). And still others who are skeptical of these diagnoses believe that CFS is all in the mind of the sufferer.

Chronic fatigue syndrome has become a new "waste can" diagnosis that many people give themselves and to which some physicians acquiesce simply when a person feels tired often. Such cases are not always correctly diagnosed since many cases of fatigue seem to be the result of poor diet, diminished sleep, mental depression, or some other disease process.

Most physicians today diagnose a person as having chronic fatigue syndrome only when he or she has not only physical and mental fatigue but also several of the following symptoms: muscle and joint pains, headaches, abdominal pains, cold extremities, lymph swelling, numbness, depression, and difficulty concentrating. Having a low white blood cell count along with several of these symptoms further suggests chronic fatigue syndrome.

Whatever the cause and whatever the actual diagnosis, homeopathic medicines are often extremely helpful. Due to the varied symptoms that people with CFS experience and because many people with CFS are seriously ill, it is generally best for them to receive professional homeopathic care. Because homeopaths base their prescriptions on a person's individual symptoms, a medicine is chosen for its ability to match all of those symptoms. This medicine tends to augment the overall state of health, thereby diminishing symptoms of illness whatever the source of the problem.

Although homeopathic medicines may help begin the healing process, this does not mean that they can or will cure every person with CFS. Improvement from CFS is often gradual. Generally, the longer the person has had this condition, the more gradually improvement will be noticed, though every homeopath has patients who have noticed significant and rapid improvement very shortly after taking the individualized homeopathic medicine. Sometimes, however, people suffering from CFS have several layers of illness that need treatment, requiring individualized remedies for each layer. (See Chapter 2 for a discussion of layers of disease.)

It is interesting to note that various nineteenth-century and early-twentieth-century homeopaths wrote about "postinfluenza syndrome." Some of the remedies they wrote about as a treatment for this condition are among the remedies that homeopaths today use to treat chronic fatigue syndrome, including **Gelsemium, Cinchona, Kali phos, Arsenicum, Pulsatilla, Sulphur,** and **Scutellaria.** There are, however, numerous other remedies that can and should be considered, depending on the person's unique pattern of symptoms.

Professional individualized homeopathic care is the preferred treatment for those with CFS, but this does not mean that homeopathic combination formulas should be ignored. Homeopathic formulas for fatigue are often effective in providing temporary improvement in energy level. Such benefit is truly appreciated by CFS sufferers. If professional homeopathic care is not available or if tangible results with it are not obtained after one year, homeopathic formulas for fatigue should certainly be considered.

People with CFS are usually not only sick and tired, they are sick and tired of being sick and tired. Homeopathic medicine may not always be the answer (because nothing is), but it can often provide a tangible improvement in health which can help people literally and figuratively get back on their feet.

RESOURCES

Few homeopathic books for the general public discuss chronic fatigue syndrome because it generally requires constitutional care from a professional homeopath. There are ultimately so many possible remedies that may be indicated for a CFS sufferer that the best ways to learn about common remedies for CFS is to obtain a repertory and several *materia medica* (see the annotated bibliography in Part IV). The following book provides an excellent review on possible causes and treatments of chronic fatigue. The author does not discuss how to treat fatigue with homeopathic medicine, but instead recommends seeing a professional homeopath.

Michael Schmidt, *Feeling Tired All the Time*. Berkeley: North Atlantic, 1995.

Sexually Transmitted Diseases

Sex is an act of giving and receiving. Unfortunately, the giving and receiving is not always just love and affection; sometimes diseases are shared as well.

Sexually transmitted diseases (STDs) are both an ancient and a modern plague. Some (herpes simplex) are relatively minor, others are potentially fatal (AIDS). AIDS is an important enough topic to warrant its own section later in this book; see page 281.

Prior to the introduction of antibiotics, syphilis was a major cause of death. Not only was there a high mortality rate linked to syphilis, it caused a wide variety of serious neurological, vascular, skeletal, dermatological, and characterological disorders in the process. This disease manifested in so many different forms that one prominent physician asserted that if a doctor understood syphilis, he understood the whole field of medicine.

Conventional physicians today believe that antibiotics can cure many STDs, and they verify this belief by clinical relief of symptoms and by normalization of laboratory tests that confirm the elimination of the infective agent.

The antibiotics may get rid of the infection, but homeopaths commonly find that people who get syphilis, gonorrhea, or any other STD tend to need at some time in the future a homeopathic nosode (a potentized dose of the offending bacterium or virus) or some other individualized homeopathic remedy to treat the remaining subtle disease. This is because while the antibiotic may kill off the vast majority of an infection, it is rarely able to completely eradicate it from the body. A pattern of subtle and not so subtle symptoms develops in the ensuing years in susceptible individuals. Homeopaths attribute these new symptoms to the STD because this pattern of symptoms fits some of the known homeopathic medicines for that STD (for more details about chronic symptoms and diseases called miasms related to STDs and other infections, see "Homeopathic Understanding of Chronic Disease," page 27).

Homeopaths certainly realize that antibiotics play an important role today in the treatment of STDs, but it should be noted that homeopaths in the nineteenth century claimed to be able to cure syphilis and gonorrhea with homeopathic medicines. Few homeopaths today have been able to verify this in modern clinical practice, mostly due to the medicolegal constraints against them which require antibiotic prescription. These same obstacles are not present in the treatment of other common STDs such as herpes and venereal warts.

HERPES

Back in the 1970s, herpes was considered the modern-day scarlet letter. Although it has since been overshadowed by AIDS, it is still as common and as infectious as it was in the years prior to the AIDS epidemic. Herpes is the result of viral infection from direct contact with another person who has an active or emerging lesion. Most often, herpes symptoms erupt on the lips and the genitals, though one can also get herpetic eruptions in the eyes and on the skin.

Self-treatment of herpes with homeopathic medicines will commonly get rid of the eruptions quickly, but professional constitutional care is recommended if one wants to reduce the frequency or intensity of eruptions and potentially eliminate them altogether.

The following are some of the common remedies for acute eruptions of herpes on the mouth. **Rhus tox** is indicated when the symptoms either start at night or are worse at night, while **Natrum mur** treats eruptions that start or are worse in the daytime. **Natrum mur** is also noted to treat eruptions at the corner of the mouth or below the corner. People who need **Hepar sulphur** have herpetic eruptions which are extremely sensitive to touch or cold. **Borax** is indicated when the person has a history of canker sores or concurrently has a hypersensitivity to noise. **Sepia** (more often given to women) and **Sulphur** (more often given to men) are indicated when the person has symptoms of these medicines' constitutional type.

The two most common remedies for herpetic eruptions on the genitals are **Natrum mur** (see above) and **Petroleum** (when symptoms are worse in the winter and better in the summer or when herpes spreads to the anus, perineum, or thighs). Other remedies to consider are **Graphites** when the person is obese, thick-skinned, and slow-thinking), **Dulcamara** (aggravation from cold, damp weather or just changes in the weather), **Hepar sulph** (see above), **Capsicum** (sores that burn like hot pepper, accompanying depression or homesickness, **Tellurium** (eruptions with concurrent back or sciatica pains), **Thuja** (for people who have a history of warts), and **Sepia** (see above).

Dose: Three doses twice a day of the 6, 12 or 30th potency should produce results. If change is not noticeable after forty-eight hours, consider another remedy.

VENEREAL WARTS

Venereal warts, also the result of viral infection, are becoming increasingly common today because of their highly contagious nature. As with herpes, one can treat oneself for acute eruptions of venereal warts, but it is preferable to seek homeopathic constitutional care to help reduce the number and frequency of eruptions. The two most common homeopathic remedies for venereal warts are **Thuja** (soreness, burning pain; warts bleed easily or may ooze, may smell offensive, may extend to the scrotum) and **Nitric acid** (for cauliflower-like warts, hypersensitive to touch, sore with burning pain; bleed easily). Other remedies to consider are **Natrum sulphur** (soft, red, and fleshy warts), **Hepar sulphur** (hypersensitive to touch and cold, may smell offensive), **Lycopodium** (dry and itching) and **Cinnabaris** (burning pain, fan-shaped warts that bleed easily).

Dose: Generally, one to four doses of individualized remedy in the 12 or 30th potency will be all that is necessary. Results are commonly observed within forty-eight hours.

CHLAMYDIA, TRICHOMONAS, AND GARDNERELLA

Chlamydia, Trichomonas, and *Gardnerella vaginalis* (previously called *Hemophilus*) infections are all STDs which lead to various genital and reproductive health problems. *Chlamydia* rarely causes noticeable symptoms initially and is often diagnosed only when a doctor performs a culture or in later stages when complications of infection create more serious inflammation in reproductive organs. These three conditions are treated conventionally with antibiotics or antimicrobials but can also be treated with homeopathic medicines.

Some of the most common medicines for these conditions are **Pulsatilla, Kreosotum, Borax, Hydrastis, Sepia, Graphites,** and **Calcarea carb** (see the section on vaginitis, page 192, in "Women's Conditions" for individualizing symptoms for these remedies).

Despite the efficacy of homeopathic medicines in treating these conditions, it is useful to seek medical attention before and after homeopathic treatment to know what infection the woman is experiencing, since some STDs remain active and contagious even when obvious symptoms disappear.

Men who are infected with *Chlamydia, Trichomonas,* or *Gardnerella* often do not have symptoms, thus making it very difficult to treat them with homeopathic medicines. Because of this, it is generally recommended that a man seek conventional medical treatment when his sexual partner has developed one of these infections. Another strategy is for the man to seek constitutional care, though he should not engage in sex until laboratory reports confirm that the infection has been resolved.

PUBIC LICE AND SCABIES

Pubic lice (crabs) and scabies can be transmitted through either sexual or casual contact. They are most effectively treated with conventional medications, though because of the toxicity of this pesticide-like treatment, some homeopaths recommend concurrent treatment with **Nux vomica** or **Arsenicum.** These remedies are thought to strengthen the liver so that it can more effectively help the body detoxify from the exposure to the conventional medications. Old homeopathic texts refer to **Staphysagria** as a remedy to help get rid of lice, but it was primarily used in exceedingly low potencies (1x), which are only available via a doctor's prescription due to the toxicity of this herb in unpotentized doses. Some herbal remedies can also be used, including eucalyptus oil, citronella oil, and wormwood oil.

Dose: Take either **Nux vomica** or **Arsenicum** in the 12 or 30th potency three times a day for two days.

RESOURCES

Susan Curtis and Romy Fraser, *Natural Healing for Women*. London: Pandora, 1991.

Thomas Kruzel, *Homeopathic Emergency Guide*. Berkeley: North Atlantic, 1992.

Andrew Lockie and Nicola Geddes, *The Women's Guide to Homeopathy*. New York: St. Martin's, 1994.

See also resources in "Women's Conditions," page 197, and "Men's Ailments," page 212.

AIDS

As horrific as the AIDS epidemic is, it has had one silver lining: it has implanted into the awareness of the medical community and the general public the importance of the body's immune system. Prior to the emergence of AIDS, few people were familiar with or cared about the immune system.

Now more than ever, the general public is interested in exploring ways to bolster immune response to prevent the progression of AIDS, as well as to reduce the number and intensity of opportunistic infections and to improve the overall state of their health. The medical community, however, has focused its AIDS resources on creating antiviral medications, which despite great hope and expectation have not achieved the results anticipated. In fact, the leading AIDS drug, AZT, has not been found to prolong the lives of people with AIDS,[1] and due to the side effects that it is known to cause, the quality of life during this time is not high.

What is yet to be understood by the medical community is that they need to direct more attention and research to ways to augment immune response, rather than ways to inhibit viral replication. By strengthening a person's own defenses, the body is best enabled to defend itself.

Homeopathy is one way to do this. Although no therapy can or will help every HIV+ person or everyone with AIDS, homeopathy is beginning to develop a reputation for helping people at varying stages of this disease. To understand what homeopathy has to offer, it is nec-

282 CAN HOMEOPATHY HELP ME?: SPECIFIC CONDITIONS

essary to learn something about a different approach to infectious disease than simply attacking a pathogen.

Louis Pasteur, who initially suggested that bacteria cause disease, later realized that, as noted previously, bacteria may not necessarily be the causes of disease as much as the results of disease.[2] Like Claude Bernard,[3] the father of experimental physiology, Pasteur came to realize that the susceptibility of the individual, the "host resistance," was a greater determinant of the development of disease than the infective agent itself.

Despite the later recanting by Pasteur, he had already set in motion a medical mind-set that focused entirely on eliminating pathogens and that ignored exploring ways to augment immune and defense response. Just as physicians and scientists are finally realizing the limitations and problems inherent in antibiotics as antimicrobial agents, antiviral drugs will inevitably suffer a similar fate. While physicians tend to know this both rationally and intuitively, they ignore these obvious problems in their clinical practice, in part because they don't know what else to do and in part because their biomedical paradigm limits their vision of alternatives to antimicrobial therapy.

As increasing numbers of physicians learn about homeopathic medicine, they will be exposed to viable alternative treatments which can play an integral role in the care and treatment of people with HIV and AIDS. A recent survey of physicians in the Netherlands verified this possibility. The survey showed that 50 percent of Dutch physicians instigated and supported the use of homeopathic and natural therapies in the treatment of people with AIDS.[4]

Preventing AIDS

The best and most certain way to prevent AIDS is to avoid exchanging bodily fluids with people who are HIV+. Exposure to these bodily fluids most commonly occurs through sexual activity, sharing needles, or receiving blood transfusions. However, just because an individual is exposed to a person with HIV does not necessarily mean that the individual will get the virus. And further, just because an individual becomes infected with HIV does not necessarily mean that he or she will get AIDS.

The various factors that influence whether exposure leads to infection and whether infection leads to disease remain unknown.

However, as with many infectious conditions, a stronger immune system reduces the chances of getting the disease or at least decreases the chances of complications from the infection. It therefore seems prudent to avoid the factors that inhibit immune response and to utilize those that augment it. The factors that inhibit immune response include an unhealthy lifestyle (i.e., smoking, poor diet, significant stress, sedentary habits) and the use of therapeutic and recreational drugs, while those that augment immune response tend to be a healthy lifestyle and utilizing natural therapeutics, including homeopathic medicines.

While the precise mechanism of action that leads to AIDS isn't known, a new and significant study suggests that homeopathic medicines may have a dramatic effect on some people with HIV. A study performed by a government research center in India with 129 asymptomatic HIV+ patients (120 male and 9 female) showed that during homeopathic treatment over a period of three to sixteen months, 13 patients changed from HIV+ to HIV−.[5] No conventional drugs of any type were prescribed to these patients.

The medical literature has on rare occasions reported individual patients who for unknown reasons converted from being HIV+ to being HIV−. This study is the first to report more than one.

It should be noted that this writer acknowledges that it does not initially make sense that people can turn from HIV+ to HIV−, because the tests that determine this status are simply evaluating a person's antibodies, not the disease itself. It is generally assumed that people who become HIV+ will remain that way throughout their lives. It therefore seems obvious that the work by the Indian researchers should be more carefully studied to evaluate this potentially significant clinical result.

It should also be noted that these researchers have elsewhere published more up-to-date data which shows significant improvement in immune panels and blood work in HIV+ and AIDS patients as the result of homeopathic treatment.[6]

These same researchers also conducted a study on the immunological status of 34 HIV+ patients.[7] After six months of individualized homeopathic treatment, 23 (67 percent) of the 34 subjects' immune profiles improved. Thirteen patients experienced a 0 to 10 percent increase in CD4 lymphocytes (a higher number of CD4 lymphocytes suggests a stronger immune response) and 10 patients experienced a greater than 10 percent increase. Because there is a tendency for people with HIV to have continually decreasing CD4 lymphocytes, this study suggests that homeopathic medicines provided a benefit to the subjects.

A San Francisco Bay Area homeopath, Laurence Badgley, M.D., reported on a six-month study of 36 patients with AIDS or HIV whom he treated with homeopathic and other natural medicines. He observed a 13 percent increase in T4 helper cells and an average weight gain of two pounds.[8] AIDS tends to have increasingly degenerating effects on the body, and improvement in the immune profile and weight gain seem to be rarely experienced under conventional medical treatment.

In addition to what homeopathy offers in the prevention of AIDS, other natural therapies that strengthen the body's own defense should also be considered. For instance, a recent study of HIV+ patients who were given only a multivitamin/mineral supplement were found to develop AIDS at a substantially slower rate than those who did not supplement their diet. If this simple addition to one's prevention program is so effective, it isn't hard to imagine what more individualized nutritional and natural medicine programs can do to slow down onset of this dreaded disease.

TREATMENT OF ACUTE ILLNESSES DURING AIDS

Because of the seriousness of this disease, the treatment of people with HIV or AIDS requires professional health care, even when their ailments are seemingly minor. Ideally, they should receive treatment from a homeopath who is an M.D., a D.O., or an N.D., but otherwise the best care is one that integrates homeopathic treatment with appropriate medical diagnosis and, in emergency situations, with appropriate medical treatment.

People with AIDS are prone to opportunistic infections due to their immunodeficient state, ranging from fungal infections in the mouth to respiratory infections. The use of conventional drugs can provide valuable temporary relief; however, occasional or repeated use of these drugs takes its own toll on their health and immune system, and thus provides short-term relief but longer-term immune complications. Safer therapies that are not as physiologically disruptive as conventional drugs are necessary for the long-term improvement of people with AIDS. Homeopathic medicines can play an important role in the treatment of these opportunistic infections.

One of the advantages of using homeopathy in treating people with AIDS is that they tend to get various unusual symptoms, diseases, and syndromes which evade immediate diagnosis. A homeopath, however, can prescribe a remedy before a definitive conventional diagnosis is made. Because homeopathic medicines are prescribed on the basis of a person's unique pattern of symptoms, a conventional diagnosis is not necessary for a curative remedy to be prescribed.

TREATMENT OF PEOPLE WITH AIDS

Despite the seemingly positive results that homeopathic medicines provide for people who are HIV+, for those with early onset of AIDS, and for those with nonextreme cases of AIDS, most homeopaths do not observe significant improvement in treating people who have advanced stages of AIDS. That said, it should also be noted that there are exceptions to this general rule, and numerous homeopaths find that select patients with advanced stages of AIDS experience dramatic improvement in their quality of life.

The experience of Bill Gray, M.D., a homeopath in Davis, California, is typical of many homeopaths. He has had thirty-three AIDS patients, only three of whom have survived. The remaining three patients were the only ones who insisted on avoiding AZT and ddI (another popular AIDS drug). Dr. Gray has also had thirty HIV+ patients for an average of five years, only one of whom developed AIDS. Although this one patient has suffered from two bouts of pneumocystis pneumonia, he is actually doing quite well under homeopathic treatment.

Dr. Gray and most homeopaths utilize classical homeopathy in the treatment of people with AIDS, using a single remedy prescribed individually to the unique pattern of symptoms experienced by the patient. This highly individualized treatment generally includes the use of homeopathic medicines which are highly potentized (usually higher than the 200th potency).

Because of the urgency of some AIDS patients' situations, some homeopaths experiment with new homeopathic remedies and with nonclassical approaches to homeopathy. For instance, Dr. Elliot Blackman, an osteopathic physician in San Francisco, occasionally prescribes cyclosporine in homeopathic doses as an intercurrent medicine (an intercurrent medicine is one that is prescribed after another medicine which is individually determined). In conventional doses, cyclosporine is an immunosuppressing drug, thus suggesting that it can be effective in homeopathic doses for treating people who have an immunosuppressed condition (this prescription is not "classical homeopathy" because each immunosuppressing drug creates its own unique pattern of symptoms, and the classical use of this drug would be more individualized).

In addition to the nonclassical approach, some homeopaths have been experimenting with giving AIDS patients homeopathically potentized doses of their own blood. The clinical benefit of this approach, however, has not yet been systematically tested.

Alan Levine, M.D., a San Francisco physician who integrates homeopathic and other natural medicines with occasional prescriptions of conventional drugs, has one patient who was so sick with AIDS that he developed dementia, a state of mental deterioration that tends to occur in late stages of AIDS. This patient refused all conventional drugs from Dr. Levine and from all other physicians. Using homeopathic medicines, acupuncture, and herbs, the patient is now very healthy, has no signs of dementia, and has not had a single opportunistic infection in several years.

This case is mentioned because, despite the small chances of surviving late stages of AIDS and despite the generally accepted experience that dementia represents an irreversible neurological change, it is inspiring to know that significant and even substantial improvement is sometimes possible.

It should be noted that people with AIDS occasionally develop a fever shortly after taking the correct homeopathic medicine. This fever is considered a beneficial response of the body to the remedy and should not be suppressed. Physiologists recognize the therapeutic value of fever as a response to infection, and homeopathic medicine seems to be one way to augment this healing response.

HOMEOPATHIC TREATMENT OF INFECTIOUS DISEASES AND IMMUNOLOGICAL DISORDERS

In order to fully appreciate the potential of homeopathic medicine in the treatment of AIDS, it is useful to get some historical perspective as well as to investigate what homeopathy has to offer in the treatment of viral and immunological disorders.

Homeopathy has an impressive history of successes in treating infectious disease, including many of the most serious and potentially fatal infectious diseases known to humankind. As noted, the significant successes of homeopathic treatment of the infectious disease that raged during the 1800s in the United States and Europe created tremendous support for this natural therapy. Death rates in homeopathic hospitals from cholera, typhoid, yellow fever, scarlet fever, and pneumonia were commonly one half to as little as one eighth those in conventional medical hospitals. Besides hospitals, prisons and insane asylums that employed physicians who specialized in homeopathy experienced a similar success rate compared to other institutions under the care of conventional physicians.

Just as homeopathy became known in the nineteenth century for its successful treatment of infectious diseases of that era, based on growing clinical and laboratory evidence, it is likely that it will become known in this era for its results in treating contemporary viral infections.

Although homeopathic medicines are not considered to have traditional antiviral action, their ability to augment the body's own defenses suggests that they have antiviral effects. One study on chicken embryo viruses showed that eight of ten homeopathic medicines tested inhibited the growth of the viruses by 50 to 100 percent.[9] A similar study done by the same researchers did find, however, that none of the four homeopathic medicines tested for their effects on a mouse virus had any effect.[10] Taken together, these studies suggest that homeopathic medicines can have significant antiviral effects, but it is necessary to find the individualized remedy for each situation.

Despite this preliminary work, it is conjectured that homeopathic medicines do not have traditional antiviral effects but have immunomodulatory effects ("immunomodulatory effects" refers to a tonification of the body's immune system—that is, an ability to augment immune response when it needs to be stimulated and to depress an already overstimulated immune system). One laboratory study showed that the homeopathic medicine **Silicea** had dramatic effects on *stimulating* macrophages, an important part of the body's immune system, by 55.5 to 67.5 percent.[11] On the other hand, another clinical trial showed the efficacy of individualized homeopathic medicines on the treatment of people with rheumatoid arthritis,[12] an autoimmune disease, which is when a person's immune system is overly active, leading the body to attack itself. This study suggests that homeopathic medicines *decreased* the overly active immune system.

Other studies have shown the immunomodulatory effects of homeopathic medicines,[13] though their description is too technical for this book. (See Bellavite and Signorini's *Homeopathy: A Frontier in Medical Science*. Berkeley: North Atlantic, 1995.)

In Summary

The history of homeopathy's successes in treating infectious disease epidemics, the research that suggests the immunomodulatory effects of homeopathic medicines, and the clinical research on HIV+ and AIDS patients that indicates beneficial response to homeopathic medicines should command attention by physicians, scientists, and public health officials. Despite this body of work, it is both surprising and depressing that homeopathic medicine has been consistently ignored as a viable part of a comprehensive program in treating HIV+ and AIDS patients.

Homeopathy is not the only alternative that is being ignored by the AIDS medical community. Even though a large number of people with AIDS, especially long-term survivors, are using one or more alternative treatments, there is little data on their use or success. The leading AIDS organizations are likewise ignoring any serious investigation of their use. Until AIDS activists, the concerned general public, and open-minded health professionals start insisting that research on alternatives be performed, potentially valuable therapies will continue to be ignored, and the AIDS epidemic will continue to devastate our society. When these alternative therapies are integrated within a comprehensive program which includes public health measures that seek to prevent infection, the AIDS epidemic will finally begin to recede.

Resources

Dana Ullman, *Discovering Homeopathy*. Berkeley: North Atlantic, 1991.

A reader of many of the above-listed difficult-to-obtain articles is available for $10 (plus California tax of 7.75 %) from Homeopathic Educational Services; see page 366.

Heart Disease

Although people tend to fear cancer more than heart disease, heart disease is the number one cause of death today in most developed countries. Over one third of deaths today in America result from heart disease. Despite this significant number, it is not an adequate representation of the health problems that heart disease creates, since stroke, which is a complication of atherosclerosis (or heart disease), is the number three killer of Americans.

High blood pressure, which is one of the risk factors for heart attacks and strokes, is an adaptive response of the body to one's diet and lifestyle as well as to various genetic and environmental factors. Drugs that simply reduce blood pressure arbitrarily but do nothing to influence the physiological processes that have adapted to and are dependent upon this increased blood pressure ultimately cause side effects which further aggravate the condition of the already ill person.

Because blood pressure–lowering drugs cause various side effects, physicians commonly prescribe other drugs to deal with the side effects, though each of these drugs tends to create its own problems.

Because of the side effects, most medical authorities today recognize that people with borderline to moderate hypertension (high blood pressure) should not be placed on drugs (borderline to moderate hypertension is defined as 140–150 systolic over 90–100 diastolic). Several studies have, in fact, shown that blood pressure–lowering drugs provide minimal benefit to people with mild to moderately high blood pressure while posing significant risks.

The same criticism of drugs that simply lower blood pressure rather than deal with the totality of physiological and psychological factors that led to high blood pressure can be made against drugs that simply reduce other heart disease risk factors such as high cholesterol. While it may make sense to consider using these drugs in cases where a person's cholesterol is extremely high, safer, more natural therapies should be considered as a first method of treatment in the majority of people with even moderately high cholesterol levels.

What Studies Say

Instead of using conventional drugs to lower blood pressure or reduce cholesterol levels, there is a growing amount of research that supports the use of a low-fat diet, exercise, stress management, and group support. There is evidence that homeopathic medicines can be helpful.

One double-blind study tested a specific homeopathic medicine in the treatment of thirty-four hypertensive subjects of both sexes, aged between fifty-two and ninety-three, who were confined to bed in two old people's homes in Italy.[1] Half of the patients who participated in the study were given **Baryta carbonica** 15c and half were given a placebo. For medicolegal reasons, conventional medical treatment was continued throughout the trial.

There were no statistically significant differences between the two groups. However, prior to the start of the study, it was determined that only eight of the subjects fit the symptomological picture of **Baryta carbonica.** After the completion of the trial, it was noted that four of these patients were given the homeopathic medicine and four were given a placebo. The four patients given the placebo experienced no observable changes. Of the four patients who were given the homeopathic medicine, three experienced a considerable drop in both systolic and diastolic blood pressure, and one experienced a complete regression of a distressing symptom that had troubled him for half a century.

Although the number of patients involved in this trial, especially those who fit the symptoms of the medicine being tested, was very small, this experiment suggests that homeopathic medicines may be effective in treating hypertensive patients, but only if the medicines are individually suited to their unique symptoms. The results of this investigation also suggest that it is critical for studies to be sensitive to the homeopathic approach in order to best evaluate efficacy of treatment.

Another study of interest to people concerned about heart disease was performed at a veterinary medical school in the Netherlands to test the ability of a specific homeopathic medicine to lower cholesterol in rabbits.[2] Rabbits were first given increased amounts of cholesterol in their diets. Then one group of rabbits were given **Chelidonium 3x,** while the other group of rabbits were given a placebo. After thirty-four days the results showed that the rabbits given the homeopathic medicine had about 25 percent less serum cholesterol than those given the placebo.

One remedy which homeopaths and herbalists alike have found to be effective in both preventing and treating many kinds of heart disease is **Crataegus oxyacantha** (commonly known as hawthorn berries). Research has shown that extracts of hawthorn berries help to reduce angina attacks and lower blood pressure and cholesterol levels.[3] This herb is best taken in nonpotentized extract doses. In America, it requires a doctor's prescription and is not available to nonphysicians as a homeopathic medicine. However, it is available in herb and health food stores as an herbal remedy.

TREATING HEART PAIN ON THE WAY TO THE DOCTOR

You can possible save a life when you know how to treat a person suffering from heart pain or even a heart attack with homeopathic medicines, though such treatment should be administered on the way to the doctor or hospital.

Aconitum is almost always indicated during a person's first heart attack, especially when the prominent symptoms include significant panic and profound fear of death. These people become extremely restless, and yet any motion tends to cause further distress. They experience a burning thirst and a hypersensitivity to noise along with their rapid heartbeat and full, hard, bounding pulse.

Cactus, reflective of the substance from which it is made, is known to benefit people who experience prickly pains in and around the heart and feel great constriction, as though there were an iron band around the heart. These people tend to experience their heart symptoms at eleven p.m. or ten to eleven a.m. and feel worse when lying on the left side. People who need **Cactus** may also experience great fear and anxiety, though not to the degree of those who need **Aconitum. Cactus** is more indicated for fear of having an incurable condition than for fear of death.

Arsenicum is useful when the person experiences burning sensations in the chest along with the pain, constriction, and fear. This person is very chilly, and his symptoms usually begin at or after midnight.

Glonoine is indicated when people have throbbing pains in the chest, rapid pulse with great force, and alternating congestive feelings in the heart and the head. These people tend to hold their chest and head due to the pain they experience. Their pains are aggravated by the sun, stooping, and heat.

Arnica is an important medicine for heart pain and is also an extremely common and important remedy for treating shock and trauma after a heart attack or stroke. Some homeopaths consider it a routine prescription at those times. It is useful for angina pain when there is concurrent severe pain in the left elbow. There also may be a sense of bruised soreness and achiness all over, with an aversion to being touched. When in shock, people who need this remedy may deny that they are ill, despite being in grave condition.

Because time is of the essence, it is more important that the correct remedy be given than the perfect potency. Whatever potency you have of the above remedies will generally be adequate. If you do have a choice, use the highest potency if you are confident in the selection of the remedy.

Dose: Use the highest potency available of the indicated remedy and give it every fifteen to thirty minutes until there is significant improvement. The time between doses can be lengthened as pain decreases.

THE STORY OF NORMAN COUSINS

The late Norman Cousins was an internationally respected journalist. He was the editor of the *Saturday Review* and adviser to several American presidents. Despite lifelong work on international peace and disarmament, he achieved his greatest fame as a result of writing *Anatomy of an Illness,* an autobiography which chronicled his experience in contracting a deadly illness and curing it. In the mid-1970s, he was diagnosed with ankylosing spondylitis, a normally incurable degenerative disease of the connective tissue of the body. What was truly remark-able about his case was that he claimed to cure himself by taking large doses of vitamin C and by experiencing frequent fits of laughter (he watched numerous TV comedy programs, including *Candid Camera* and *I Love Lucy*).

Several years later he suffered a severe heart attack. He was treated conventionally except for one thing; his wife, who was a serious stu-dent of homeopathic medicine, gave him several doses of **Cactus**. Despite having had a massive heart attack (and without taking vitamin C or watching any comedy programs), he was sitting up in bed read-ing and writing within a couple of hours.

Many conventional physicians remain skeptical about the curative power of vitamin C and laughter in treating ankylosing spondylitis, and perhaps their skepticism is justifiable. The fact that Cousins' wife prescribed homeopathic medicines for him during both illnesses might better explain his remarkable recoveries.

THE HOMEOPATHIC ORIGINS
OF AN IMPORTANT HEART MEDICINE

One of the classic drugs for heart pain used in conventional medicine for over a century has been nitroglycerine. This drug was actually dis-covered by a homeopath.[4]

Constantine Hering, M.D., the father of American homeopathy, was the first physician to use nitroglycerine in medicine. He con-ducted a proving of it to see what symptoms it caused in overdose in order to determine what it could treat in homeopathic microdoses. Hering conducted these experiments on himself and his colleagues between 1847 and 1851. He discovered that nitroglycerine caused powerful symptoms, including palpitation of the heart, stabbing pain in the heart region, labored action of the heart with a sense of oppres-sion, violent throbbing of the head, and a confused state. **Glonoine** (nitroglycerine) has been used in homeopathic doses for these symp-toms ever since.

Contemporary editions of the *Merck Index* and the *Physicians' Desk Reference* list similar symptoms. Modern texts also note that alco-hol use further aggravates the symptoms that nitroglycerine causes (that's why doctors discourage alcohol use by patients who are taking it), which was an observation also made by Hering over a century ago.

It wasn't until 1858 that nitroglycerine was first mentioned in conventional medical journals.

Physicians note that over 50 percent of patients who take nitroglycerine experience headaches as a "side effect"; typically, they arbitrarily differentiate between the main effect of a drug and its side effects. Conventional physicians commonly emphasize the value of knowing the mechanism of action of their drugs, and they describe the benefits from nitroglycerine as the result of its ability to dilate the heart's blood vessels and reduce the heart's demand for oxygen. Homeopaths go one step farther and explain the underlying reason *why* it has these effects: nitroglycerine reduces heart pain because it *causes* heart pain in overdose. Homeopaths' perspective of pharmacological action will soon play a significant role in helping physicians and pharmacologists understand their own drugs.

In Summary

Heart symptoms and heart disease require the attention of a professional homeopath. Considering the vast sums of money presently being spent on heart disease research, it is sad that no moneys are devoted to studying potentially useful but inadequately tested treatments for heart disease such as homeopathic medicines. Such research requires individualized care, for serious ailments like heart disease require the best care possible. Individualizing a medicine to a person's unique symptoms is the homeopath's way to get to the heart of heart disease.

Resources

Note: There are few books that provide information to the general public about the homeopathic treatment of heart disease. Professional homeopaths generally obtain their information from *materia medica* and repertories.

Andrew Lockie, *The Family Guide to Homeopathy*. New York: Fireside, 1993.

Prakash Vakil, *Diseases of the Cardiovascular System: A Textbook of Homeopathic Therapeutics*. Bombay: Vakil, 1982.

Cancer

Two of the prominent conventional treatments for people with cancer are radiation and chemotherapy. The irony to homeopaths is that radiation and many chemotherapeutic drugs are known to *cause* cancer. This does not, however, suggest that these are homeopathic treatments, for their dosage is given in anything but homeopathic quantities.

Ever since cancer was first discovered as a disease, there have been two distinct schools of medical thought about it. One school has assumed that cancer is a local manifestation due to a local irritation. The other school has believed that cancer is a systemic disorder of the whole organism that manifests in various localized symptoms, including tumors.

The first school of thought gave rise to conventional medical treatments, including surgery, radiation, and chemotherapy, all of which seek to excise or kill cancer cells.

In contrast, various natural therapies, including homeopathic medicines, are prescribed to augment a person's overall immune and defense system so that the body can effectively reestablish health on its own. Natural therapies, however, are not the only type of intervention that follows this approach. In fact, the recent interest in immunotherapy in conventional cancer treatment indicates a change in the conventional medical approach from methods that seek to attack a tumor to ones that seek to strengthen the cancer patient. Immunotherapy is an investigational and still unproven treatment that uses either a vaccine or some other drug that boosts the patient's ability to make anti-bodies or that mobilizes lymphocytes and other cells to kill cancer cells.

BCG (a weakened strain of a TB vaccine), monoclonal anti-bodies, interleukin, and tumor necrosis factor are some of the drugs considered a part of immunotherapy. It is interesting to note that oncologists typically prescribe very small doses of these substances. However, they are not as small as doses commonly used in homeop-athy, and because of this, immunotherapeutic drugs create various side effects.

The Homeopathic Approach to Cancer

Although homeopathy's founder, Samuel Hahnemann, practiced in the early 1800s, he had a sophisticated understanding of cancer causa-tion. He recognized that poor or inappropriate diet and chronic poi-soning were factors that led to many cancers. He also acknowledged the influence of mental and emotional states on precancerous and can-cerous conditions. And he knew there was a genetic component to cancer causation (see discussion of miasms in Chapter 2). Hahnemann even recognized the value of surgery in cancer treatment, but he also warned against its overuse.

It seems that every month or so new studies are published declar-ing that a common substance or activity causes cancer: smoking, too much meat or fat in the diet, pesticides, radon, electrical appliances, etc. The truth of the matter, however, is that most of these supposed causal factors lead to cancer in only a very small number of people. The individual's personal susceptibility to cancer plays a primary role as co-factor in the development of cancer. This susceptibility is based on a person's genetics, the diseases he or she has had, how these dis-eases have been resolved, and his or her psychological state. Homeo-paths theorize that symptoms and diseases that are suppressed lead to increasingly more serious conditions, including cancer.

To understand the homeopathic approach to treating people with cancer, we must first clarify that homeopathic medicines do not treat the cancer but the person with the cancer. The natural remedies indi-vidually prescribed on the basis of the totality of a person's physical and psychological symptoms reduce that person's susceptibility to dis-ease. If he or she already has cancer, the remedies are thought to strengthen the body so that it can effectively heal itself. Sometimes, however, the disease is too strong and/or the body is too weak to regain health.

Early-twentieth-century American physician and homeopath Stuart Close once eloquently stated, "That the treatment and cure of cancer is definitely within the scope of possibilities of homeopathy has long been known and proved. The first thing to do after one has made and substantiated a pathological diagnosis of cancer is to forget it. Thenceforth, if one expects to succeed, he will treat not cancer, but a cancer patient."

These words do not just describe an idealized concept. Indeed, homeopathic constitutional care provides a specific and practical model for treatment that seeks to reduce a person's susceptibility to illness and augment his or her body's response to disease.

Although there is a shortage of controlled studies in the homeopathic treatment of cancer, there is also a shortage of studies proving the effectiveness of conventional therapies. Despite the vast amount of resources available for conventional cancer treatments (the National Cancer Institute spent $2 billion in 1994), various leading experts openly acknowledge that modern medicine has lost the war on cancer. According to a review of conventional cancer treatment in *Scientific American,* medical treatment today prevents deaths from cancer in only about 5 percent of people with the disease, primarily people with childhood leukemia, Hodgkin's disease, testicular cancer, and the rare cancer of the placenta.[1] There has been little improvement in curing cancers of the lung, breast, bowel, or prostate, which account for more than one half of cancer deaths in the United States. In fact, an extensive review of cancer statistics has shown that overall death rates from cancer increased by 7 percent from 1975 to 1990.[2]

These statistics may seem completely wrong to the average person, in part because physicians and cancer organizations commonly distort cancer statistics by bragging that people with cancer are surviving five years after diagnosis at a greater rate than in the past; however, they don't mention that new technologies are enabling physicians to diagnose cancer at its earlier stages, and people are not necessarily living longer as a result of modern medical treatment than those who are not receiving this treatment. Part of the reason for the ineffectiveness of conventional treatment of cancer is the pervasive use of powerful drugs and radiation which are toxic not only to malignant cells but to normal cells as well. And while modern surgery for cancer patients can be a godsend, it usually provides only temporary relief and rarely cures the underlying condition.

People with cancer need a different approach than one that simply attacks the cancer. They need therapies that strengthen their own defenses, and homeopathy is one such method that accomplishes this goal.

The Homeopathic Treatment of People with Cancer

Despite the shortage of controlled studies, several leading homeopaths have had considerable experience in treating people with cancer. A. H. Grimmer, M.D., a Chicago homeopath who often wrote in homeopathic journals from 1920 to 1950 about his experiences in such treatment, described his clinical results:

"In my own practice of over fifty years, my records will show a high percentage of cures. These include incipient cases and advanced and terminal ones. The percentage of cures in incipient [early-onset] cases is 80%, 10% in late and terminal ones. . . . The more I study cancer, the more I prescribe for cancer, the more I am convinced that the earlier we start prescribing for cancer the better our results will be. Sometimes the results we get in very late cases are astonishing, but these are the exceptions."[3]

More recent experiences of homeopaths have confirmed some good results in treating people with early-onset cancer, though no one has yet quantified any results.

Vincent Speckhart, M.D., an oncologist and homeopath in Norfolk, Virginia, is one of the more experienced contemporary homeopaths treating people with cancer. Dr. Speckhart commonly has observed his patients with early onset of many kinds of cancer to be free of all tumors in about a year. He usually sees a patient every sixty days, except in aggressive types of cancer, where visits every twenty to thirty days are more common. He finds low-potency medicines are most effective on people with large tumors; the smaller the tumor, the higher the potency he uses.

He finds that people with breast and prostate cancer tend to be the easiest to treat. He is not certain why this is true, though he speculates that the chemotherapeutic drugs for these types of cancer are not as toxic as others. He has also observed that patients who have used conventional therapies tend to heal from their cancer more slowly than those who use only natural therapies.

Dr. Speckhart practices an innovative type of homeopathy in which he uses a Voll Electro-acupuncture machine (described in Chapter 8). He finds that it is generally more effective to prescribe several medicines to be taken concurrently than to prescribe a single remedy, and these medicines need to be taken repeatedly until the next visit. He also uses herbs as an adjunct to keep the patient's health progressing. Some of the herbs he most often prescribes are burdock, slippery elm, red clover, sheep sorrel, and turkey rhubarb root.

Dr. Speckhart refuses to specify which homeopathic medicines he uses, because his care is too individualized and the list of remedies is too long.

One of the striking observations that Dr. Speckhart has made about his use of homeopathic medicines in treating people with cancer is that chemotherapeutic drugs do not necessarily inhibit the action of homeopathic medicines, even though they are toxic to the human body and create their own complex set of symptoms and syndromes. He doesn't prescribe them himself because of the serious diseases they create, but he doesn't consider people who use them incurable. He assumes that the drugs work on a different level than the energetic homeopathic medicines. Dr. Speckhart does, however, sometimes prescribe homeopathic doses of the chemotherapeutic drugs that his patients are taking, as a way to decrease their side effects. Some Belgian researchers have confirmed through laboratory experiments the protective effect that potentized doses of carcinogens can have.[4] Other researchers at UCLA have used homeopathic doses of conventional immunotherapy drugs, such as tumor necrosis factor, to reduce some of the side effects of its crude doses.[5]

Not only do some homeopaths use potentized doses of chemotherapeutic drugs to reduce the side effects of their crude doses, they also prescribe certain homeopathic medicines to reduce the side effects of radiation treatment. Recent laboratory research has suggested that homeopathic remedies are beneficial in providing protection from radiation.[6]

Dr. Grimmer's most frequent remedy for antidoting the side effects of radiation was **Cadmium iodatum.** He used many cadmium salts for various stages of cancer, and he encouraged professional homeopaths to learn about them if they wanted to achieve the best results.

While actual cure of a person with cancer is not always possible, homeopathic medicines can improve not only the quality but also the length of life. One case study published in a conventional medical journal, *Thorax,* discussed a patient suffering from small-cell lung cancer, a notoriously aggressive type of cancer with an average survival time of six to seventeen weeks.[7] The patient was treated with radiotherapy but refused chemotherapy, instead opting for homeopathic care; he was prescribed various individually chosen homeopathic medicines (not disclosed in the article) along with an extract of *Viscum album* (mistletoe). He survived for five years and seven months after diagnosis of the cancer. The authors acknowledge that this case does not prove that the homeopathic medicines used were effective, though they also note the extreme rarity of survival beyond several months in patients suffering from small-cell lung cancer.

It should be noted that clinical and laboratory research has shown the homeopathic medicine **Viscum album** to be an effective immunostimulant and an inhibitor to cell proliferation *in vitro.*[8]

Advice for People with Cancer

People with cancer should not attempt to treat themselves with homeopathic remedies but should seek professional homeopathic care. Even when these individuals have acute symptoms such as indigestion, fatigue, or headaches, covered elsewhere in this book, professional care is generally required in order to treat the underlying chronic ailment which is manifesting in various acute symptoms.

While chemotherapy, as noted, will not always interfere with the action of homeopathic medicines, the chemotherapeutic agents change a person's symptoms significantly enough that it is considerably more difficult to find the correct remedy. Also, because radiation reduces immune response, it inhibits the potential for healing. If a person with cancer who is presently undergoing conventional treatment seeks care from a classical homeopath, it may be difficult, though not impossible, to find the correct remedy for the person. Dr. Speckhart and others who use some of the experimental electronic devices believe they are better able to treat patients who are concurrently undergoing conventional treatment, because these practitioners do not base their prescriptions on the person's symptoms, as do classical homeopaths, but on the readings from their instruments, which are presumably less influenced by toxic drugging.

No matter what kind of homeopathic care they receive, people with cancer should recognize that homeopathy should be only one part of their treatment. Proper diet, stress management, fitness, and psychological and social support are important adjuncts to obtaining the best possible results in the most expedient manner. People with cancer would also benefit from learning what conventional medical treatment offers so that they can make the most informed choices in dealing with this serious and too often fatal disease.

In Summary

"Despite frantic efforts, the causes of cancer, of arteriosclerosis, of mental disorders, and of other great medical problems of our time remain undiscovered. It is generally assumed that these failures are due to technical difficulties, and that the cause of all disease can and will be found in due time by bringing the big guns of science to bear on the problems. In reality, however, search for the cause may be a hopeless pursuit, because most disease states are the indirect outcome of a constellation of circumstances rather than the direct result of single determinant factors." René Dubos, in *The Mirage of Health.*

Whether a person's cancer is the result of a single or a multifactorial cause, simply getting rid of it does little to change the factors that led to it in the first place. Recurrence of cancer is extremely common. A new and different approach to treating people with cancer is needed.

Homeopathic medicines are not the only alternative, and they are best utilized in conjunction with other natural therapies. But with an individualized comprehensive program that includes homeopathic treatment and may also utilize conventional medical therapies when truly indicated, we may finally have a better chance at healing. The "big C" may someday stand for the big Cure, rather than the big Cancer.

Resources

P. L. Benthack, "Definite Indications for Ten Remedies in Malignancy," *Homeopathic Recorder,* March 1937, 99–106.

Michael Lerner, *Choices in Healing: Integrating the Best of Conventional and Complementary Approaches to Cancer.* Cambridge: MIT Press, 1994.

Andrew Lockie, *The Family Guide to Homeopathy*. New York: Fireside, 1993.

Robin Murphy, *Cancer I and II* (audiotapes). Available from Homeopathic Educational Services; see page 366.

Psychological Conditions

Two hundred years of homeopathic clinical experience verifies the value of homeopathic medicines in treating psychological as well as physiological conditions. Charles Frederick Menninger, the founder of the famed Menninger Clinic, which is considered one of this country's leading mental health institutions, acknowledged the benefits that homeopathic medicines can provide in treating psychological problems, stating, "Homeopathy is wholly capable of satisfying the therapeutic demands of this age better than any other system or school of medicine."[1] Though he wrote this in 1897 when he was the head of his local homeopathic society, his words may be equally valid today.

Typically, conventional physicians and psychiatrists tend to oversimplify psychological conditions, not recognizing the interaction between body and mind. One of the reasons why homeopaths commonly experience good results in treating a wide variety of emotional and mental ailments is that homeopathy is an integrated system which heals physical and psychological problems concurrently.

BODY-MIND INTERCONNECTEDNESS

In *The Alchemy of Healing*, homeopath and psychiatrist Edward C. Whitmont criticizes modern scientific understanding of mental illness: "Scientists' methods of reducing soul and spirit to purely physiochemical and neurological phenomena remain the only valid approaches to 'truth.' Mind is viewed as though it were only an epiphenomenon or even a 'byproduct' of organic brain function, produced in a way similar to how the stomach produces acid and digestive enzymes. Psychological problems or illnesses are then reduced to 'nothing but' a chemical imbalance in the brain."[2]

There are over 10 trillion nerve cells in the brain that govern sensing, thinking, and feeling. Each cell works synergistically with others, creating a complex network that is impossible to comprehend completely. Author Lyall Watson said it well, "If the brain were so simple that we could comprehend it, we would be so simple that we couldn't."

Homeopaths honor conventional scientists for laying out a sophisticated road map of the human mind and body. However, while conventional scientists have focused their attention on the road map itself, homeopaths have directed theirs to understanding basic principles underlying the road map and to the invisible but tangible connections between mind and body. And while conventional psychiatrists have tended to get confused by the chicken-and-egg question—Which comes first, the psychological problem or the physical problem— homeopaths answer this nagging question by asserting that mind and body cannot be separated. Dr. Whitmont notes, "We operate as body-minds." The psychological and the physical manifest at the same time even when one may be more predominant than the other. Just as the body is susceptible to certain physical symptoms, a person's psychological state is susceptible to psychological symptoms. And just as the body is influenced by psychological aberrations, the mind is influenced by physical aberrations. Body and mind immediately and directly affect each other.

Homeopaths do not pretend to understand how or why people have unique constellations of seemingly disparate psychological symptoms. However, homeopaths do have a way to treat people based on the principle of similars. The homeopaths' approach to treating a person experiencing psychological problems is the same approach as to treating any illness. Rather than prescribing drugs that seek to control or suppress brain and body chemistry, homeopaths prescribe microdoses of substances that in overdose would cause similar symptoms to what the sick person is experiencing. Because symptoms of the body-mind are always the best adaptation and response to the entire organism based on its present capabilities, homeopathic medicines augment the person's ability to restore internal balance, vitality, and health.

While homeopathic medicines are prescribed on the basis of the principle of similars, conventional drugs are generally prescribed on the basis of their capacity to alter physiochemical processes that can reduce specific symptoms. In so doing, however, conventional drugs create various side effects, not just physical but psychological as well. For instance, antihistamines are known to create anxiety and hallucinations. Oral contraceptives tend to cause depression. Anticonvulsant drugs cause agitation, delirium, and hallucinations. And there are numerous other examples. Homeopaths theorize that conventional medications suppress physical ailments, pushing the disease deeper into the person's psyche, which can cause serious problems in both mind and body. Because of the powerful effects of conventional drugs, all competent physicians and psychologists should carefully review whatever medications their patients are taking, to determine if any psychiatric condition is drug-induced.

EFFECTS OF TREATMENT

Contrary to common assumptions, the majority of drugs used for chronic psychological conditions have not been proven to be effective. According to *Consumer Reports*, most anxiety-reducing drugs, for instance, have only been found to be effective in treating acute anxiety attacks, not long-term anxiety disorders.[3] What's more, these drugs tend to be effective for only a month and then lose their efficacy. In addition, once the patient stops taking the drug, a rebound effect tends to occur, and there is a significant increase in the number and intensity of anxiety and panic attacks.

Evidence of the efficacy of homeopathic treatment of people with mental illness is drawn from homeopathy's history. In 1874, the first publicly financed homeopathic hospital for the mentally ill was opened in Middletown, New York. The successes that this hospital experienced were significant enough that numerous similar public institutions were developed in New York and in several other states. The rate of discharge from Middletown and other homeopathic mental institutions was often twice that of conventional mental institutions. Even the death rate in the homeopathic asylums was one third of that in conventional asylums.[4]

Besides being used to treat people with psychiatric problems, homeopathic medicines can also be useful in helping people get off conventional psychiatric medications. One study which showed the efficacy of using homeopathic medicines for this purpose was con-ducted in France.[5] A thirty-day study was conducted with four groups of fifty patients being treated with benzodiazepines (tranquilizers) for chronic anxiety. One group was given a homeopathic formula, an-other group was given a different homeopathic formula, a third group was given hydroxyzine dihydrochlorate (a conventional drug popu-larly known as Atarax), and the final group was given a placebo. The study showed that almost all of the patients treated with the homeo-pathic medicines were able to be weaned off benzodiazepines within thirty days without side effects. The study also showed that almost three times as many patients given the conventional drug or the placebo dropped out of the study due to side effects or ineffective treatment as those given a homeopathic medicine.

Withdrawal from conventional drugs can be extremely difficult and painful, but homeopathic medicines can play an important role in helping people taper and get off these medications with greater ease.

THOUGHTS ON THE HOMEOPATHIC APPROACH
TO SCHIZOPHRENIA

A fascinating fact about people who experience schizophrenic epi-sodes is that whatever chronic physical symptoms they normally expe-rience disappear during their episodes of mental breakdown.[6] By conventional standards they may seem physically healthy during these times, even though psychologically they are deeply ill.

Homeopaths make sense of this phenomenon by assuming that these individuals experience so much mental confusion and so many identity problems that their immune and defense systems experience a similar type of disorientation. Their immune system becomes unable to differentiate "self" from "nonself," and therefore they are unable to respond to and defend against pathogens or physical stresses, making them less likely to have any physical symptoms.

As people who experience schizophrenic episodes come out of their mental breakdown, they begin to reexperience their normal physical ailments. Sadly yet predictably, their physicians ultimately prescribe conventional medications again to control their physical symptoms and suppress their disease deep into the mental level. The cycle of mental and physical disease continues to spin an increasingly complicated and tangled web.

One interesting fact of psychiatric history is that prior to the out-lawing of LSD, this drug was used therapeutically to treat schizophren-ics and others suffering from delusional states. Since LSD causes delusional and hallucinatory states, it makes sense from a homeopathic perspective that it could be a good medicine for these psychiatric con-ditions, though homeopaths recommend taking it in significantly smaller doses than have been used in the past. However, homeopaths have not been able to use or test this potentially useful remedy because the FDA has outlawed LSD even in the homeopathic doses which cannot create any hallucinatory symptoms.

Because it is extremely difficult to treat people with schizophrenia outside an institutional setting and because there are presently few psy-chiatrists who are homeopaths working in such settings, there has not been much recorded experience in treating this mental condition. It is therefore unknown how successful homeopathic medicines can be in treating schizophrenia.

TREATING PSYCHOLOGICAL PROBLEMS

The vast majority of psychological problems require treatment by a professional homeopath. However, there are a small number of acute emotional conditions that can be treated at home. The following remedies are useful not only for emotional trauma but also for the concurrent physical ailments that may be encountered. The list of remedies is by no means complete. Readers are encouraged to review the books listed in the *Resources for Self-Treatment* on page 310. These remedies may provide significant relief, though concurrent individual or group therapy can also be beneficial.

If one experiences **acute grief,** there are three remedies most commonly prescribed.

Ignatia is more commonly given to women than men and is in-dicated when someone experiences sudden grief—i.e., a breakup in a close relationship or a death of a loved one. Although these people may have temporarily tried to hold their emotions back, they can't do this for long and ultimately sob uncontrollably, sometimes hysterically mixing laughter and crying. When they are able to catch their breath, their sadness manifests in frequent sighs, a lump in the throat, and sometimes either anorexia or bulimia. **Ignatia** is usually indicated in nervous, sensitive, and romantic women who invest all their emotions in an idealized relationship.

Natrum mur is useful for people who are easily hurt but don't show it, who feel betrayed, and who tend to hold grudges against anyone who has ever hurt them in any way at any time in their life. These people try not to display their emotions. They rarely cry in public, but instead may do so privately, their held-back emotions erupting in loud sobbing until someone breaks their privacy. Their condition is aggravated by efforts to console them as they try to bear the burden of their emotional traumas alone.

Staphysagria should be considered when a person experiences strong emotions of grief, anger, and indignation, especially when these emotions have long been suppressed, as in someone who has been trying to get out of or away from an abusive relationship, from either a lover or one's parents. These people have long stewed about their problems and may finally explode with rage. They feel humiliated, embarrassed, and disgraced from their relationship, and now they may tremble, throw things, lose their voice, or suffer from various physical complaints—e.g., migraines, psoriasis, indigestion, and urinary complaints. **Staphysagria** is also commonly indicated after a rape or any type of physical or mental abuse.

Dose: Take the 6, 12, or 30th potency (though the 30th potency is most preferred), one to six doses over a two-day period, stopping as soon as symptoms abate.

When a person experiences ailments after **anger,** the following are four of the most common remedies to consider.

Staphysagria is one of the primary medicines to consider (see symptoms mentioned above).

Nux vomica is indicated for Type A people, that is, those who are high-strung, competitive, hard-driving, and impatient. These argumentative people will quarrel over the slightest offense. They are very critical of others and demand that others be as hardworking as they are. Restless and irritable, they tend to use various stimulants (coffee, tea, amphetamines) to help them maintain their energy, and they also commonly use alcohol and drugs to help them cope with their stressful life. Their nature and their lifestyle lead them to insomnia, digestive complaints, constipation, and nervous complaints.

Colocynthis is a key remedy given to infants and children who experience temper tantrums. These children complain constantly. They are irritable and impatient, and are offended easily. They want to be left alone and refuse to talk to anyone. Typically, they develop vomiting, diarrhea, and/or stomach cramps.

Chamomilla is another key remedy for infants and children, though it is also given to adults who are drug abusers. Like these who need **Colocynthis,** these children throw temper tantrums. Nothing provides any relief except being rocked or carried. When they are given what they demand they refuse it. They cry, scream, throw things, and may even bang their head against the wall. These symptoms are commonly experienced during episodes of teething or colic. The use of **Colocynthis** in adults tends to be for people who become exceedingly irritable during stages of drug withdrawal. They are extremely restless and inconsolable, cannot bear to be looked at, and easily fly into a rage.

Dose: Take the 6, 12, or 30th potency (though the 30th potency is most preferred), one to six doses over a two-day period, stopping as soon as symptoms abate.

Anxiety prior to an examination or performance is another condition which people can self-treat, and three remedies are most commonly used. **Gelsemium** is indicated when they feel and/or act cowardly and are unable to face any challenge. Physically, they feel weak and may tremble, especially in the knees. They tend to become chilly, experience a hollow feeling in the chest, and are relieved by moving about. **Argentum nitricum** is useful when people feel very anxious and nervous, with great anticipation about what will happen. Physically, they tend to experience diarrhea or flatulence. **Lycopodium** is helpful when people have low self-esteem and a deep fear of failure, particularly of appearing foolish or incompetent. Although these people may sometimes feign great self-confidence, they know underneath that they are faking it.

Dose: Take the 6, 12, or 30th potency (though the 30th potency is most preferred), once the night before the event, another dose in the morning, and if necessary, one dose just before and after the event.

The Bach flower remedies, a tangent of homeopathy, are nonpotentized microdoses of thirty-eight different flowers, each of which is used to treat specific emotional states. This psychopharmacological system was developed by a bacteriologist and homeopath, Dr. Edward Bach.

Bach performed a proving on himself using these flowers, imbibing each flower essence and feeling its effects. He described a different set of emotions with each flower he tested. Although this system is quite simplistic, tens of thousands of Europeans and Americans regularly experience benefit from taking the remedies.

In the 1980s, several new varieties of flower essences became available for the treatment of emotional and mental conditions. Among the more popular are the California flower essences, Australian flower essences, and Perelandra flower essences. They are indicated for a wide range of psychological and spiritual conditions, though there is a need for formal testing to verify their effectiveness.

RESOURCES

Jonathan Davidson, "Psychiatry and Homeopathy: Basis for a Dialogue," *British Homeopathic Journal,* April 1994, 83:78–83.

Resources for Self-Treatment

Edward Bach, *The Bach Flower Remedies.* New Canaan: Keats, 1931.

Peter Chappel, *Emotional Healing with Homeopathy.* Rockport, MA: Element, 1994.

Luis Detinis, *Mental Symptoms in Homeopathy.* Beaconsfield: Beaconsfield, 1994.

Trevor Smith, *Homeopathic Medicine for Mental Health.* Rochester, VT: Healing Arts, 1989.

Keith Souter, *Homeopathy: Heart and Soul.* Saffron Walden, England: C. W. Daniel, 1993.

Resources for Learning about the Homeopathic Constitutional Types

Philip Bailey, *Homeopathic Psychology: Personality Profiles of the Major Constitutional Remedies.* Berkeley: North Atlantic, 1995.

Catherine Coulter, *Portraits of Homeopathic Medicines* (2 volumes). Berkeley: North Atlantic, 1986, 1988.

Edward C. Whitmont, *Psyche and Substance: Essays on Homeopathy in the Light of Jungian Psychology.* Berkeley: North Atlantic, 1991.

Drug, Alcohol, and Nicotine Addiction

Neuroscientists have discovered that the human brain creates its own opiate chemicals called endorphins. These endorphins tend to reduce the sensation of pain after an injury, provide a sense of exhilaration from exercise, and even envelop us in feelings of love.

Many recreational drugs create similar effects, and because people wish to experience these good feelings as often as possible, it is predictable that some would tend to abuse substances that artificially create these feelings. The problem with these drugs, however, is that their effects are short-lived, they tend to create addiction, and they cause a host of physical and psychological side effects. Generally speaking, the higher the high a person experiences, the lower the low that is created. Light tends to create shadow.

Homeopaths define health as physical, emotional, and mental freedom. Addiction to any substance, except those things that bring nourishment to the body, limits this freedom. One can be addicted not only to recreational drugs or alcohol, but also to tobacco, stimulants such as coffee and tea, and conventional therapeutic drugs.

While politicians and the media have tended to focus on the problems of recreational drugs and alcohol abuse, they have often ignored the serious health problems created by addiction to therapeutic drugs. In part because politicians and the media know so little about viable alternative therapies to conventional medications, they tend to rationalize addictions to tranquilizers, painkillers, antihistamines, and other commonly prescribed drugs as a "necessary evil."

Therapeutic drugs are sometimes more addictive than recreational drugs, and the symptoms of withdrawal can be extremely strong. Some people become addicted without knowing that the prescribed drug has addictive properties and only realize the problem when they try to stop taking it.

Conventional treatment for addictions is recognized as woefully inadequate and ineffective. The best treatments have tended to develop outside the conventional medical model. The various support groups, including Alcoholics Anonymous and other twelve-step programs, are recognized as considerably more effective than medical treatment.

Still, social support is often not enough. It is becoming widely known that acupuncture is effective in helping people break addictions. Not as well known is the fact that homeopathic medicine can also be extremely helpful in dealing with various stages of addiction recovery.

The Homeopathic Perspective of Addiction

Conventional physicians have begun to recognize that addiction is a disease. Some evidence has indicated that there are certain differences in brain chemistry in alcoholics, though it must be emphasized that it is uncertain whether the chemistry creates the behavior of addiction or the behavior creates the brain chemistry.

Homeopaths don't treat disease. Homeopaths treat the *person* with the disease. Likewise, homeopaths don't treat addiction; they treat people who, among various physical and psychological states, are also addicted to something. Homeopathic medicines don't change people's habits, but they will change people so that they can change their habits themselves.

The approach to treating an addicted person with homeopathic medicine is the same as the approach to treating any other person. Through a detailed interview process, the homeopath individualizes a medicine based on the totality of symptoms being presently experienced. The key words here are "totality of symptoms" and "presently experienced." The symptoms of a person going through withdrawal will be considerably different than during his or her normal state, and therefore the present symptoms require the appropriate remedy. Then, as the person goes through a detoxification stage, a different remedy will be needed to treat the changing symptoms experienced. As he or she moves on through the recovery stage, a still different remedy will usually be necessary.

Homeopaths will rarely prescribe a constitutional medicine during the time they are treating addiction recovery, unless the remedy just happens to fit the present stage the patient is experiencing. Only in these unusual cases will the same remedy be indicated at different stages of addiction recovery.

When seeking out constitutional medicines for patients who are *not* necessarily addicted, some homeopaths ask them how they act when they are intoxicated. Because mind-altering substances tend to reduce a person's inhibitions, they can uncover key underlying personality traits which can shed light on an appropriate deep-acting remedy.

As part of the process of finding these deeper-acting medicines, homeopaths inevitably make note of any and all addictive tendencies. From a homeopathic point of view, one does not have to be addicted to an actual drug to have an addictive personality. People are commonly addicted to TV, shopping, chocolate and other sweets, food, fame, money, and even love. None of these things are necessarily bad or considered unhealthy in and of themselves, but they can create disease when dependence upon them and obsession with them reaches certain heights.

HOMEOPATHIC MEDICINES FOR TREATING ADDICTION

There is presently no book on the homeopathic treatment of addiction, though there is a real need for one. It is impossible to cover this subject in a chapter; at best this chapter will provide a *Cliff Notes* version of the common remedies to consider for the most frequently experienced symptoms of addictive states and the process of recovery. People who try to treat themselves with the information in this chapter may get some benefits, but the best results in treating the various stages of addiction come from professional homeopathic care.

Homeopathic medicines can effectively decrease the physical addiction, but the greater the social pressure, the greater the difficulty in breaking the addiction. For instance, a homeopathic medicine may reduce a person's addiction to cocaine or alcohol, but if he is influenced by social pressures to share a line or a drink with others, homeopathic treatment will not always be enough.

Dealing with the social pressures of habit is where group support from the various twelve-step and other recovery programs is invaluable. Addiction treatment programs of the future will hopefully integrate these programs with good homeopathic and acupuncture treatment.

Two of the most common homeopathic medicines used for various stages of the withdrawal, detoxification, and recovery process are **Nux vomica** and **Staphysagria.**

Nux vomica is indicated for people who are nervous, irritable, angry, and impatient. Physically, they experience various muscle spasms, tremblings, and twitchings. As they move out of the acute withdrawal stage, they develop digestive disorders, including cramps and fitful but unfruitful urgings to eliminate a stool. These people are driven, compulsive, competitive, and easily offended. They cannot stand the pain or bear light, noise, touch, or music. They can get violent, though they are the type of people who become very apologetic afterward.

Staphysagria is useful in extremely angry individuals, especially when they have earlier suppressed whatever feelings they had. These people tend to have been abused physically, sexually, or psychologically and are now in a state of rage. Like a volcano, they are now erupting. They may throw things, break things, and slam doors. **Staphysagria** is more commonly indicated for women, though it can certainly be useful in treating men who have been abused and/or seriously humiliated.

In addition to the above two remedies, please read the following sections for additional remedies to consider for specific stages of the withdrawal and detoxification process.

Dose: Follow the dosage recommendations based on the stages of addiction and recovery that are discussed later in this chapter.

ACUTE WITHDRAWAL

Acute withdrawal needs acute remedies. Los Angeles homeopath Janet Zand has likened the intensity of the withdrawal experience to the intensity and shock experienced by a woman during labor. Fear, restlessness, delirium, anger, irritability, and even uncontrollable behavior may be experienced during withdrawal as well as birth. She notes that homeopaths use similar remedies to treat both experiences.

Acute withdrawal can often create serious and extreme symptoms which generally require professional attention. Description of the following remedies is provided primarily for informational and not self-care use, except by trained professionals. Homeopathic medicines will not immediately "cure" people's symptoms of withdrawal, but can ease their emotional and physical symptoms so that they are better able to go through this healing process.

For some, the acute withdrawal phase may require **Aconitum,** as when the person is acutely fearful, restless, anxious, and consciously aware of his heart palpitations. A key feature of people who need **Aconitum** is that they tend to be fearful of death and may think they are going to die. They have great fear that they will be unable to stop their addiction, and they may become highly irritated and angry about having to stop. This remedy is particularly common for cocaine users.

Arnica is indicated when the whole body becomes hypersensitive. These people have a bruised feeling and do not want to be touched. They fear touch and will be fearful of anyone nearby. They want and may demand to be left alone.

Chamomilla is the remedy of choice when the person is hyper-irritable, impatient, restless, demands something but then refuses it when it is offered, and is extremely sensitive to light, noise, touch, slight drafts, and the slightest pain. Like **Chamomilla** infants who feel better when rocked, addicts who need this remedy feel compelled to rock themselves back and forth. They may experience stomach pains that cause them to double over.

Aurum met is an important medicine when people become extremely despondent. They feel utterly worthless and are very self-condemning, have a disgust for life and may talk about and even try to commit suicide, and are oversensitive to noise and excitement.

Arsenicum is effective when people become extremely restless and agitated, and despair of recovering. This despair drives them from place to place. They are reluctant to be left alone because they are afraid they will hurt or kill themselves. Despite their great agitation, they are obsessive about order and will insist that wherever they are have some degree of tidiness. **Arsenicum** is commonly given to people withdrawing from marijuana, especially those people who are restless and agitated and feel they need marijuana to relax them.

Stramonium is suggested when people ceaselessly talk, earnestly beseeching others to stay with them and save them from darkness. They laugh, cry, sing, swear, and experience hallucinations, especially of animals and insects. They are extremely fearful of water and shiny objects, which may cause spasms in various parts of the body. They may become violent or lewd. This state is most common in alcoholics.

Another remedy that is useful during violent stages of withdrawal is **Belladonna.** These people suffer from hallucinations, usually of a fantastic nature, including monsters and hideous faces. They may sing, dance, laugh, and whistle, while frequently moaning. They seem to live in their own world. Physically, they may have a high fever, a flushed face, dilated pupils, and throbbing pains.

Dose: Due to the intensity of symptoms common during the withdrawal process, homeopathic medicines for this condition generally require frequent repetition, sometimes as often as every hour, though some homeopaths recommend only one to four doses of a high-potency medicine. Some homeopaths will prescribe high-potency remedies (200c, 1M, 10M), but only when they are very confident about the accuracy of the prescription. Repetition of these higher potencies is not as frequent as with the lower potencies. Less experienced individuals should consider using 6, 12, or 30th potencies frequently (every hour or every other hour) during intense symptoms and four times a day toward the end of the withdrawal phase.

DETOXIFICATION

Detoxification refers to the time when the person is no longer experiencing the powerful symptoms of withdrawal and no longer has strong cravings for these addictive substances. The detoxification process is the body's efforts to heal itself from the damage caused by the addictive substance. People who take the addictive substance during detoxification will slow down the body's efforts to heal itself. While the addictive substance may temporarily reduce some symptoms of detoxification, it will simply prolong the process of healing.

Homeopathic medicines for detoxification vary depending on the symptoms that the person is experiencing. These symptoms tend to differ based on the addictive substance.

Because alcohol and drugs have damaging effects on the liver, remedies that are known to restore and improve liver function are commonly indicated during the detoxification process. Also, remedies for healing the nervous system and addressing the physical and psychological symptoms that accompany neurological dysfunction, such as headache, digestive distress, and hyperirritability, are useful.

Nux vomica and **Staphysagria,** described earlier, are key remedies for detoxification because of their dramatic healing effects on neurological and liver functions.

Arsenicum, described earlier, is also effective. Physically, these people experience morning vomiting, fruitless retching, chronic gastric irritability with heartburn and various burning pains in the abdominal region, and great weakness. They have a great thirst but for only sips of water at a time.

Lycopodium is indicated when people experience much gas, bloating, and indigestion. Their appetite may vary; at one time they will experience abdominal fullness after only a small amount of food and at other times have a ravenous appetite and feel increasingly hungry while eating. Their worst symptoms occur between four and eight p.m. and after midnight.

Chelidonium is the remedy of choice when people experience pain in the liver region that radiates back to the right scapula. They have abdominal pain which is relieved by eating, by drinking very hot drinks, and by lying on the left side with legs drawn up. They may have jaundice or at least the face will look pale.

Carduus marianus is effective in treating people with liver pains that are aggravated by breathing deeply or by any motion and when they are lying on the left side (note that people who need **Chelidonium** are better lying on their left side). It is thought to be particularly helpful for alcoholics who have a history of heart disease.

Zincum is more useful for nervous symptoms than digestive complaints. These people are restless, have abnormal or involuntary movements, twitches, and sometimes convulsions. During detoxification they may become very irritable and complain intensely or may experience mental dullness, depression, and possibly suicidal thoughts. **Zincum** is also valuable in treating the alcoholic who has an allergy to alcohol, when ingesting even small amounts leads to intoxication, great fatigue, headache, and/or indigestion.

Ignatia successfully treats people, most often women, who experience depression during the detoxification stage. Some type of disappointed love or failed romance is a common precursing event. They become easily offended and hurt and usually brood about their emotional pain. Characteristically, they tend to sigh frequently. They may experience contradictory and alternating emotional states. Physically, they may have twitches and spasms and a lump in the throat.

Gambogia is a little-known but invaluable medicine for treating the cocaine addict. Characteristically, these people experience a cold sensation at the edge of their teeth. They also tend to have dry mucous membranes and burning and dryness of the mouth and throat. They may have severe diarrhea with a sudden gushing of a stool and concurrent diarrhea and vomiting.

Dose: Compared with the withdrawal process, the symptoms of detoxification are not nearly as acute. There are different schools of thought on the dose and potency. Some will recommend frequent repetitions of 6, 12, or 30th potencies, ranging from doses every two hours to three times a day for up to seven days, while others will recommend a single or a couple of doses of a higher potency.

RECOVERY

After detoxification, people who were addicted to alcohol or drugs either reexperience their previous (prior to addiction) complex of symptoms or have a new set of symptoms that supersede the old ones.

The new symptoms are generally the result of the damaging effects of the addictive substance and overall addictive lifestyle. The homeopath will prescribe based on the person's present symptoms and then work his or her way back through the various layers of disease the person has experienced (see the discussion on Hering's guidelines in Chapter 2 for more information on this healing process; page 18).

There is a school of thought in addiction research that posits that once an addict, always an addict. This does not mean that the person will always be addicted to something, but that addicts are extremely vulnerable to becoming readdicted to their previous drug of choice or to a new one. The assumption is that there is a certain addictive personality and once people become addicts, they must work to avoid addiction one day at a time for the rest of their lives. It may be true that addicts who stop their addiction to one substance may not be curing their underlying addictive personality; however, this point of view assumes that one cannot change oneself or be changed in a significant way by any therapeutic modality. The homeopathic perspective and experience on this issue is that homeopathic medicines can profoundly change a person so that addictive tendencies are truly cured.

Because constitutional homeopathic care is oriented toward strengthening a person's overall physiopsychological state, homeopathic medicines can play a major role in treating addicts, during both the addiction stage and the recovery process. Although homeopathic medicines will not stop a person from an addictive behavior, they can influence and improve the person's physical and psychological state so that he or she may be less likely to develop addictive behaviors.

There have been few formal studies on the homeopathic treatment of addiction, but one from India merits attention. This double-blind study was of sixty heroin addicts, of whom half were given individualized homeopathic medicines and half were given placebos. The number and intensity of the symptoms during withdrawal and detoxification were significantly less in patients given an individualized homeopathic medicine than those given a placebo. Further evidence of the benefits received from the homeopathic medicines was the fact that 35 percent of patients on the placebo left the study prior to its completion due to lack of therapeutic benefit, while only 5 percent of those taking the homeopathic medicine left the study.[1]

The empirical and research results using homeopathic medicines for treating addicts is so significant that several police stations in India have integrated homeopathic medicine into their drug abuse treatments. From 1987 to 1993, over three thousand addicts have been detoxified with homeopathic medicines as their primary method of treatment.

Clinical experience with homeopathic medicines provides additional evidence of the benefits from these natural medicines. Jack Cooper, M.D., a now deceased psychiatrist and homeopath who served as chief psychiatrist for seventeen years at New York's Westchester County Prison and Jail, commonly treated inmates who were going through withdrawal. Besides experiencing good results from using homeopathic medicines to treat withdrawal and detoxification, he consistently found better results when the jailed patients did not know they were receiving treatment. While such care without consent may not be ethical today, its practice several decades ago suggests that homeopathic medicines offer benefits beyond the placebo effect and beyond the awareness that patients were even being treated.

NICOTINE ADDICTION

There is now a strong body of evidence that nicotine in tobacco is an addictive substance. It makes sense that nicotine patches, a homeopathic-like product, have become a common prescriptive product which some people have found invaluable in helping their nicotine addiction. Although these patches utilize small doses of nicotine, homeopaths commonly use even smaller doses.

Similar to the use of the patches, homeopaths have sometimes found that homeopathic doses of tobacco **(Tabacum)** can help people break their addiction to smoking. Homeopaths have found other remedies to be helpful also, including **Nux vomica, Arsenicum,** and **Caladium.** However, they strongly believe that concurrent homeopathic constitutional care is invaluable to help treat the underlying addictive personality that created the problem in the first place.

Tabacum should be given if none of the following remedies is obviously indicated.

Nux vomica is useful for Type-A people who are highly competitive, irritable, and impatient. They crave stimulants of various kinds to help them maintain their desired hyperactive state. They even smoke rapidly. **Arsenicum** is good for nervous, anxious individuals who have various obsessive-compulsive behaviors, including a fastidiousness in which they are very careful not to get their tobacco ashes anywhere other than an ashtray. **Caladium** is indicated when the person is addicted to cigarettes and is impotent, or at least has difficulty getting an erection. Headache, forgetfulness, and sensitivity to noise are other common symptoms for this medicine.

Dr. Francisco Eizayaga, a respected Argentinian homeopath, recommends the use of **Tabacum fumar** (tobacco smoke) as his favorite remedy to help ease addiction to nicotine, but this remedy is difficult to obtain in the United States.

It should be said that these remedies should be tried only if the person genuinely wants to stop smoking. Homeopathic remedies will not stop someone from putting a cigarette in his mouth, though they can reduce the desire for it. Thus some type of support group and/or behavioral training program is important as a conjoint treatment with homeopathic medicines.

In addition to treating addiction to smoking, homeopaths commonly treat the various symptoms that smoking is known to aggravate. Besides obvious symptoms such as coughing, smoking can cause headaches, diarrhea, dyspepsia, nausea, insomnia, poor circulation, high blood pressure, and lung cancer. The homeopath prescribes according to the person's unique symptoms.

Although homeopathic medicines may help relieve some of the symptoms that smoking causes, the best results will remain elusive until the person stops smoking. Homeopaths commonly acknowledge that one must remove the "obstacle to cure" in order for a significant curative process to occur.

Dose: To help reduce the addiction to nicotine, use the 6, 12, or 30th potencies whenever you feel a strong urge to smoke, though you should not take a dose more than eight times a day. The length of time to take a remedy varies on the success of the remedy in treating one's cravings, and one's efforts to reduce the frequency of the remedy. The basic idea is to take the remedy as often as necessary but as seldom as possible. Continue to take the remedy if it provides relief of symptoms but try to continually decrease the dose until no more doses are necessary. If you have not completely stopped smoking and remedy taking after two months, seek professional homeopathic care.

Resources

Note: There is no good single source of information on the homeopathic treatment of addiction. Generally, homeopaths use their repertories and *materia medica* texts to individualize care.

J. P. Gallavardin, *How to Cure Alcoholism: The Non-Toxic Homeopathic Way.* New Delhi: B. Jain (reprint from the nineteenth century).

Andrew Lockie, *The Family Guide to Homeopathy.* New York: Fireside, 1993.

Andre Saine, *The Homeopathic Treatment of Alcoholism* (two cassettes).*

Janet Zand, *Using Homeopathy to Alter Habitual Patterns* (cassette tape).*

---

*Available only through Homeopathic Educational Services; see page 366.

Conditions of
Travel and Recreation

Mark Twain once said, "Travel is fatal to prejudice, bigotry, and narrow-mindedness." While travel may be beneficial to the human mind and spirit, it is not always so kind to the body.

Because stress is recognized as any change, positive or negative, which requires a person to adapt, travel is inherently stressful.

In addition to the various digestive disturbances from new and unusual microorganisms that travel can bring, there are other travel-related stresses that can result in minor or serious illness. Because recreation and travel are often one and the same, the ailments related to both will be discussed in this chapter, along with homeopathic medicines commonly effective in treating them.

Finding the homeopathic medicines you may need is not always easy during travel or recreation. Because of this, it is worthwhile to put together your own homeopathic travel kit which includes remedies that treat possible problems that may arise during your particular kind of trip or sport. Such preparation may not only allay pain and suffering, it may save your vacation or help you finish the game.

JET LAG

The human organism has evolved over hundreds of thousands of years, yet it is only in the last few decades that humans have to travel to distant places on the globe within a day. The fact that some people cannot easily adapt to rapid travel and significant time zone changes is certainly understandable. There are, however, some homeopathic medicines that can strengthen a person's body so that modern travel has less stressful effects.

The primary remedy for jet lag is **Arnica,** known for its ability to deal with shock or trauma of injury. While jet lag is not exactly an injury, it is a stress to the system, and **Arnica** helps to relieve it. **Gelsemium** should be used if exhaustion is so strong that the person has difficulty raising the eyelids fully and the limbs feel limp. If nausea predominates and persists, **Ipecacuanha** should be given. If nausea and vertigo are experienced together, **Cocculus** is the remedy of choice.

Dose: If jet lag is commonly experienced and one wishes to prevent it, take the 6, 12 or 30th potency of the remedy just prior to boarding, once every four hours of flight, and if necessary, every four hours for the next twenty-four. To treat jet lag, take the 6, 12, or 30th potency every two hours for intense symptoms and every four hours for mild discomfort.

Motion Sickness

The nausea and dizziness of motion sickness can be felt in a car, boat, train, or plane. Although anyone can get motion sickness, it tends to be more common in children.

The primary remedy for motion sickness is **Cocculus.** It is particularly indicated when the person feels vertigo and nausea. Typically, there is a sensation of hollowness or emptiness in the head or other parts. **Cocculus** is more commonly effective in treating people of mild and sluggish temperament than irritable and hyperactive types of people.

If a person experiences the greatest symptoms of motion sickness during downward motions of a plane or boat, this is an indication for **Borax. Tabacum** is useful when there is nausea, giddiness, vomiting, pallor, icy coldness, and sweat. Typically, vertigo is worse upon opening the eyes. **Theridion** has many of the same symptoms as **Tabacum,** but these people feel vertigo upon closing the eyes. **Ipecacuanha** is useful when there is persistent nausea which is not relieved after vomiting. One homeopathic medicine which is also a known herbal remedy is **Zingiber** (ginger). Homeopaths recommend taking this remedy in tincture (unpotentized form), five to ten drops every two hours. If you are uncertain about which remedy to take, this one or **Cocculus** should be considered.

In addition to these individualized remedies, there are various homeopathic combination formulas available for motion sickness. In fact, there is some good research performed by a leading ear, nose, and throat specialist which shows that a homeopathic formula can be very effective in treating nausea and vertigo.[1]

Dose: Take the 6, 12, or 30th potency every thirty minutes during intense symptoms and every two or four hours during mild symptoms. To prevent motion sickness, people who commonly experience it should take one dose prior to departure and one dose approximately every two hours during travel, except during long-term ship travel, where a couple of doses a day until they sense that they have adapted to the motion is all that is generally necessary.

ILL EFFECTS OF SUN AND HEAT

Like most things, the sun can be healing as well as a source of disease. And like everything else, its effect is primarily a matter of quantity. Because people tend to spend more time in the sun on vacation and during recreation than at other times, overexposure is a common problem for them.

Too much sun can lead to relatively mild ailments such as sunburn or heat exhaustion, or medical emergencies such as heatstroke. (Remedies for sunburns are discussed in "Skin Conditions" in the section on burns, page 254.)

Heat exhaustion is a fairly common condition in which the person experiences fatigue, coldness and clamminess of the skin, headache, nausea and vomiting, dizziness, and muscle cramps. **Veratrum album** is the most common remedy for heat exhaustion. It is indicated when people experience great weakness, profuse and clammy sweat, faintness, chilliness, pallor, nausea, and cramps in the extremities. They may have had diarrhea prior to and/or after the heat exhaustion. People who need **Cuprum metallicum** have similar symptoms, though the most prominent ones are cramps, with possible jerking in the muscles and/or convulsions. They are aggravated by movement and touch. **Carbo veg** is useful when people become so exhausted they are in a state of collapse. They feel so tired that they hardly seem to have enough energy to breathe and may request that people nearby fan them to help give them air. They may also demand that all windows be kept open.

Heatstroke (also called sunstroke) is a rarer condition. It is a medical emergency which results from dehydration and a disruption in the heat-regulating mechanisms of the body. There is a rise in bodily temperature, a diminution of sweat, and increased urination. These factors lead to a fast and forceful pulse, visual disturbances, convulsions, confusion, stupor, and loss of consciousness.

On the way to emergency medical care, **Belladonna** and **Glonoine** are the two remedies to consider. Both of these remedies are known to treat people who have a flushed red face, a throbbing headache, and delirium. **Belladonna** tends to be indicated when the person is radiating heat from the whole body and may be experiencing hallucinations. He or she will primarily feel heat emanating from the head and may experience some general relief from bending it backward, keeping it uncovered, and sitting quietly. People who need **Glonoine** will feel pulsations not only in the head but all over the body. They will have a sensation that the head is extremely large, and their symptoms are aggravated by bending it backward and by applying cold water, and are relieved by uncovering the head and being in the open air.

Dose: Use the highest potency available every fifteen to thirty minutes during the crisis period and every other hour during milder symptoms. If no obvious improvement is observed after two hours, consider changing the medicine.

High Altitudes

Travel to high elevations stresses the body as it must adapt to increasingly thinner air. Extreme or prolonged exposure to high elevations, whether it be while skiing, mountain climbing, or simply visiting mountainous areas, can lead to altitude sickness. Symptoms of altitude sickness include headache, weakness, drowsiness, pallor, nausea and vomiting, breathing difficulties, and blueness of the lips and skin. In more serious situations, altitude sickness can cause wheezing and rattling of fluids in the chest, great confusion, and unconsciousness.

The remedies to consider for altitude sickness include **Arnica, Aconitum, Carbo veg, Silicea,** and **Calcarea carb. Arnica** and **Aconitum** are indicated in the early stages of this condition. **Arnica** is useful when the person is weak, confused, and may be unaware that anything is wrong (a state of shock). **Aconitum** is helpful when the person is restless, fearful, and anxious, with a concern that she might die. People who need **Carbo veg** experience weakness, chilliness, pallor, blueness of the lips and skin, bloating, and breathing difficulties (they feel a need to be fanned). **Silicea** is indicated in thin, often frail people who become easily exhausted and chilled. **Calcarea carb** is usually effective in treating fair-skinned, overweight, chilly people who have poor stamina and a fear of heights.

Dose: Take the 6, 12, or 30th potency every thirty to sixty minutes during the first couple of hours and then every two to six hours, depending on the intensity of the symptoms. If obvious change has not occurred after two hours, consider another remedy. To prevent altitude sickness, **Arnica 30** can be taken three times a day.

FROSTBITE

Jack Frost does not just nip at your nose; he can nip at your toes, your fingers, and any parts of your body that are left exposed to cold for prolonged periods of time. Mountain climbers, backwoods skiers, and snow backpackers should be especially cautious of lengthy exposure to cold, which can lead to frostbite. Not all types of frostbite require medical attention, unless pain persists for more than a couple of hours.

Homeopathic medicines can be helpful, though they should be used in conjunction with standard practices of first aid. **Agaricus** is the primary remedy for frostbite. Typically, the person experiences burning, itching, redness, and swelling. **Carbo veg** should be considered when someone who has these symptoms is in a state of collapse, has difficulty breathing with a need to be fanned, and may even faint. **Silicea** is indicated for frostbite experienced by thin, frail, faint-hearted, normally chilly type of people who become easily tired. These people may develop infected and pus-filled wounds, either on frostbitten or nonfrostbitten parts.

The experience of frostbite not only affects localized parts but can be a shock to the whole system as well. If a person who has previously been frostbitten develops any new symptoms after the experience, it is highly recommended to seek professional medical and homeopathic care.

Dose: Take the 6, 12, or 30th potency every hour for the first six doses and then every two to four hours for the next couple of days. Stop taking the remedy if there is significant progress in healing.

GASTROINTESTINAL PROBLEMS

Traveling to faraway and foreign lands gives you the chance to see new sights, experience new experiences, taste new foods, and ingest bacteria, parasites, and other microorganisms that your body has never previously consumed, thus disrupting digestion and health.

Homeopathic medicines can often be effective in helping the body rid itself of these microorganisms,[2] though admittedly, some bacteria and parasites can be resistant to conventional and homeopathic treatment.

Some of the most common homeopathic remedies for travelers' diarrhea and its attendant symptoms are **Arsenicum, Podophyllum, Chamomilla, Mercurius, Sulphur,** and **Veratrum album.** See the section on acute diarrhea, page 243, in "Digestive Disorders" for details about how to individualize homeopathic remedies for these complaints.

Because parasites can cause a wide variety of symptoms for which there are a large number of potentially useful medicines, and because many of these symptoms are serious, it is generally recommended to seek the care of a professional homeopath for their treatment. Professional homeopathic care should definitely be sought if some obvious relief from self-care is not experienced within forty-eight hours. Medical care is also highly recommended so that laboratory analysis can help provide an appropriate diagnosis.

IMMUNIZATIONS

Citizens who travel abroad to certain countries are required to get certain immunizations if they wish to return to their country of origin. While there are such alternatives as "homeopathic immunizations," they are not recognized by any government as a legal alternative to conventional immunizations.

"Homeopathic immunizations" refer to the presently experimental use of potentized doses of pathological agents (bacteria or viruses) which are thought to immunize against the disease they cause. For instance, **Pertussinum 200** is given by a small group of homeopaths in an effort to prevent whooping cough (*Pertussis* is the bacteria known to cause this disease). There is, however, inadequate evidence that these homeopathic immunizations are effective.

Some classical homeopaths tend to question whether homeopathic immunizations make sense from a homeopathic point of view. These homeopaths assert that the microdoses won't have any effect unless a person has similar symptoms to those they cause. Giving a homeopathic medicine as prevention to people who do not have any symptoms does not fit this approach. These homeopaths prefer to prevent ailments by prescribing constitutional medicines, since they commonly find that these deep-acting remedies strengthen a person's overall defenses.

Although there is controversy as to whether homeopathic medicines can prevent diseases, there is no controversy about their ability to reduce the side effects that inoculations can cause, some of which are acute, such as fever and diarrhea, and others of which are chronic, including certain neurological syndromes. Some homeopaths recommend taking the potentized dose (usually the 30 or 200th potency) of the immunization in the morning before the treatment and one dose shortly afterward (these remedies tend to require a doctor's prescription in the United States). Some of the classically oriented homeopaths do not recommend any treatment unless the person actually develops symptoms, at which time the homeopath will prescribe a remedy according to the patient's unique symptoms.

Resources

Colin B. Lessell, *The World Traveller's Manual of Homeopathy*. Saffron Walden, England: C. W. Daniel, 1993.

Injuries

Conventional medicine is at its best in the treatment of injuries, especially serious injuries. Standard medications can eliminate or at least significantly reduce pain and discomfort. Sophisticated medical technologies can literally be lifesaving, and modern surgery can help to repair many injuries that nature itself could not always accomplish. In addition, modern orthopedic devices can protect the injured part from further injury and thereby aid in its recovery.

While conventional medicine can perform miracles when a person is seriously injured, it has less to offer for the everyday, less serious injury. In fact, some of what contemporary medicine offers for the treatment of injuries actually slows down the healing process.

For instance, aspirin and ibuprofen products may effectively reduce the pain of injury; however, they block the production of prostaglandin, a bodily chemical that is essential for muscle repair. Aspirin creates additional complications because it reduces blood clotting factors, which can lead to bleeding problems for people with deep external cuts or internal bruises. Aspirin also increases sweat and urination, which can lead to dehydration, a problem that can be exacerbated by exercise.

Some people who are injured resort to corticosteroid drugs ("steroids") to reduce inflammation as a result of injury. Although these drugs seem to perform miracles due to their ability to rapidly reduce pain and swelling, they also inhibit the body's immune system and natural defenses. Prolonged use of steroids can lead to serious disease, and if the steroid is injected into the muscle, it can weaken it, increasing the chances of future injury.

Homeopathy has much to offer for the treatment of injury and trauma. That is not to say that homeopathic care should replace standard first-aid practices or conventional medical care. In fact, homeopaths honor the various standard first-aid practices in use today as well as many lifesaving medical procedures. Homeopathic medicine can and should be used in conjunction with conventional treatments, with the exception of some of the above-described drugs which require special care in use.

Treating injuries with homeopathic medicines is often very easy. Whereas the healing of disease requires individualized treatment of a person's unique pattern of symptoms, people who are injured usually experience similar symptoms and generally require a similar curative process to heal their injuries. Because of this, there are certain homeopathic medicines which are used considerably more often than others for the treatment of certain injuries.

The use of homeopathic combination formulas makes a lot of sense in the treatment of injuries. When injured, people commonly traumatize various tissues, including muscle, connective tissue, nerves, and bone, and it is often necessary to take one remedy for injury to the muscle, another for injury to connective tissue, another for injury to nerves, and so on. Combination remedies for injuries often contain all of these different remedies.

The treatment of injuries sometimes benefits from the use of homeopathic external applications. Robert Becker, M.D., a respected orthopedic surgeon, was particularly impressed with the healing ability of external applications of **Arnica,** and asserted that its healing effects are "far more effective than those of any standard pharmacological agent."[1] Dr. Becker did, however, warn that relief from pain was noticeably reduced immediately after washing off the application. Homeopaths recommend that people reapply external applications after every wash, if not more frequently.

Like internally taken homeopathic medicines, homeopathic external applications are composed of single-ingredient remedies as well as combination formulas. External remedies, both single and formulas, contain primarily unpotentized tinctures of the homeopathic medicines.

Shock of Injury

Effective treatment of injuries requires treatment for the shock and trauma of the injury. In fact, standard first-aid treatment emphasizes that a seriously injured person must be treated for shock as soon as possible. "Shock" refers to a disorder in which blood flow is reduced below the levels needed to maintain vital functions. Because the nervous system's reaction to an acute injury can alter blood flow, someone in shock may not have adequate blood flow to the brain, leading to the possibility of the death of brain cells which cannot be replaced.

In addition to standard first-aid practices (having the person lie down with feet slightly elevated, protecting her from the extremes of heat or cold, loosening clothing, letting her sip fluids if she is conscious), there are two common homeopathic medicines that one should consider to help a person recover from shock.

Arnica is by far the most common remedy for shock of injury. It is particularly indicated when the person has the classic symptoms of shock: pale face, confusion, dizziness, and sweating. Typically, someone who needs **Arnica** is not thinking clearly and may not even recognize that injury has occurred.

Aconitum is another remedy to consider for shock, though unlike people who need **Arnica,** people who need **Aconitum** realize that they are injured and may experience great fear and anxiety as a result of the injury. These people may think that they are going to die or may be very anxious about their condition. People who have injuries to the eye experience so much pain that **Aconitum** is commonly indicated.

The average person in shock may not have symptoms as obvious as in either of the extreme cases described here. In such instances, **Arnica** is most effective.

Please also note that some people can go into shock from experiencing a close call or near injury. **Arnica** is recommended in these cases.

Dose: Use the 6, 12, 30th, or even higher potency (preferably the 30th or higher) as soon as possible after injury. Repeat as needed, usually every thirty minutes for the first couple of doses, and if more is necessary, increase by one hour the time in between doses (at first it will be every two hours, then every three hours, and so on).

CUTS

Standard first-aid procedures recommend that measures to stop bleeding be given high priority in injuries. Pressure on the injured part or just above the injured part can help stop bleeding. Homeopathic medicines can also help stop bleeding and augment healing of the cut.

Minor cuts are best treated externally. External applications of **Calendula** will effectively heal the cut faster than just letting nature take its course. **Calendula** is so effective in closing up wounds that it is not recommended for use in deep cuts because it can close a wound too rapidly and lead to an abscess. External applications of **Hypericum** are preferred for the treatment of deeper cuts. Internally, **Hypericum** should be given for deep cuts or for wounds that are hypersensitive to touch. **Millefolium** is a key internal or external remedy for wounds causing significant bleeding or for wounds that are slowly bleeding without adequate clotting.

There are various homeopathic formulas for external application which include **Calendula, Hypericum,** and other remedies. These formulas can be particularly effective. However, if one has a deep or open wound, one should avoid applying any external formula containing **Arnica** because it can sometimes increase bleeding.

Dose: Externally, tinctures, gels, ointments, or sprays are all effective. However, if using a tincture, dilute it with water because the high alcohol content can cause stinging. Internally, take the 6, 12, or 30th potency only if pain is significant enough to warrant it. For deep wounds, take every two hours at first, and then increase the time in between doses to four or six hours.

PUNCTURE WOUNDS

Depending on where and how deep a puncture or stab wound is, it may require medical attention. Also, because bacteria or some foreign material may be on the stabbing instrument, medical care may be necessary to prevent infection.

The most common homeopathic remedy for stab wounds is **Ledum.** It is particularly useful if the injured part feels cold or numb and/or is relieved by cold applications. It is also valuable when there are no strong indications for using any other remedy. **Hypericum** is useful for wounds that are hypersensitive to touch, especially if any part of the body richly supplied with nerves is injured, such as the back, fingers, feet, or eyeballs. **Staphysagria** is indicated for stab wounds to the abdomen or back (not for wounds to the spine, which are best treated with **Hypericum).**

If a puncture wound is serious enough to bring the person to a state of shock, internal doses of **Arnica** (the highest potencies possible) are recommended.

External applications of **Hypericum** should be considered at first, and toward the end of the healing, **Calendula** should be externally applied.

Dose: Take the 6, 12, or 30th potency every other hour for the first four doses and four times a day after that time, but generally not for more than three days.

BRUISES AND CONTUSIONS

Black-and-blue bruises are perhaps the most common type of injury, whether they result from falling, getting hit with a blunt object, or from medical instrumentation (getting your blood withdrawn or having an IV inserted).

Arnica is the number one homeopathic remedy for bruises. It helps strengthen blood vessels and aids in the absorption of blood. It is effective when used either internally or externally, though one will get the best results when using both approaches. However, **Arnica** should not be externally applied over an open wound; instead, it should be applied near it. One can also consider similarly applying one of the many injury or "sports injury" homeopathic external formulas which contain **Arnica.**

Ledum is the second most common remedy for bruises and is indicated when the bruise is relieved by cold applications. It is also a leading remedy for black eyes. **Hypericum** is useful for contusions to the fingers, toes, back, or anywhere there are many nerves. **Millefolium** is effective for bruises that are accompanied by persistent bleeding. **Bellis perennis** is helpful for injuries to deeper tissues, as is common from blows to the abdomen or the genitals, or from surgery. Like **Arnica,** it affects the blood vessels and helps to reduce swelling. It also helps to reduce near and remote effects of an injury. **Sulphuric**

acid is valuable for treating spontaneous bruising without injury, especially when accompanied by great fatigue.

Dose: Take the 6, 12, or 30th potency every four hours for one or two days. Reapply external applications after every washing or at least once a day.

BURNS

There are different degrees of burns: first, second, and third degree. First degree burns are the common minor burns that can result from briefly touching a hot pan or from overexposure to the sun. Second degree burns cause blistering of the skin. Third degree burns involve charring of the skin when all layers of the skin are burned. Second degree burns that cover an area larger than one's hand or any third degree burn require medical attention. Electrical, chemical, and radiation burns also require medical attention.

Following standard practices of the first-aid treatment of burns (including cleaning the wound and keeping it sterile) is essential, and homeopathic medicines can further aid the healing. For first degree burns, **Calendula** should be applied externally, and if the pain is significant, **Urtica urens** should be taken internally. For second degree burns, **Calendula** or **Hypericum** (or both) can be applied externally, and **Hypericum** or **Causticum** should be taken internally. For third degree burns, **Cantharis** should be taken internally.

External combination formulas for burns are very effective for healing various types of burns.

Because a person who gets a second or third degree burn inevitably experiences shock, internal doses of **Arnica** (the highest potencies possible) are recommended as the first homeopathic remedy.

Dose: Reapply external application with the changing of the burn's dressing. Take the 6, 12, or 30th potency every other hour at first, and then four times a day when the pain has significantly diminished.

SPRAINS AND STRAINS

Conventional treatment for sprains and strains is RICE (Rest, Ice, Compression, and Elevation). While this certainly makes sense, homeopaths prefer to add homeopathic medicines to make the treatment even more effective.

Arnica is an extremely common remedy for injuries to muscles and connective tissue. It is particularly useful for injuries from overuse. Even if another remedy is recommended internally, **Arnica** or a homeopathic combination formula that contains it should be applied externally to the sprain or strain.

Another common homeopathic medicine for sprains and strains is **Rhus tox.** The symptom complex that this remedy is known to treat effectively is called the "rusty gate" syndrome—that is, when people feel pain and stiffness upon initial motion, then limber up and feel decreasing amounts of pain and stiffness until they rest or sleep, and then are like a rusty gate on first moving again.

Bryonia is indicated for sprains and strains that are aggravated by any minor motion. It is particularly indicated for injuries to the chest and for frozen shoulder (another remedy that should be considered for frozen shoulder if **Bryonia** doesn't work is **Thiosinaminum**). **Bryonia** is also an important remedy for injured or tight hamstring muscles, especially if the muscle cannot take any motion without great pain.

Ruta is useful for torn ligaments, wrenched tendons, or bruised periosteum (bone covering). It is most effective after **Arnica** and/or **Rhus tox** has reduced the initial swelling. Injuries to the knee, shinbone, or elbow (including tennis elbow) are commonly relieved by this remedy. **Ruta** is also the leading remedy for runner's knee (chondromalacia), which includes symptoms of wobbly knees when walking or running.

In addition to the above remedies for the acute sprain or strain, the following remedies should be considered for recurrent sprains. **Ledum** is useful for people whose ankle pain is aggravated by applications of heat and relieved by cold applications. **Strontium carb** is helpful for people with chronic sprains who have persistent swelling and frequently icy cold feet, especially in the evening. **Natrum carb** is indicated in people with chronically weak ankles, who easily twist or dislocate their ankles, who tend to have an aversion to exercise, and who feel increased ankle pain from slight changes in weather.

Dose: Take 6, 12, or 30th potencies every two hours for the first several doses and then a dose four times a day for several days, if necessary.

Apply **Arnica** or external formulas that contain it in gel, ointment, or spray form after every washing or at least once a day.

INJURIES TO THE BONES

Fractures require medical attention to set the bones together; however, there are no conventional medical treatments available that augment bone healing. Homeopathic medicines can help in this regard.

One should first take **Arnica** for the shock and trauma of the fracture. After the initial state of shock is over, the most common homeopathic remedy for treating fractures is **Symphytum.** This remedy should not be given until the fracture has been set.

Ruta is a leading remedy for injuries to the bone (the periosteum), especially injuries to the elbow, the knee, and the shinbone, including old injuries to these parts.

Hypericum should be given along with other remedies if there is a compound fracture. Because **Hypericum** is so helpful for injuries to the nerves and because a compound fracture will inevitably cause nerve damage, this remedy is invaluable.

Bryonia is a leading remedy for fractured ribs.

If bones are slow to heal, **Calcarea phos** should be considered.

Dose: **Arnica** should be taken first in the highest potency available. Take it every hour for the first several doses. After six hours or so, use the 6, 12, or 30th potency of the indicated remedy every two hours during the first twenty-four hours, every four hours for the next twenty-four, and then four times a day for the next ten days.

HEAD INJURIES

Benjamin Spock once said that a child who never bumps his or her head is being watched too closely. Most of the time, head traumas aren't serious, even some that result in "goose egg" bumps. However, damage to the brain is possible from head injuries, since they can lead to bleeding or swelling underneath the skull or within the brain. Medical attention should be considered, especially when there has been a severe head injury or any subsequent symptoms.

Head injuries that are severe enough to injure the brain are called concussions, contusions, or hematomas, depending on the severity of the injury. A concussion includes a temporary loss of brain function, usually without permanent damage or bleeding in the brain. A contusion refers to a condition in which brain tissue is actually bruised, and a hematoma, the most serious of brain injuries, refers to a collection of blood as a result of broken blood vessels in the brain.

Any head injury that results in noticeable symptoms requires professional medical attention. In addition to such care, the following remedies will help decrease the possibility of complications from head injury. **Arnica** is the first remedy to consider for the acute pain, shock, and trauma felt immediately after any type of head injury. Typically, people who need this remedy are in a state of mild or severe shock. They may not think that anything is wrong and will tend to be confused and in a fog. **Arnica** is effective in treating people who are in a coma as a result of head injury as well as people who had a head injury several years ago but still experience some symptoms as a result of it. **Cocculus** is the leading remedy for people who experience dizziness after a head injury. The whole world seems to spin, forcing them to lie down. Nausea may be felt upon attempting to get up. **Cicuta** should be considered if a person develops epilepsy or convulsions after a head or spinal injury. It is also useful if the head injury was significant enough to lead to mental retardation.

Natrum sulph is the leading remedy when people have experienced symptoms as a result of head trauma in the past, even the distant past. After a head injury a wide range of both physical and psychological symptoms may be experienced which indicate this remedy, including headache with sensitivity to light and excessive salivation, depressive states with a suicidal disposition, and a worsening of health during wet weather. **Aurum** is useful for people who experience great depression as a result of head injury. Their physical and psychological pain may be significant enough that they contemplate suicide. This remedy commonly heals the head pain, depression, and suicidal thoughts. **Helleborus** is indicated when a person experiences stupefaction and mental dullness after a head injury. These people talk very slowly and with great effort, and their minds are almost completely blank. **Hypericum** is indicated for head injuries in which the person experiences sharp and/or shooting pains.

A constitutional remedy or an individualized acute remedy may be necessary for some people who develop idiosyncratic symptoms. If the injured individual does not fit any of the above-described remedies and if **Arnica** has not provided adequate relief, seek professional homeopathic care.

Dose: Take the 6, 12, or 30th potency every fifteen or thirty minutes during the first couple of hours after an injury. After this, a dose every two hours is recommended for those in severe pain or discomfort and every four hours for less severe pain. Stop doses once pain is mild or nonexistent. People who are treating an old head injury should take the 30th potency three times a day for two days, or fewer doses if the symptoms disappear.

INJURIES TO THE BACK

Back injuries can range from being minor traumas to being totally incapacitating. They are so common that back pain is one of the leading causes of missed work days. Homeopathic medicines do not take the place of appropriate physical therapy, chiropractic treatment, or massage, but the following remedies can help to reduce the pain and discomfort commonly experienced.

Arnica is indicated for the immediate shock and trauma of the injury. It is also useful for backaches where there is a generalized bruised sensation. **Hypericum,** which is sometimes called "the **Arnica** of the nerves," should be given alternating with **Arnica** shortly after the injury. It is most commonly prescribed for sharp and shooting back pains.

If a person still experiences pain a couple of days after the injury, **Rhus tox** should be given, especially if he or she has the "rusty gate" syndrome (aggravation of symptoms upon initial motion and then loosening up after continued motion). People who need **Rhus tox** may also experience an aggravation of their symptoms at night or during cold or cold, wet weather. It is useful not only for backaches but for neck pains as well.

Bryonia is a common remedy for injuries to the back or neck, especially when the problem is aggravated by any motion of the injured parts. People who need **Bryonia** are immobilized. They are even aggravated by deep breathing. **Colocynthis** is indicated for sudden, gripping, cramping pains in the back that are relieved by strong pressure and heat.

Besides the various internal remedies, external **Arnica** or external formulas that include it should be applied concurrently.

Dose: Take the 6, 12, or 30th potency (preferably the 30th) every hour immediately after injury, extending this to every other hour after the first six doses (or a night's rest, whichever comes first). If you choose to alternate **Arnica** and **Hypericum,** you can either take them together or take one remedy at one dosage time and the other at the next. External applications should be reapplied after every washing or at least two times a day.

CARPAL TUNNEL SYNDROME

Carpal tunnel syndrome is a relatively recently diagnosed injury which is in part the result of our industrial and postindustrial world. It is caused by compression of the median nerve in the wrist, usually the result of repetitive motions of the wrist, and increasing numbers of people are experiencing its debilitating effects. This condition is particularly common in people who spend many hours a day at a computer.

The most common homeopathic medicine for carpal tunnel syndrome is **Ruta.** Even before the recognition of this condition, homeopaths have known that **Ruta** is a primary remedy for wrist injuries, especially from overuse or flexing the wrist over edges. The wrist feels stiff and bruised, whether one is using it or not.

Rhus tox is helpful when the wrist has the "rusty gate" syndrome (pain on initial motion and reduced pain on continued motion). It is also useful when the pain is aggravated in cold or cold, wet weather. **Hypericum** should be considered if one experiences sharp or shooting pains extending from the wrist.

Causticum is indicated for chronic carpal tunnel syndrome, when a person not only feels bruised, burning, and drawing pains but also has great stiffness, constriction, and weakness in the wrist. Heat and warm applications provide some relief of discomfort, while cold aggravates the condition. **Guaiacum** is another remedy for the chronic stages of this condition. People who need this remedy experience a feeling of heat from the wrist. Their stiffness and pain is aggravated by heat and relieved by cold applications. And despite their stiffness, they feel compelled to stretch the wrist in order to keep it from becoming stiff.

In addition to the above internal remedies, external applications of **Arnica** or various combination formulas that include it is a useful adjunctive treatment.

Dose: Take the 6, 12, or 30th potency four times a day when experiencing pain. If no relief is observed for two days, consider another medicine. If the remedy provides relief but the condition continually returns, seek professional homeopathic care for a constitutional remedy that will strengthen the body's overall health.

MISCELLANEOUS INJURIES

Injuries to nerves: One generally knows that nerve injury has occurred when the pain is particularly sharp or shooting. **Hypericum** is the leading remedy for nerve injuries.

Phantom limb pain: Phantom limb pain refers to the pain experienced in limbs which have been amputated. **Hypericum** is the most common remedy for this condition.

Injuries to the eyeball: **Aconitum** is generally necessary to deal with the shock and trauma of injuries to the eyeball, while **Symphytum** is useful after the first six hours to help heal the injury itself. Medical care should be concurrently sought.

Joint dislocations: **Arnica** internally and externally helps to relieve the pain of a dislocation and helps to strengthen the connective tissue to reduce the chances of recurrent dislocations.

Dose: Take the 6, 12, or 30th potency every two hours in intense pain and every four hours in less intense pain. If significant pain or discomfort lasts more than a couple of days, seek medical attention.

RESOURCES

Stephen Cummings and Dana Ullman, *Everybody's Guide to Homeopathic Medicines.* Los Angeles: Tarcher, 1991.

Asa Hershoff, *Homeopathic Medicines for Musculoskeletal Problems.* Berkeley: North Atlantic (forthcoming).

Luc de Schepper, *Musculoskeletal Diseases and Homeopathy*. Santa Fe: Full of Life, 1994.

National Safety Council, *First Aid Handbook*. Boston: Jones and Bartlett, 1995.

Steven Subotnick, *Sports and Exercise Injuries*. Berkeley: North Atlantic, 1992.

Pre- and Postsurgical Treatment

Surgery represents conventional medicine at its best and its worst. On the one hand, surgery demonstrates incredibly sophisticated informational and technical advancement, yet on the other hand, it often indicates the inability of physicians and patients to prevent this invasive treatment of last resort.

Like other health professionals, homeopaths honor the special role that surgery and surgeons have in health care. Homeopaths are not against surgery, because certain conditions are simply not treatable without it. At the same time, however, surgery is often performed unnecessarily. It is performed when other, safer measures can be effectively used. It is performed too early when the body can sometimes heal itself. And it is performed inappropriately, primarily because surgeons only know surgery and don't know what else to do (the law of hammers pervades many professions: when you are a hammer, everything becomes a nail).

Even when surgery is successful, this does not necessarily mean that the person is "cured." Surgery may, for instance, remove an abscess, a tumor, kidney stones or gallstones, or other diseased parts, but because this removal doesn't change the underlying pathological processes that created them in the first place, it is understandable and even predictable that people tend to reexperience their ailment.

Even if the ailment seems to have disappeared, homeopaths do not believe that a curative process has always taken place. While the initial complaint may have been eradicated, sometimes more serious pathology develops shortly after the surgery. Although doctors tend to believe that this is a "new" disease, homeopaths theorize that the surgery probably suppressed the original ailment.

This critique of surgery is not meant to devalue its appropriate use in treating various congenital deformities, structural problems, severe injuries, or life-threatening pathological conditions. As previously stated, homeopaths are not against the judicious use of surgery.

When possible, homeopaths first attempt to see if treatment with an individualized homeopathic medicine can prevent the need for surgery. Patients and even homeopaths are sometimes surprised and impressed at the significant results that homeopathic medicines can provide—not that they can do the impossible, but they can often elicit a healing response when conventional therapeutics cannot.

The integration of homeopathic medicines with surgical care uses the best of both worlds to create comprehensive and ultimately more effective health care.

HOMEOPATHIC MEDICINES
BEFORE AND AFTER SURGERY

Once it is determined that surgery is medically necessary, homeopathic medicines can reduce complications of surgery and augment healing so that people can recover more quickly afterward.

Surgeons commonly ask patients not to take any food, drink, or drugs prior to surgery. While it makes sense to avoid food, drink, and conventional drugs, there have never been any reported problems from taking homeopathic remedies prior to surgery.

Some homeopaths recommend **Ferrum phos 6,** four times a day for two days, prior to surgery in order to prevent infection and hemorrhaging.

Homeopathic medicines can also help people deal with the various emotions they are experiencing prior to surgery. **Gelsemium 6** or **30** is a common remedy for the person who experiences great anxiety, apprehension, weakness, and trembling prior to surgery. **Aconitum 6** or **30** is indicated when the person is terrified about surgery and thinks that he will die from it.

Take either **Gelsemium** or **Aconitum** the night before the surgery and another dose upon waking in the morning. If fear and/or anxiety is felt after surgery, take one to three more doses.

One double-blind, randomized trial on fifty children who underwent surgery showed that 95 percent of those given the homeopathic medicine **Aconitum** experienced significantly less postoperative pain and agitation.[1] **Aconitum** was chosen because it is a common remedy for ailments in which sudden and violent onset of shock or trauma is a primary indication, as well as symptoms of fear and anxiety, which are especially common emotions experienced by children prior to surgery.

Arnica is another common homeopathic medicine given to people before and after surgery because of its ability to reduce surgical shock and minimize bleeding. Surgical shock is a condition that trauma or surgery can cause in which all the capillaries and small blood vessels are filled with blood at the same time. A randomized, placebo-controlled, crossover study showed that **Arnica** significantly decreased bleeding time.[2]

The late British homeopathic physician Donald Foubister recommended **Arnica 30** the night before surgery, another dose the morning of the surgery, another dose just prior to the surgery, and different medicines afterward, depending upon the type of surgery and the symptoms the patient feels.

Homeopathic medicines can also be beneficial for patients who undergo long-term intravenous (IV) therapy. Frequent insertion of an IV commonly causes phlebitis (inflammation of the vein) and hematoma (the pooling of blood under the skin); a double-blind study using **Arnica 5c** found that it can effectively reduce and prevent such problems.[3] The study showed significant benefits from **Arnica,** including reduced pain. Besides subjective improvement, there were also objectively measured increases in blood flow and in blood coagulation factors.

While **Arnica** is the primary remedy to be taken just prior to the majority of surgeries, there are a certain number of operations for which Dr. Foubister commonly recommended other remedies. For surgery involving cartilage and periosteum, as often occurs in the knee or elbow, it is recommended to take **Ruta 30** the evening before, the morning of the operation, and immediately afterward. For hemorrhoidal surgery, it is recommended to take either **Staphysagria 30** or **Aesculus 30** in a similar pattern as described for **Ruta.** And for circumcision, **Staphysagria 30** and **Arnica 30** should be given similarly as above.

The following are common recommendations for after surgery. Please note that the length of time of treatment can and should be different with each patient, depending upon the intensity of symptoms. Doses should generally be taken as long as pain persists, though they should not be taken for more than a couple of days, unless the person is still in pain and the remedy is providing obvious relief. **Arnica 6, 12,** or **30** should be given for at least two doses after surgery, approximately one hour apart. In addition to this remedy, the following remedies should be given one hour after the last dose of **Arnica:**

- gynecological surgery

  dilation and curettage: **Belladonna 30,** every six hours

  hysterectomy: **Causticum 30,** three times a day (some homeopaths recommend **Staphysagria 6** or **30,** three times a day)

  cesarean section or episiotomy: **Staphysagria 30** or **Bellis perennis 30,** three times a day

  abortion or miscarriage: **Ignatia 30,** every four hours

- plastic surgery on the breast: **Bellis perennis 6** or **30,** three times a day

- removal of the breast or a lump: **Hamamelis 30,** every four hours

- circumcision: **Staphysagria 30** and **Arnica 30,** every four hours for a day

- prostate surgery: **Staphysagria 30,** three times a day

- abdominal surgery: **Staphysagria 30** or **Bellis perennis 30,** three times a day

- appendectomy: **Rhus tox 30,** three times a day

- gastrectomy: **Raphanus 30,** three times a day

- gallbladder surgery: **Lycopodium 30,** three times a day

- eye surgery: **Ledum 30,** every four hours

- tonsillectomy and adenoidectomy: **Rhus tox 30,** every four hours

- orthopedic surgery

  involving cartilage or periosteum: **Ruta 30,** every four hours

  involving the spine: **Hypericum 30,** every four hours

- surgery for bullet wounds and/or stab wounds: **Staphysagria 30,** four times a day
- plastic surgery: **Arnica 30** (internally) and **Calendula** (externally), four times a day
- amputation: **Hypericum 30,** every four hours
- hemorrhoids: **Staphysagria 30** or **Aesculus 30,** every four hours for two or three days
- varicose veins: **Ledum 30,** three times a day
- dental surgery: **Hypericum 30** and **Ruta 30,** alternating every two to four hours

HOMEOPATHY FOR SPECIFIC AILMENTS AFTER SURGERY

Readers who experience symptoms or syndromes discussed elsewhere in this book should review those chapters. For instance, if you have urinary symptoms after surgery, which is common when catheterization takes place, consult the section on bladder infection in "Women's Conditions," page 191 (even if you are a man). If you are now suffering from acute insomnia, consult "Insomnia," page 268.

Some common conditions after surgery for which homeopathic medicines are often effective include the following:

Fear of Death

Aconitum 30 is indicated (every hour for up to four doses).

Bleeding

Arnica 30 helps to slow or stop bleeding after surgery. **Phosphorus 30** is the primary remedy for helping to stop bleeding when **Arnica** does not work adequately. **Ipecacuanha 30** is indicated when there is much bleeding of bright red blood, often accompanied by nausea. **Secale 30** is effective in treating uterine bleeding that is aggravated by heat and relieved by cold. **Cinchona 30** is helpful for people whose bleeding and general loss of fluids lead them to feel weak and faint and have ringing in the ears. This remedy is sometimes indicated several weeks, months, or years after much fluid has been lost, after either an illness or an operation. **Arsenicum 30** is useful when profuse bleeding leads to great weakness, burning pains, restlessness, anxiety, and fear, along with a characteristically large thirst for only sips at a time.

Dose: Take the remedy every hour until bleeding stops, not more than four doses. If bleeding has not significantly slowed, consider another remedy. The next day, take one more dose of whichever works to reduce the possible complications of blood loss.

Trauma to Tissue

Arnica topically and **Arnica 6** or **30** are useful when the muscle feels bruised or swollen and when there is any pooling of blood under the skin. **Hamamelis** topically and **Hamamelis 6** or **30** are effective when the person has weak veins, passive hemorrhage, bleeding hemorrhoids, or varicose veins. Capillaries are enlarged and congestion is marked. **Calendula** in external application (gel, ointment, tincture, spray) is indicated to heal wounds or incisions. **Bellis perennis 6** or **30** is a remedy for use after abdominal surgery and when deep internal tissue has been traumatized.

Dose: Apply external remedies at least once a day, and apply again if bathing washes them off. Generally, only two to eight doses of the internal remedy over a two-day period will be necessary to complete the healing process.

Wound Infection

External applications of **Calendula** and **Hypericum,** either alone or preferably together, help to both prevent and treat infection of surgical wounds. If pus has developed and caused hypersensitivity of the wound, **Hepar sulphur 30** is recommended. Because **Hepar sulphur** is an effective remedy for helping to push out splinters, pieces of glass, and various foreign objects that get stuck under the skin, it also has a tendency to push out surgical stitches. Thus it is not recommended to use this remedy when there are stitches, except toward the end of the healing process, when their removal is part of the healing. If the wound becomes purplish, **Lachesis 30** or **Gunpowder 30** is indicated. If there is much burning in the wound or wound area, **Sulphur 30** is helpful.

Dose: Apply external remedies at least once a day, and apply again if bathing washes them off. Take internal remedies every two to four hours during the first twenty-four hours and four times a day for two to five more days.

Scarring and Adhesions

Apply **Thiosinaminum** tincture externally or use an external combination formula that also contains **Calendula** (some injury gels include these ingredients). Take **Graphites 12** internally.

Dose: Apply external remedies at least once a day, and apply them again if bathing washes them off. You may need to do this for several week or months. Internal remedies should be taken three times a day for two days, and if necessary, repeated one month later.

Constipation

Raphanus 6 or **30** is indicated when there is constipation with no urgings for a stool and/or when there is painful gas; see also "Digestive Disorders," page 240, for other potential medicines for constipation.

Dose: Take this remedy three times a day for up to four days.

Nausea and Vomiting

Nux vomica 6 or **30** is good for violent retching, especially when there is generally ineffectual retching that does not lead to vomiting. **Phosphorus 6** or **30** helps to prevent or treat nausea after surgery; it is indicated when the patient has a strong thirst for ice drinks; he or she may also have a concurrent headache. **Ipecac 6** or **30** is effective for persistent nausea with vomiting, when vomiting does not provide relief. **Arsenicum 6** or **30** treats violent and incessant vomiting which is made worse by drinking water, especially cold water, or eating. There may also be burning pain in the stomach. See also "Digestive Disorders."

Dose: Take a remedy every two hours during intense symptoms and every four hours during less intense discomfort. If improvement is not obvious after twenty-four hours, consider another remedy.

Gas

Carbo veg 6 or **30** helps people who suffer from great distension and offensive gas, who get some relief from release of gas, and who desire carbonated drinks because they seem to help them release gas. **Cinchona 6** or **30** is useful when there is more pain than distension, frequent rumbling in the abdomen, and no relief from releasing gas. **Raphanus 6** or **30** is a common remedy for people who have a distended abdomen but are unable to expel gas. Because this condition is extremely common after surgery, especially abdominal surgery, this remedy is often indicated. **Colocynthis 6** or **30** is effective when there is more pain than distension, and also cramps that are relieved by bending over.

Dose: Take a remedy every two hours during intense pain and every four hours during mild discomfort. If improvement is not obvious after twenty-four hours, consider another remedy.

Bedsores

See the section in "Conditions of the Elderly," page 218, for details.

Homeopathic Resources

This book cannot possibly include all the important information that one needs to know about homeopathy. The following books, organizations, manufacturers, schools and training programs, journals and newsletters, and study groups will provide valuable information for those people who want to know more about using homeopathic medicines for themselves and their family, as well as for those who are interested in pursuing a career in the field.

Homeopathic Books: An Annotated Bibliography

Homeopaths believe in the power of small doses, but they also believe in large doses of homeopathic books. (An asterisk indicates a particularly good book.)

INTRODUCTORY AND FAMILY GUIDEBOOKS

Nancy Bruning and Corey Weinstein, *Healing Homeopathic Remedies.* New York: Dell, 1995. This book provides a basic overview of homeopathy and practical applications of the remedies.

*Dale Buegel, Blair Lewis, and Dennis Chernin, *Homeopathic Remedies for Health Professionals and Laypeople.* Honesdale, PA: Himalayan, 1991. This book has several unique features not found in other self-care books. In addition to the conventional listing of remedies for common conditions, the authors list under each condition the important questions to ask in order to find the best remedy. Also, there are fifteen computer-created charts which cross-index common symptoms of each ailment with those medicines known to cure it. This feature helps the reader to use remedies more precisely.

Miranda Castro, *The Complete Homeopathy Handbook*. New York: St. Martin's, 1990. No single homeopathy book can ever be "complete," but this handbook covers seventy common ailments, with special chapters on case taking and homeopathic external applications. The chapters on case taking provide examples of what symptoms should be collected from a sick person and how to figure out which remedy to give.

Trevor Cook, *Homeopathic Medicine Today*. New Canaan: Keats, 1989. Written by a homeopathic pharmacist, this book gives a good introduction to homeopathy's history, basic principles, and pharmacy (its strongest chapter), along with short chapters on research and on practical applications of select homeopathic remedies.

*Stephen Cummings and Dana Ullman, *Everybody's Guide to Homeopathic Medicines*. Los Angeles: Tarcher, 1991. This is presently the most popular homeopathic family guidebook in the United States. Distinct from many homeopathic guidebooks which provide too little information about how to properly individualize remedies, this book gives adequately detailed and useful information about key remedies. One of the book's unique features is that each chapter on specific ailments provides a detailed protocol for when medical care should be sought and when it is safe to use homeopathic or other home care measures.

Harold Gaier, *Encyclopedic Dictionary of Homeopathy*. London: Thorsons, 1991. This 601-page book provides historical and contemporary information about important homeopathic concepts, famous homeopaths, controversial topics, and clinical issues.

*Richard Grossinger, *Homeopathy: An Introduction for Beginners and Skeptics*. Berkeley: North Atlantic, 1993. Grossinger focuses on the philosophical, sociological, and anthropological implications of various modes of medical care. He immerses himself in the mystery of the phenomenon of healing and in the paradigm of healing that homeopathy presents. This is a sophisticated, intellectual overview of homeopathy and its meaning for society. Grossinger is more interested in the paradoxes that homeopathy creates and the dialogue that ensues than he is in the research itself.

Robin Hayfield, *Homeopathy for Common Ailments*. Berkeley: North Atlantic, 1993. This is a useful guidebook, though it does not provide as much useful information as most other guidebooks; it has some magnificent photographs of common homeopathic medicines which are not in any other homeopathic book. Some people use it as a coffee table book.

*Thomas Kruzel, *Homeopathic Emergency Guide*. Berkeley: North Atlantic, 1992. This book is not for beginners but for people who want the next step up. Initially written for practitioners, it teaches the reader how to be a more sophisticated user of homeopathic medicines for acute ailments. Kruzel describes more medicines and in more detail than any other family medicine guidebook, though he does not teach how to find the remedy or how to choose the correct potency or dosage.

Andrew Lockie, *The Family Guide to Homeopathy*. New York: Fireside, 1993. This book, for better and for worse, tries to do it all. It describes homeopathy, discusses how to find the correct remedy, and teaches how to treat virtually every disease (both acute and chronic). Because it is so ambitious, it does not always provide an adequate amount of information to help the reader find the correct remedy, and it encourages self-treatment for many serious and life-threatening conditions which should receive professional attention. Still, when used in accompaniment with other books and with some common sense, this book has much useful information.

Maesimund Panos and Jane Heimlich. *Homeopathic Medicine at Home*. Los Angeles: Tarcher, 1980. Written in a wonderfully folksy way, this popular book describes how to use homeopathic medicines to treat common ailments. It contains some useful charts to make the selection of the correct remedy easier.

Barry Rose, *The Family Guide to Homeopathy*. Berkeley: Ten Speed, 1993. This beautifully illustrated coffee table book is also a useful and practical guidebook. It is also a great gift book.

*Dana Ullman, *Discovering Homeopathy*. Berkeley: North Atlantic, 1991. This book not only helps readers understand homeopathy and the homeopathic approach to a wide variety of diseases, it also helps them better understand the modern conventional model of healing. Written for the advocate or skeptic of homeopathy, it reviews homeopathic research and presents a strong case for why homeopathy should become integrated within a comprehensive health care system.

George Vithoulkas, *Homeopathy: Medicine for the New Man*. New York: Arco, 1979. This short book is a good, though somewhat dated, introduction to homeopathy. One unique feature is that it includes descriptions of five homeopathic remedies and their bodymind pattern of symptoms.

*Edward C. Whitmont, *The Alchemy of Healing*. Berkeley: North Atlantic, 1993. Written by an internationally respected Jungian psychiatrist and homeopath, this is one of the most brilliant books about healing presently available. Although the first chapter focuses on homeopathy and the subject is mentioned in various parts of the book, it covers a much broader area than homeopathy. The author integrates new physics, Jungian and depth psychology, homeopathy, and alchemy.

Robert Wood, *Homeopathy: Medicine that Works*. Pollock Pines, CA: Condor, 1990. This book describes homeopathy from the point of view of a homeopathic patient. Although the author idealizes homeopathy and homeopaths, his personal experiences provide some insights into this healing method not available in other books.

SPECIALIZED SELF-CARE BOOKS

Miranda Castro, *Homeopathy for Pregnancy, Birth and Your Baby's First Year*. New York: St. Martin's, 1993. For a time in their lives when women need to avoid taking conventional drugs, this book provides specific information about which homeopathic medicines should be considered for common ailments during birth and pre- and postpregnancy. It is an excellent complement to Dr. Moskowitz's book (described below).

Peter Chappel, *Emotional Healing with Homeopathy*. Rockport, MA: Element, 1994. This is the best self-help manual to using homeopathic medicines to treat emotional problems, though it is not a simple guide, since no good book can provide simple answers to the complexities of psychological problems.

Susan Curtis and Romy Fraser, *Natural Healing for Women*. London: Pandora, 1991. This book discusses various natural therapies for treating women's ailments. Homeopathic medicines and botanical remedies are the two most thoroughly described treatments, though nutrition and aromatherapy are also included. Discussions of personal and spiritual awareness are integrated throughout the book. The authors provide more detailed information on homeopathic medicines than other books listed in this section, although it isn't as easy to use as Lockie and Geddes's book.

Colin B. Lessell, *The World Traveller's Manual of Homoeopathy*. Saffron Walden, England: C. W. Daniel, 1993. This book is an impressively comprehensive guide to homeopathic as well as general home-remedy treatment of common travel-related ailments. It is published with rounded corners and a strong and flexible spine, allowing for ease in travel.

*Andrew Lockie and Nicola Geddes, *The Women's Guide to Homeopathy*. New York: St. Martin's, 1994. This is the most comprehensive book on the subject presently available. Like Dr. Lockie's book described earlier, it is ambitious in attempting to teach the reader how to treat a wide variety of acute and chronic ailments. The same benefits and limitations of Dr. Lockie's other book apply to this one.

*Richard Moskowitz, *Homeopathic Medicine for Pregnancy and Childbirth*. Berkeley: North Atlantic, 1992. If you want only a single book on the subject, this should be it. Dr. Moskowitz's book provides the most information about how to use homeopathic medicines for pregnancy and childbirth. He describes how to find the right medicine to use, and he spices up his descriptions of each medicine with interesting case histories.

*Michael A. Schmidt, *Healing Childhood Ear Infections: What Conventional and Alternative Medicine Offers*. Berkeley: North Atlantic, 1996. This is the most comprehensive book on ear infections presently available. It reviews the conventional medical literature as well as the alternative health literature. It discusses the benefits and limitations of antibiotics and ear tubes. It also describes how to use nutrition, herbs, homeopathic medicines, and acupressure to treat ear problems.

Keith Souter, *Homoeopathy for the Third Age*. Saffron Walden, England: C. W. Daniel, 1993. This book tries to simplify using homeopathic medicines for psychological problems, and although it does so with the aid of interesting graphs, it is best used in concert with homeopathic *materia medica* and repertories.

*Steven Subotnick, *Sports and Exercise Injuries: Conventional, Homeopathic, and Alternative Treatments*. Berkeley: North Atlantic, 1991. This instructive and well-illustrated book provides much practical advice on how to treat various injuries, integrating whatever therapies work, with special emphasis on the use of homeopathic medicines.

*Dana Ullman, *Homeopathic Medicine for Children and Infants*. Los Angeles: Tarcher, 1992. This is the most detailed book on the homeopathic treatment of acute conditions of children. Although it is primarily directed at the treatment of pediatric conditions, the vast majority of ailments and the remedies for them can be directly applied to adults. This book actually has more information about homeopathic medicines than Cummings and Ullman's *Everybody's Guide to Homeopathic Medicine,* though not as much general health information.

*Robert Ullman and Judyth Reichenberg-Ullman, *The Patient's Guide to Homeopathic Medicine.* Edmunds, WA: Picnic Point, 1995. This book describes homeopathy clearly and answers common questions about what to expect from professional homeopathic care.

*Janet Zand, Rachel Walton, and Bob Rountree, *Smart Medicine for a Healthier Child.* New York: Avery, 1994. This A-to-Z guidebook provides information about almost every common pediatric ailment and the recommended homeopathic, nutritional, herbal, and conventional medical treatments for them. The authors then give their personal recommendations on which therapies to use first.

PHILOSOPHY AND METHODOLOGY

Note: Books on philosophy and methodology are primarily for students or practitioners of homeopathy, though anyone with a serious interest in the healing process can learn much from them.

M. L. Dhawale, *Principles and Practice of Homoeopathy.* Bombay: D. K. Homoeopathic Corporation, 1967. This book provides a good overview of the homeopathic methodology to selecting an individualized remedy and analyzing its efficacy.

*Samuel Hahnemann, *Organon of Medicine.* New Delhi (reprint); also Blaine, WA: Cooper Publishing. This seminal book by homeopathy's founder is essential reading for serious students and practitioners of homeopathy because it lists each postulate/principle of the homeopathic method. Although written in the 1830s and 1840s, the book was ahead of its time and it is in the forefront of medicine today.

*James Tyler Kent, *Lectures on Homoeopathic Philosophy.* Berkeley: North Atlantic, 1979 (reprint). Originally written in 1900, this book sought to update Hahnemann's *Organon.* Like the *Organon,* it is considered essential reading because both lay the foundation for understanding homeopathic philosophy and methodology.

Gerhard Koehler, *The Handbook of Homeopathy.* Rochester, VT: Healing Arts, 1987. This is a popular textbook with good chapters on case taking, different ways to find the correct medicine, and how to use the repertory.

H. A. Roberts, *The Principles and Art of Cure by Homoeopathy.* New Delhi: B. Jain (reprint). This book updates Kent's book, described above, and is easier to read and to understand.

*Rajan Sankaran, *The Spirit of Homeopathy.* Bombay: Homeopathic Medical, 1991. This is not a comprehensive review of all the important methodological issues involved in homeopathic practice, but it is an exceptional and insightful book for those subjects dealing with case taking and case analysis that it covers. Sankaran is particularly known for special insights into using a person's psychological characteristics to find the correct homeopathic medicine.

*George Vithoulkas, *The Science of Homeopathy.* New York: Grove, 1980. Written by a leading contemporary homeopath, this book is an overview of homeopathy and the homeopathic method. It also includes good information for anyone interested in real healing, as is evidenced by the first several chapters, which include a detailed discussion on the definition of health.

MATERIA MEDICA AND REPERTORIES

Note: Most of these books are useful primarily for professional homeopaths, though most people will be able to understand and use them. By adding a *materia medica* and a repertory to your library, you can be more precise in the selection of an individualized remedy. (A *materia medica* is a book that lists homeopathic medicines and the various symptoms and syndromes they are know to cure. A repertory is a listing of symptoms and the various medicines that have been found to cause them in overdose and cure them in homeopathic doses. It is common for people to have several *materia medica* and at least one repertory.)

H. C. Allen, *Keynotes and Characteristics of the Materia Medica.* New Delhi: B. Jain (reprint). This book provides short summaries of the key features of common remedies. Although the symptoms are simply listed without elaboration, the book provides useful skeletal information about remedies.

*Philip Bailey, *Homeopathic Psychology: Personality Profiles of the Major Constitutional Remedies.* Berkeley: North Atlantic, 1995. This important work briefly describes thirty-five key homeopathic constitutional types, with primary focus on each type's psychological char-

acteristics. The author provides insight into the most significant behavioral patterns, emotional tendencies, internal conflicts, and spiritual issues that each typology faces.

*William Boericke, *Pocket Manual of Materia Medica with Repertory.*
Santa Rosa: Boericke and Tafel (reprint). Owned by virtually every
homeopath, this book is also useful to any layperson interested in improving his or her prescribing for acute ailments. This is the only book
presently available that includes a *materia medica* and a repertory. Although these two sections are abbreviated to fit them into one book,
the summary information is excellent.

John Clarke, *Dictionary of Practical Materia Medica* (3 volumes). Saffron Walden, England: C. W. Daniel. Reprint. Mostly useful to the
practicing homeopath, this three-volume text provides detailed information about most remedies presently available.

*Catherine Coulter, *Portraits of Homoeopathic Medicines* (2 volumes). Berkeley: North Atlantic, 1986, 1988. The author is a homeopath with a graduate degree in European literature. She describes the
homeopathic typologies in light of famous authors and characters
from novels. Each volume covers nine constitutional types.

*D. M. Gibson, *Studies of Homoeopathic Remedies.* Beaconsfield,
(England): Beaconsfield, 1987. This excellent *materia medica* describes
the key symptoms of over a hundred remedies in clear, modern language. Rather than listing symptoms according to parts of the body,
the author describes them according to systems of the body (i.e., respiratory, circulatory, endocrine).

Constantine Hering, *Guiding Symptoms of Our Materia Medica* (10
volumes). New Delhi: B. Jain (reprint). For the practicing homeopath,
this set of books is the best multivolume text. Although it does not
cover as many remedies as Clarke's three-volume set, it provides more
information about those remedies it does cover.

*Paul Herscu, *The Homeopathic Treatment of Children: Pediatric
Constitutional Types.* Berkeley: North Atlantic, 1991. Eight of the most
common constitutional types of children are vividly described, with
specific references to how different types of children behave in a doctor's office and within family situations.

*James Tyler Kent, *Lectures on Homoeopathic Materia Medica.* New
Dehli: B. Jain (reprint). Considered a classic, this book is vital for
learning about homeopathic medicines. It is known for its useful and
reliable information about the constitutional features of remedies.

*————, *Repertory of Homeopathic Materia Medica.* New Delhi: B.

Jain (reprint). This repertory is the *standard* text that homeopaths use to look up a person's symptoms. It is also very helpful to nonpractitioners who wish to improve the quality of their home use of homeopathic remedies.

*Roger Morrison, *Desktop Guide to Keynotes and Confirmatory Symptoms.* Berkeley: Hahnemann, 1993. Written by one of America's leading homeopaths primarily for fellow practitioners, this book provides information about more than three hundred remedies, mostly for constitutional care.

*Robin Murphy, *Nature's Materia Medica.* Pagosa Springs, CO: HANA, 1995. This excellent *materia medica* (1,000+ pages) integrates information from the classical and modern texts. The author provides information about both constitutional and acute care.

———, *Homoeopathic Medical Repertory:* Pagosa Springs, CO: HANA, 1993. This book adds many common modern symptoms and syndromes to Kent's *Repertory.* The author has also reordered the chapters by alphabetical listing, making it easier to use than other repertories.

E. B. Nash, *Leaders in Homoeopathic Therapeutics.* New Delhi: B. Jain (reprint). This book provides key information about a hundred or so common remedies, primarily for constitutional prescribing.

Rajan Sankaran, *The Substance of Homeopathy.* Bombay: Homeopathic Medical, 1994. This fascinating book describes how to use the mineral remedies in homeopathy for constitutional care. The author discusses the nature of each element, its place on the chemical chart used in chemistry, and the implications of this in homeopathic care.

F. Schroyens, *Synthesis Repertorium.* London: Homeopathic Book Publishers, 1993. This new repertory is the most detailed repertory presently available in a single volume.

Margaret Tyler, *Drug Pictures.* Saffron Walden, England: C. W. Daniel, 1952. The author provides quotes from the past masters of homeopaths describing how they used a hundred or so common medicines. She then discusses her own experiences with treatment, and describes the symptoms that each medicine is best known to treat.

Leon Vannier, *Typology in Homoeopathy.* Beaconsfield: Beaconsfield, 1992. The author describes homeopathic typologies in reference to archetypes from Greek and Roman mythology.

Roger Van Zandvoort, *The Complete Repertory* (3 volumes). Leidschendam, the Netherlands; IRHIS, 1994. This is the most complete repertory in a multivolume text.

Frans Vermuelen, *Concordance Materia Medica*. Haarlem, the Netherlands, 1994. This book attempts to update Boericke's *materia medica* by emulating its style but integrating the writings of past and present masters of homeopathy into its 1,000+ pages.

*Edward C. Whitmont, *Psyche and Substance: Essays on Homeopathy in the Light of Jungian Psychology*. Berkeley: North Atlantic, 1991. A brilliant book, half of which is devoted to describing homeopathy in light of Jungian psychology, new physics, and alchemy, and half devoted to describing thirteen homeopathic medicines for constitutional care.

*Ananda Zaren, *Core Elements of the Materia Medica of the Mind* (2 volumes). Gottingen: Burgdorf, 1993, 1994. The author writes with special insight into primary psychological issues in people's lives and describes homeopathic medicines in light of them.

SCIENCE AND RESEARCH

*Paolo Bellavite and Andrea Signorini, *Homeopathy: A Frontier in Medical Science*. Berkeley: North Atlantic, 1995. This book provides the most comprehensive review of homeopathic research presently available. Besides covering laboratory and clinical research, it provides sound, up-to-date, even cutting-edge theoretical foundations for homeopathic microdoses. An exceedingly important book.

Harris L. Coulter, *Homoeopathic Science and Modern Medicine: The Physics of Healing with Microdoses*. Berkeley: North Atlantic, 1980. Though this book is dated, it contains some valuable references to old homeopathic research as well as to microdose research in other fields.

M. Doutremepuich (ed.), *Ultra-Low Doses*. Washington, D.C./London: Taylor and Francis, 1991. Like *Ultra High Dilution,* this book consists of specific studies, including those in experimental pharmacology, biophysics, biochemistry/toxicology, cell biology, and clinical pharmacology.

*P. C. Endler and J. Schulte (eds.), *Ultra High Dilution: Physiology and Physics*. Dordrecht: Kluwer Academic, 1994. This work consists of scientific studies and theoretical expositions by respected researchers in the various scientific fields. While the Bellavite and Signorini book is the best for describing the various studies, this book includes the studies themselves (no clinical studies are provided; only basic science work is included).

Dana Ullman, *Monograph on Homeopathic Research* (2 volumes). Berkeley: Homeopathic Educational Services, 1981, 1986. These monographs contain reprinted articles on homeopathic research and on theoretical discussions of their possible mechanism of action.

Roeland van Wijk and Fred A. C. Wiegant. *Cultured Mammalian Cells in Homeopathy Research: The Similia Principle in Self-Recovery.* Utrecht: University of Utrecht, 1994. This technical book describes a body of laboratory studies performed by professors of molecular cell biology which not only verify the biological effects of homeopathic microdoses but also provide evidence for the homeopathic principle of similars as an effective pharmacological methodology.

History of Homeopathy

Trevor Cook, *Samuel Hahnemann: His Life and Times.* Wellingborough: Thorsons, 1981. The author describes the life and times of homeopathy's founder.

*Harris L. Coulter, *Divided Legacy: A History of the Schism in Medical Thought* (4 volumes). Berkeley: North Atlantic, 1975, 1977, 1981, 1994. These four volumes provide a history of Western medicine from Hippocrates to the present, describing two prominent schools of medical thought: the rational and the empirical. While modern medicine today developed from the rational school, homeopathy developed from the empirical. Of special interest to people interested in the history of homeopathy is volume 3: *Divided Legacy: The Conflict Between Homoeopathy and the American Medical Association.*

*Rima Handley, *A Homeopathic Love Story.* Berkeley: North Atlantic, 1990. The author describes the relationship between homeopathy's founder and his second wife, an artist and feminist, age thirty-four, when he married at seventy-nine. The book also provides much new information about the way Hahnemann practiced during the last ten years of his life.

Matthew Wood, *The Magical Staff: The Vitalist Tradition in Western Medicine.* Berkeley: North Atlantic, 1992. This fascinating book provides biographical vignettes about seven leading Western physician/healers whose work popularized concepts of energy in healing.

Homeopathic Tapes

Individual tapes from lectures at conferences and sets of tapes from specialty workshops are available from select homeopathic resources.

Dana Ullman, *Homeopathic Healing: An Introduction to Homeopathic Medicine* (set of six tapes). Boulder: Sounds True, 1995. This set of tapes provides an overview of homeopathy and its approach to health and disease. Listeners are taught how to use over thirty homeopathic remedies for common acute ailments and injuries.

Dr. Robin Murphy is a naturopath who specializes in homeopathy. He offers over thirty different sets of tapes on various subjects (each set contains six to twelve tapes), including children's health care, women's ailments, psychological problems, dermatology disorders, fevers and infectious diseases, nervous disorders, musculoskeletal problems, and gastroenterology problems. These tapes are not on an introductory level, but they are useful to anyone who wishes information on specific topics.

Edward C. Whitmont, *Homeopathy and Jungian Psychotherapy* (seven tapes). The first half of this set of tapes is a brilliant presentation on homeopathy in light of Jungian psychotherapy, new physics, and alchemy. The second half focuses on dream analysis from a Jungian perspective.

Homeopathic Software

Homeopathy has entered the computer age, with programs for both the general public and the professional homeopath.

The Homeopath. This DOS software is designed for the layperson and is simple to use. Twenty common ailments are a part of the program, including colds, flu, sore throat, cough, earache, headache, indigestion, urinary problems, and various injuries. The program asks the users specific questions, and after receiving the answers, recommends a remedy. Information on fifty-nine different remedies is provided.

CARA. This excellent DOS- or Window-based program is designed for the practicing homeopath. Although not as elaborate as the *MacRepertory,* it still provides access to several major repertories and *material medica,* and it is quite cost-friendly.

The MacRepertory. Designed for the practicing homeopath, this program is the most sophisticated presently available. Comprising several modules, it gives users access to virtually every known repertory and *materia medica,* and a new program provides access to hundreds of old homeopathic journals. Available for MacIntosh and IBM.

Radar. This excellent IBM-based program provides access to several repertories and *materia medica* and includes an expert system developed by Greek homeopath George Vithoulkas.

Homeonet. Homeonet is not a software program but a computer network of professional homeopaths and serious students of homeopathy who converse about homeopathy. You can access up-to-date information about upcoming conferences, seminars, media coverage of homeopathy, research, and numerous other discussion topics. There is a monthly fee to access Homeonet. For further information, contact: Institute for Global Communications, 18 De Boom Street, San Francisco, CA 94107, (415) 442-0220.

Source of Homeopathic Books, Tapes, and Software

Homeopathic Educational Services
2124 Kittredge Street
Berkeley, CA 94704
(510) 649-0294

Note: Many of the sources of homeopathic medicines listed later in this section also sell homeopathic books.

Homeopathic Organizations

National Center for Homeopathy
801 North Fairfax, #306
Alexandria, VA 22314
(703) 548-7790

This is the most important American homeopathic organization. It publishes a monthly magazine, maintains an active network of homeopathic study groups, holds annual conferences and short summer training programs for laypeople and health professionals, and provides spokespersons to the media.

International Foundation for Homeopathy
2366 Eastlake Avenue East #325
Seattle, WA 98102
(206) 324-8230

This organization specializes in training homeopaths. It also publishes a bimonthly magazine and organizes an annual conference for serious students and practitioners of homeopathy.

American Institute of
Homeopathy
1585 Glencoe Street, #44
Denver, CO 80220
(303) 321-4105

Founded in 1844 and the oldest national medical society in the country, this organization admits only medical doctors and osteopaths as voting members. It publishes a journal and sponsors or co-sponsors an annual conference. It also interfaces with government bodies on issues relating to the homeopathic profession.

Foundation for Homeopathic
Education and Research
2124 Kittredge Street
Berkeley, CA 94704
(510) 649-8930

This organization seeks to educate the medical community and the general public about research in homeopathy. It provides speakers on homeopathic research to hospitals, medical schools, industry, and community groups.

Homeopathic Academy of
Naturopathic Physicians
14653 South Graves Road
Mulino, OR 97042

This is the organization of naturopathic physicians who specialize in homeopathy. They certify qualified naturopaths, and they publish a professional journal.

American Homeopathic
Pharmacists Association
P.O. Box 174
Norwood, PA 19074

One of two homeopathic pharmacist trade organizations

American Association of
Homeopathic Pharmacists
P.O. Box 11280
Albuquerque, NM 87192

One of two homeopathic pharmacist trade organizations.

Sources of Homeopathic Medicines

The following companies either manufacture homeopathic medicines or provide a mail order service for them. Homeopathic medicines are also commonly available at health food stores and pharmacies, though the following list of companies provides a more extensive assortment of homeopathic remedies.

Biological Homeopathic
Industries
11600 Cochiti S.E.
Albuquerque, NM 87123
(505) 293-3843

Boericke and Tafel
2381 Circadian Way
Santa Rosa, CA 95407
(707) 571-8202

Boiron-Bornemann, Inc.
6 Campus Boulevard, Building A
Newtown Square, PA 19073
(610) 325-7464
also:
98c West Cochran
Simi Valley, CA 93065
(805) 582-9091

Dolisos
3014 Rigel Road
Las Vegas, NV 89102
(702) 871-7153

Homeopathic Educational
Services
2124 Kittredge Street
Berkeley, CA 94704
(510) 649-0294

Hahnemann Pharmacy
828 San Pablo
Albany, CA 94706

Luyties Pharmacal
4200 Laclede Avenue
St. Louis, MO 63108
(314) 533-9600

Medicine From Nature
10 Mountain Springs Parkway
Springville, UT 84663
(801) 489-1500

Standard Homeopathic
Company
204-210 West 131st Street
Los Angeles, CA 90061
(310) 321-4284

Homeopathic Training Programs

Note: With the exception of the naturopathic medical schools (see page 372) which provide full-time instruction, all other training programs are primarily two to four days per month of instruction. In addition to course hours, students are usually expected to study from one to three hours a day.

Hahnemann Medical Clinic
828 San Pablo
Albany, CA 94706
(510) 524-3117

An excellent high-level three-year training in classical homeopathy led by leading homeopaths. This program is open only to licensed professionals.

Pacific Academy of
Homeopathic Medicine
1678 Shattuck, #42
Berkeley, CA 94709
(510) 389-8065

A three-year program is open to both laypeople and professionals.

International College of
Homeopathy and Bio-Dynamic
Studies
8306 Wilshire Boulevard, #728
Beverly Hills, CA 90211
(213) 734-4798

A 400-hour course plus 200 hours of clinical instruction (in India) over a thirty-two-month period is offered. Only licensed health care professionals are admitted. Affiliated with New York Chiropractic College (continuing education credit for chiropractors is provided).

British Institute of
Homoeopathy
520 Washington Boulevard,
#423
Marina del Rey, CA 92092
(310) 306-5408

A three-year course is offered to either health professionals or laypeople.

Institute of Classical
Homeopathy
1336-D Oak Avenue
St. Helena, CA 94574
(707) 963-2022.

The primary teacher of this course, located north of San Francisco, is Nikki Henriques, a student of British homeopath Sheilagh Creasy.

Training in Clinical
Homeopathy
556 Ocean View Avenue
Santa Cruz, CA 95062
(408) 425-1422

Respected homeopath and author Ananda Zaren teaches five three-day weekend seminars over a one-year period. One course is in Santa Barbara and the other is in Boston.

Academy for Classical
Homeopathy
7549 Louise Avenue
Van Nuys, CA 91406
(818) 776-8040

Dr. Linda Johnston, a physician and homeopath, offers a one-year training program to licensed health professionals only. Training available in Dallas, Minneapolis, Philadelphia, and selected other cities.

Colorado Institute for Classical
Homeopathy
1441 York Street, #301
Denver, CO 80206
(303) 329-6345

A two-year program open to health professionals and the general public.

Hahnemann Academy of North
America
P.O. Box 358
Pagosa Springs, CO 81147
(303) 264-2460.

Well-known homeopath/naturopath Robin Murphy, N.D., offers training programs.

New England School of
Homeopathy
356 Middle Street
Amherst, MA 01002
(203) 253-5041

Famed homeopath/naturopath Paul Herscu, N.D., offers training programs in Massachusetts, Northern Virginia, and occasionally other locations.

The Northwestern Academy of
Homeopathy
10700 Old County Road, #15
Minneapolis, MN 55441
(612) 593-9458.

A three-year program is offered
to either health professionals or
laypeople.

Five Elements Center
115 Route 46 West, Building D,
#29
Mountain Lakes, NJ 07046
(201) 335-1755

Introductory level courses are offered to all interested parties.

Atlantic Academy of Classical
Homeopathy
209 First Avenue, #2
New York, NY 10003
(718) 518-4593

A three-year program for health
professionals and laypeople is offered. Students can obtain some
credit for instruction at other
schools or training programs.

National Center for
Homeopathy
801 North Fairfax #306
Alexandria, VA 22314
(703) 548-7790

The National Center for Homeopathy (NCH) offers one- and
two-week summer courses for
health professionals and laypeople. They also offer courses for
dentists and veterinarians.

International Foundation for
Homeopathy
2366 Eastlake Avenue East, #301
Seattle, WA 98102
(206) 324-8230

A three-year training program is
provided for licensed professionals only.

Homeopathic Master Clinician
Course
F–31
Bowen Island, B.C. V0N 1G0
Canada

Louis Klein, RSHom, leads an
advanced training program in
various cities, including San
Francisco, Los Angeles, Vancou-
ver, Boston, and Orlando.

NATUROPATHIC MEDICAL SCHOOLS

National College of
Naturopathic Medicine
11231 S.E. Market
Portland, OR 97216
(503) 255-4860

Bastyr University
144 N.E. 54th Street
Seattle, WA 98105
(206) 523-0595

Southwest College of
Naturopathic Medicine
6535 East Osborn Road
Scottsdale, AZ 85251
(602) 990-7424

Ontario College of Naturopathic
Medicine
60 Berl Street
Toronto, Canada

Admission to these quality naturopathic medical schools requires
similar premedicine undergraduate course work as medical
school. The first two years are
primarily basic medical sciences,
while the last two focus on clinical naturopathic training, including homeopathic medicine.

SPECIALIZED TRAINING PROGRAMS

National Dental Seminars
P.O. Box 123
Marengo, IL 60152

Special training for dentists is offered.

Academy of Veterinary
Homeopathy
1283 Lincoln Street
Eugene, OR 97401
(503) 342-7665

Training in veterinary homeopathy is provided

Correspondence Courses

There are two responsible correspondence courses presently available.

The School of Homoeopathy
c/o Homeopathic Educational
Services
2124 Kittredge Street
Berkeley, CA 94704
(510) 649-0294

to devote two and a half hours a day, five days a week. Additional course work in *anatomy and physiology* as well as *disease and pathology* is also available via correspondence.

This course is also available from:
Center for Preventive Medicine
and Homeopathy
111 Bala Avenue
Bala Cynwyd, PA 19004
(610) 667-2927

Primarily taught by British homeopath Misha Norland, this course integrates taped instruction, written material, books, and homework. To complete in two years, students are expected

The British Institute of
Homeopathy
520 Washington Boulevard,
#423
Marina del Rey, CA 90292
(310) 306-5408

This course takes approximately two years and integrates written material, books, and several audio and video tapes. The primary teacher is Trevor Cook, a homeopathic pharmacist.

For People Interested in Traveling Abroad

Royal London Homoeopathic
Hospital
Great Ormond Street
London WC1N 3HR, England

This course offers training programs for medical doctors and pharmacists.

Society of Homoeopaths
2 Artizan Road
Northampton NN1 4HU,
England

There are numerous four-year (on weekends) training programs in England that are open to anyone interested in the serious study of homeopathy. Contact the Society for a list of these schools.

Glasgow Homeopathic Hospital
1000 Great Western Road
Glasgow G12 ONR, Scotland

This program is the most popular post-graduate medical training in the United Kingdom.

University of Oxford Department of Continuing Education
c/o HPTG
22 Farndon Road
Oxford OX2 6RT, England

This course offers training programs for medical doctors and pharmacists.

University of Western Sydney
Bourke Street
Richmond NSW 2753, Australia

A new program in homeopathy has developed within this conventional university.

Australian College of Natural Medicine
362 Water Street
Fortitude Valley, Brisbane 4006, Australia

A three-year full-time program in natural medicine, with a specialty in homeopathy.

Oceanic Institute of Classical Homoeopathy
404 Great Eastern Highway
West Midland 6056, Western Australia

The Foundation for Homeopathic Research
8-5-Giriraj, Neelkanth Valley
Ghatkopar, Bombay 400 077, India

Founded by one of Rajan Sankaran's leading students, this school offers a month-long course specifically designed for American and European students/practitioners.

Homeopathic Certification

American Board of Homeotherapeutics
801 North Fairfax, #306
Alexandria, VA 22314

This board certifies M.D.s and D.O.s, awarding them a D.Ht.

Council on Homeopathic Certification
P.O. Box 157
Corte Madera, CA 94976

The CHC provides certification to *any licensed or unlicensed individ-*

ual who has graduated from one of the accredited training programs in homeopathy. Although this certification has only just begun, it has already developed an excellent reputation of high quality. In other words, the test is quite difficult.

Homeopathic Academy of
Naturopathic Physicians
P.O. Box 69565
Portland, OR 97201

This board certifies naturopathic physicians, awarding them a D.H.A.N.P.

National Board of Homeopathic
Examiners
8306 Wilshire Boulevard, #720
Beverly Hills, CA 90211

The NBHE provides certification to *any licensed or unlicensed individual* who has graduated from one of the accredited training programs in homeopathy.

North American Society
of Homeopaths
17700 Old County Road 15
Minneapolis, MN 55441

NASH certifies only *unlicensed practitioners.* To obtain certification one must have completed an approved training program and clinical internship and pass a comprehensive examination in homeopathy. Although this certification does not grant legal right to practice homeopathy, it is beginning to lay the groundwork for a distinct profession of homeopaths.

Homeopathic
Journals and Newsletters

British Homoeopathic Journal
Headley Brothers
The Invicta Press
Ashford, Kent TN24 8HH,
England

This quarterly journal contains more research than any other journal. It also has an excellent section that reviews major articles from other homeopathic journals internationally.

Journal of the American Institute of Homeopathy
1585 Glencoe Street
Denver, CO 80220

Primarily for professional homeopaths, this quarterly journal mainly includes articles on homeopathic clinical practice.

Homeopathy Today
National Center for Homeopathy
801 North Fairfax, #306
Alexandria, VA 22314

This monthly magazine is useful for people new to homeopathy or not and is provided free with membership in the NCH. It is an excellent resource for information on American homeopathy, news from the National Center, details of upcoming events, and interesting articles.

Resonance
International Foundation for Homeopathy
2366 Eastlake Avenue East, #301
Seattle, WA 98102

This bimonthly magazine is for people new to homeopathy or not and is free with membership in the IFH. It is an excellent newsletter that keeps people up to date on various developments in homeopathy, as well as trainings and conferences in classical homeopathy.

Simillimum
Homeopathic Academy of Naturopathic Physicians
P.O. Box 69565
Portland, OR 97201

Primarily directed at students or practitioners of homeopathy, this quarterly journal has excellent articles, mostly on *materia medica* and case histories.

New England Journal of Homeopathy
356 Middle Street
Amherst, MA 06082

Directed at students and practitioners of homeopathy, this excellent quarterly journal provides articles on case histories and *materia medica*.

The Prover
5627 Atlantic Boulevard, #2
Jacksonville, FL 32207

This bimonthly magazine is written mostly by and directed to chiropractors who integrate homeopathy in their practice.

The American Homeopath
1550 Huston Road
Lafayette, CA 94549

Published once a year, this journal is oriented toward the serious student or practitioner of classical homeopathy.

Tiger Tribe
1407 East College Street
Iowa City, IO 52245

This great bimonthly magazine focuses on the homeopathic and natural treatment of cats.

Natural Pet
P.O. Box 351
Trilby, FL 33593-0351

Like the above magazine, this bimonthly publication focuses on natural treatments for animals, though it generally does not have as many articles on homeopathy.

The Homoeopath: The Journal of the Society of Homoeopaths
2 Artizan Road
Northampton NN1 4HU, England

This excellent quarterly publication is directed at students and practitioners of homeopathy. Besides quality articles on homeopathic practice, articles on philosophical issues involved in healing are frequently published.

Health and Homoeopathy
Hahnemann House
2 Powis Place
Great Ormond Street
London WC1N 3HT, England

This glossy quarterly magazine is directed primarily toward lay-

people. It includes many personal statements about homeopathy and homeopathic successes and has information about homeopathy in England.

Homeopathic Links
Bantigerstrasse 37
CH 3006 Bern, Switzerland

This superb and sophisticated quarterly journal of classical homeopathy is oriented toward students and practitioners of homeopathy.

Homeopathy International
243 The Broadway
Southall, Middx UB1 11NF
England

This quarterly magazine is published by the U.K. Homeopathic Medical Association for laypeople and health professionals.

European Journal for Classical Homeopathy
P.O. Box 56603, 8601 Warden A
Markham, Ontario L3R OM6, Canada

Edited by George Vithoulkas, this excellent quarterly journal focuses on clinical and research issues.

JOURNALS IN FRENCH, GERMAN, AND SPANISH

Les Annales Homéopathiques Françaises, 64800 Arros-Nay, C.C.P. 2594-63, Bordeaux, France

Revue Belge d'Homoeopathie, av. Cardinal Micara 7, 1160 Brussels, Belgium

Cahiers de Biothérapie, Société Médicale de Biothérapie, 71, rue Beaubourg, 75013 Paris, France

Allgemeine Homöopathische Zeitung, Karl F. Haug Verlag, Fritz-Frey-Str. 21, Postfach 10 28 40, D-6900 Heidelberg 1, Germany

L'Homéopathie Française, 16, rue Mumont d'Urville, 75116 Paris, France

Zeitschrift für Klassische Homöopathie, Karl F. Haug Verlag, Fritz-Frey-Str. 21, Postfach 10 28 40, D-6900 Heidelberg 1, Germany

L'Homéopathie Européene, 1–3, rue du Départ, 75014 Paris, France

La Homeopatía de México, Mirto 26 y 28, México 06400, D.F.

MISCELLANEOUS

Many medical school libraries carry new and old homeopathic journals. Some medical schools are treasure houses of this literature. Make certain to check the "closed stacks" departments of these libraries. Some of the good older journals are the *Homoeopathic Recorder,* the *Medical Advance,* the *North American Journal of Homoeopathy,* and the *Homoeopathic Physician.*

Homeopathic Educational Services sells a special index of the *Homoeopathic Recorder* and the *Proceedings of the International Hahnemannian Association* (1881–1958). This authoritative index lists authors, titles, remedies, and subjects covered. Of additional special interest, Dr. Maesimund Panos, who helped compile this impressive index, will make any article listed in this book available at reasonable prices (her address is listed in the book).

Homeopathic Study Groups

The National Center for Homeopathy coordinates over a hundred homeopathic study groups throughout North America. These groups of from ten to two hundred people meet usually once or twice a month to study homeopathy together and share information. Though consisting mostly of women and mothers, the groups are open to anyone interested in learning about homeopathy.

The National Center's *Directory* has a listing of these study groups, as well as regional study group leaders. This *Directory* is available directly from the National Center (801 North Fairfax, #306, Alexandria, VA 22314) or from Homeopathic Educational Services (2124 Kittredge Street, Berkeley, CA 94074).

HOMEOPATHIC MEDICINES AND THEIR COMMON NAMES

The following list of homeopathic medicines contains those remedies mentioned in one or more chapters in this book. Homeopathic medicines are typically described by their Latin names in order for homeopathic manufacturers and practitioners to be precise with the specific plant, mineral, or animal species.

The first listing is the formal Latin name of the medicine. It is followed by one or more frequently used abbreviations of the name. In parentheses is the common name for the substance from which the medicine is derived.

Aconitum napellus/ Aconitum/Aconite (monkshood)

Aesculus (horse chestnut)

Aethusa (fool's parsley)

Agaricus muscarius/Agaricus (fly agaric)

Allium cepa (onion)

Aloe socotrina/Aloe (aloe)

Ambra grisea/Ambra (ambergris)

Anacardium orientale/ Anacardium (marking nut)

Anas barbariae hepatis et cordis extractum/Anas barbariae (duck heart and liver)

Antimonium crudum/ Antimonium crud (antimonous sulfide)

Antimonium tartaricum/ Antimonium tart (tartar emetic)

Apis mellifica/Apis (honey bee)

Argentum metallicum/ Argentum met (silver)

Argentum nitricum (silver nitrate)

Arnica montana/Arnica (leopard's bane)

Arsenicum album/Arsenicum (arsenious acid)

Arum triphyllum/Arum trip (jack in the pulpit)

Asafoetida (asafoetida)

Aurum metallicum/Aurum (gold)

Avena sativa (oat)

Baryta carbonica/Baryta carb (carbonate of baryta)

Belladonna (deadly nightshade)

Bellis perennis (daisy)

Berberis (barberry)

Borax (borate of sodium)

Bryonia alba/Bryonia (white bryonia)

Cactus grandiflorus/Cactus (night-blooming cactus)

Cadmium iodatum (cadmium iodine)

Caladium (arum)

Calcarea carbonica/Calc carb (calcium carbonate)

Calcarea phosphorica/Calc phos (calcium phosphate)

Calendula (marigold)

Cantharis (Spanish fly/blistering beetle)

Capsicum (red pepper)

Carbo vegetabilis/Carbo veg (vegetable charcoal)

Carduus marianus (St. Mary's thistle)

Castor equi (thumbnail of the horse)

Caulophyllum (blue cohosh)

Causticum (potassium hydrate)

Chamomilla (chamomile)

Chelidonium (greater celandine)

Chimaphilla umbellata (pipsissewa)

Cicuta virosa (water hemlock)

Cimicifuga (black snakeroot)

Cinchona (Peruvian bark)

Cinnabaris (mercuric sulfide)

Clematis erecta/Clematis (upright virgin's bower)

Cocculus (Indian cockle)

Coffea (crude coffee)

Colchicum autumnale (meadow saffron)

Collinsonia (stoneroot)

Colocynthis (bitter apple)

Conium maculatum/Conium (hemlock)

Crataegus oxyacantha/Crataegus (hawthorn)

Croton tiglium (croton oil seed)

Cuprum metallicum/
Cuprum/Cuprum met (copper)

Cyclamen (sowbread)

Drosera rotundifolia/Drosera
(sundew)

Dulcamara (woody nightshade)

Equisetum (scouring rush)

Eupatorium perfoliatum/Eup
perf (boneset)

Euphrasia (eyebright)

Ferrum phosphoricum/Ferrum
phos (phosphate of iron)

Gambogia (garcinia morella)

Gelsemium (yellow jessamine)

Gingko biloba/Gingko (gingko)

Ginseng (ginseng)

Glonoine (nitroglycerine)

Graphites (black lead)

Guaiacum (lignum sanctum)

Gunpowder (gunpowder)

Hamamelis virginica/Hamamelis
(witchhazel)

Helleborus (snowrose)

Hepar sulphuricum/Hepar sulph
(sulfide of calcium)

Histaminium (histamine)

Humulus lupulus (hops)

Hydrastis (goldenseal)

Hypericum (St. John's wort)

Ignatia (St. Ignatius bean)

Ipecacuanha/Ipecac (ipecac root)

Iris versicolor/Iris (blue flag)

Kali bichromicum/Kali bic
(potassium dichromate)

Kali bromatum/Kali brom
(bromide of potassium)

Kali carbonica/Kali carb
(potassium carbonate)

Kali muriaticum/Kali mur
(potassium chloride)

Kali phosphorica/Kali phos
(potassium phosphate)

Kali sulphuricum (potassium
sulfate)

Kreosotum (kreosote)

Lachesis (venom of the
bushmaster)

Lacticum acidum (lactic acid)

Ledum palustre/Ledum (marsh
tea)

Lycopodium (club moss)

Magnesia phosphorica/Mag phos
(magnesium phosphate)

Medorrhinum (gonorrhea
bacteria)

Mercurius (mercury)

Mercurius corrosivus/Merc corr
(mercury bichloride)

Millefolium (yarrow)

Natrum carbonica/Natrum carb
(sodium carbonate)

Natrum muriaticum/Natrum
mur (sodium chloride)

Natrum sulphur/Natrum sulph (sodium sulfide)

Nitricum acid/Nitric acid (nitric acid)

Nux vomica (poison nut)

Opium (opium)

Passiflora incarnata/Passiflora (passion flower)

Pertussinum/Pertussis (pertussin)

Phosphoricum acid/Phosphoric acid (orthophosphoric acid)

Phosphorus (yellow phosphorus)

Phytolacca decandra/Phytolacca (poke)

Plantago major/Plantago (plantain)

Podophyllum (podophyllin)

Psorinum (fluid from scabies lesion)

Pulsatilla (windflower)

Raphanus sativus/Raphanus (black radish)

Rhus toxicodendron/Rhus tox (poison ivy)

Rumex crispus/Rumex (yellow dock)

Ruta graveolens/Ruta (rue)

Sabadilla (cevadilla seed)

Sabal serrata (saw palmetto)

Sabina (savine)

Sanguinaria (bloodroot)

Sarsaparilla (sarsaparilla)

Scutellaria lateriflora/Scutellaria (skullcap)

Secale cornutum/Secale (rye ergot)

Selenium metallicum/Selenium (selenium)

Sepia (cuttlefish)

Silicea/Silica (silica)

Spigelia anthelmia/Spigelia (pink root)

Spongia tosta/Spongia (roasted sponge)

Staphysagria (stavesacre)

Stramonium (jimson weed)

Strontium carbonicum/ Strontium carb (strontium carbonate)

Sulphur (sulfur)

Sulphuricum acid/Sulphuric acid (sulfuric acid)

Symphytum (comfrey)

Tabacum (tobacco)

Tellurium metallicum/Tellurium (tellurium)

Theridion (black spider of Curacao)

Thiosinaminum (thiosinamine)

Thuja occidentalis/Thuja (white cedar/arbor vitae)

Tuberculinum tubercle bacillus)

Urtica dioica (stinging nettle, small size)

Urtica urens (stinging nettle, large size)

Veratrum album (white hellabore)

Verbascum thapsus/Verbascum (mullein)

Viscum album (mistletoe)

Wyethia helenioides/Wyethia (wyethia)

Zincum metallicum/Zinc (zinc)

Zingiber (ginger)

NOTES

Part I. Introduction to Homeopathic Medicine

1. HOMEOPATHY: A MODERN VIEW

1. Linn Boyd, *The Simile in Medicine*. Philadelphia: Boericke and Tafel, 1936. This difficult-to-obtain book is a fascinating and brilliant review of the law of similars in Western medical history. **2.** *Homeopathic Pharmacopoeia of the United States*. Washington, D.C.: Homeopathic Pharmacopoeia Convention of the United States, 1995. This text is legally recognized as the source for specific guidelines homeopathic manufacturers are to use in making homeopathic medicines. A good book on homeopathic pharmacy is: D. D. Banerjee, *Textbook of Homoeopathic Pharmacy*. New Delhi: B. Jain, 1986. **3.** Richard Haehl, *Samuel Hahnemann: His Life and Work*. New Delhi: B. Jain (reprint), 322. **4.** V. Droscher, *The Magic of the Senses*. New York: Harper and Row, 1969, 98–99. **5.** *Ibid.*, 114. **6.** Diane Ackerman, *A Natural History of the Senses*. New York: Vintage, 1990, 12. **7.** James Gleck, *Chaos*. New York: Penguin, 1987. Also, Paolo Bellavite and Andrea Signorini, *Homeopathy: A Frontier in Medical Science*. Berkeley: North Atlantic, 1995. **8.** K. C. Cole, *Sympathetic Vibrations*. New York: Bantam, 1985, 265. **9.** Thomas Maugh, "Magnetic Particles Found Through the Human Brain," *San Francisco Chronicle*, May 12, 1992. See also: Science, 256, May 15, 1992.

2. HEALING DISEASE VERSUS SUPPRESSING SYMPTOMS

1. George Vithoulkas, *The Science of Homeopathy*. New York: Grove, 1980. **2.** *Ibid.* Also, Andre Saine, "Hering's Law: Law, Rule or Dogma," *Simillimum*, Winter 1993, 6, 4: 34–52. This article provides an excellent review and critique of Hering's laws and suggests that they be called "Hering's guidelines." **3.** Vithoulkas, *op. cit.* See also: George Vithoulkas, *A New Model of Health and Disease*. Berkeley: North Atlantic, 1991. **4.** Harris L. Coulter. *Divided Legacy*, volume 2. Berkeley: North Atlantic, 1988, 677. **5.** *Pediatric News*, 23, 1, 1989. **6.** "Pediatricians Urge Confirmatory Test for Suspected Strep Throat," *Medical World News*, January 12, 1987, 42. **7.** *Ibid.* **8.** As quoted in S. Russell, "Childhood Herpes Linked to Immunities," *San Francisco Chronicle*, October 7, 1992. See also; *JAMA*, October 7, 1992. **9.** U.S. Department of Health and Human Services, *Child Health USA 93*. Washington, D.C.: U.S. Government Printing Office (ISBN: 0-16-043116-6), 26. **10.** R. G. Gibson, S. Gibson, A. D. MacNeill, et al., "Homoeopathic Therapy in Rheumatoid Arthritis: Evaluation by Double-blind Clinical Therapeutic Trial, *British Journal of Clinical Pharmacology*, 1980,

9:453–59. **11.** E. Davenas, B. Poitevin, and J. Benveniste, "Effect on Mouse Peritoneal Macrophages of Orally Administered Very High Dilutions of Silica," *European Journal of Pharmacology*, 1987, 135: 313–19. **12.** M. Bastide, V. Daurat, M. Doucet-Jabeuf, *et.al.*, "Immunomodulatory Activity of Very Low Doses of Thymulin in Mice," *International Journal of Immunotherapy*, 1987, 3:191–200. See also M. Bastide, "Immunological Examples on Ultra High Dilution Research," in P. C. Endler and J. Schulte (eds), *Ultra High Dilution: Physiology and Physics*. Dordrecht: Kluwer Academic, 1994. **13.** Samuel Hahnemann, *The Chronic Diseases* (2 volumes). New Delhi: B. Jain (reprint). See also: H. Choudhury, *Indications of Miasms*. New Delhi: B. Jain, 1988.

3. THE HOMEOPATHIC RENAISSANCE

1. Harris L. Coulter, *Divided Legacy: The Conflict Between Homoeopathy and the American Medical Association*. Berkeley: North Atlantic, 1975. **2.** *Ibid.* See also *Transactions of the American Institute of Homoeopathy*, 1908, 128. **3.** Coulter, *op. cit.*, 314. **4.** "Riding the Coattails of Homeopathy," *FDA Consumer*, March 1985, 31. **5.** "Market Report: Herbal and Homeo," *OTC Market Report Update USA*, July 1994, 217–28. **6.** M. V. Nelson, G. R. Railie, and H. Areny, "Pharmacists' Perceptions of Alternative Health Approaches: A Comparison Between U.S. and British Pharmacists," *Journal of Clinical Pharmacy and Therapeutics*, 1990, 15:141–46. **7.** "Market Report," 226. **8.** L. Spigelblatt, "The Use of Alternative Medicine by Children," *Pediatrics*, December 1994, 811–14. **9.** Alternative Medicine/Alternative Medical Market." Frost and Sullivan Ltd. Report E874, London, 1986. **10.** *L'Homéopathie en 1993*. Lyons: Syndicat National de la Pharmacie Homéopathique, 1993 (Quoting COFREMCA and IFOP public opinion surveys). **11.** Richard Wharton and George Lewith, "Complementary Medicine and the General Practitioner," *British Medical Journal*, June 7, 1986, 292: 1498–1500 **12.** Nelson, *op. cit.* **13.** Steven Kayne, "Homeopathic Pharmacy: Education, Research and Optimism," *British Homoeopathic Journal*, October 1993, 225. **14.** British Medical Association, *Complementary Medicine: New Approaches to Good Practice*. Oxford: Oxford University, 1993. **15.** Universal News Services, June 16, 1994. **16.** Wharton and Lewith, *op. cit.* Also, E. Anderson and P. Anderson, "General Practitioners and Complementary Medicine," *Journal of the Royal Academy of General Practitioners*, 1988, 38:511–14. **17.** David Taylor Reilly, "Young Doctors' Views of Alternative Medicine," *British Medical Journal*, 1983, 287:337–39. **18.** *Marketing Herbal and Homoeopathic Remedies in Germany*. Essex, England: Nicholas Hall, July 1992. **19.** Peter Fisher and Adam Ward, "Complementary Medicine in Europe," *British Medical Journal*, July 9, 1994, 309:107–10. **20.** F. Clines, "With Medicine Itself Sick, Russians Turn to Herbs," *New York Times*, December 31, 1990. **21.** Sandra M. Chase, "The Status of Homeopathy in the World," Presentation at the National Center for Homeopathy Conference, April 7, 1995. **22.** Jugal Kishore, "Homoeopathy: The Indian Experience," *World Health Forum*, 1983, 3:107. **23.** J. Siegel-Itzkovich, "Homeopathy: Quacks Need Not Apply," *Jerusalem Post*, March 13, 1994.

4. SCIENTIFIC EVIDENCE FOR HOMEOPATHIC MEDICINE

1. A.R.D. Stebbing, "Hormesis: The Stimulation of Growth by Low Levels of Inhibitors," *Science of the Total Environment*, 1982, 22;:213–34. Also, *Health Physics*, May 1987. This entire issue was devoted to the increased effects of low doses. **2.** M. Oberbaum and J. Cambar, "Hormesis: Dose Dependent Reverse Effects of Low and Very Low Doses," in P. C. Endler and J. Schulte (eds.), *Ultra High Dilutions*. Dordrecht: Kluwer Academic, 1994. **3.** Oberbaum and Cambar, Stebbing, *op. cit.* **4.** J. Kleijnen, P. Knipschild, and G. ter Riet, "Clinical Trials of Homoeopathy," *British Medical Journal*, February 9, 1991, 302:316–23. **5.** Because much research on homeopathy has been performed by homeopaths who are primarily clinicians and are not adequately trained in research, they predictably committed errors in research design, analysis, and description of their studies. **6.** David Reilly, Morag Taylor, Neil Beattie, *et al.,* "Is Evidence for Homoeopathy Reproducible?" *Lancet,* December 10, 1994, 344:1601–6. **7.** Jennifer Jacobs, L. Margarita Jimenez, and Stephen S. Gloyd, "Treatment of Acute Childhood Diarrhea with Homeopathic Medicine: A Randomized Clinical Trial in Nicaragua," *Pediatrics,* May 1994, 93, 5:719–25. **8.** Bruno Brigo and G. Serpelloni, "Homeopathic Treatment of Migraines; A Randomized Double-blind Controlled Study of 60 Cases," *Berlin Journal on Research in Homeopathy,* March 1991, 1, 2:98–106. **9.** E. de Lange de Klerk, J. Blommers, D. J. Kuik, *et al.,* "Effect of Homoeopathic Medicines on Daily Burden of Symptoms in Children with Recurrent Upper Respiratory Tract Infections," *British Medical Journal,* November 19, 1994, 309:1329–32. **10.** R. G. Gibson, S. Gibson, A. D. MacNeill, *et al.,* "Homoeopathic Therapy in Rheumatoid Arthritis: Evaluation by Double-blind Clinical Therapeutic Trial," *British Journal of Clinical Pharmacology,* 1980, 9:453–59. **11.** P. Fisher, "An Experimental Double-Blind Clinical Trial Method in Homeopathy: Use of a Limited Range of Remedies to Treat Fibrositis," *British Homoeopathic Journal,* 1986, 75:142–47. **12.** P. Fisher, A. Greenwood, E. C. Huskisson, *et al.,* "Effect of Homoeopathic Treatment on Fibrositis," *British Medical Journal,* August 5, 1989, 299:365–66. **13.** J. Paterson, "Report on Mustard Gas Experiments, *Journal of the American Institute of Homeopathy,* 1944, 37:47–50, 88–92. **14.** R.M.M. Owen and G. Ives, "The Mustard Gas Experiments of the British Homeopathic Society: 1941–1942. *Proceedings of the 35th International Homeopathic Congress,* 1982, 258–59. **15.** D. Zicari, *et al.,* "Valutazione dell'Azione Angioprotettiva di Preparati di Arnica nel Trattamento della Retinopatia Diabetica," *Bolletino di Oculistica,* 1992, 5:841–48. **16.** J. P. Ferley, D. Zmirou, D. D'Admehar, *et al.,* "A Controlled Evaluation of a Homoeopathic Preparation in the Treatment of Influenza-like Syndrome," *British Journal of Clinical Pharmacology,* March 1989, 27:329–35. **17.** Christopher Day, "Control of Stillbirths in Pigs Using Homoeopathy," *Veterinary Record,* March 3, 1984, 114, 9; 216. Also, *Journal of the American Institute of Homeopathy,* December 1986, 779, 4:146–47. **18.** M. Shipley, H. Berry, G. Broster, *et al.,* "Controlled Trial of Homoeopathic Treatment of Osteoarthritis," *Lancet,* January 15, 1983, 97–98. **19.** David Reilly, Morag Taylor, C. McSharry, *et al.,* "Is Homoeopathy a Placebo Response? Controlled Trial of Homoeopathic Potency, with Pollen in Hayfever as Model," *Lancet,* October 18, 1986, 881–86. **20.** P. Dorfman, M. N. Lasserre, and M. Tetau, "Preparation a l'accouchement par Homéopathie: Experimentation en double-insu versus Placebo," *Cahiers de Biotherapie,* April 1987, 94:77–81. **21.** P. Eid, E. Felisi, and M. Sideri, "Applicability of Homoeopathic Caulophyllum thalictroides during Labour," *British Homoeopathic Journal,* 1993, 82:245. **22.** P. Eid, E. Felisi, and M. Sideri, "Super-placebo ou action Pharmacologique? Une Etude en Double Aveugle, Randomisée avec un Remède Homéopathique (Caulophyllum thalictroides) dans le Travail de l'accouchement," *Proceedings of the 5th Congress of the O.M.H.I.* (International Organization for Homeopathic Medicine), Paris, October 20–23, 1994. **23.** J. Zell, W. D. Connert, J. Mau, *et al.,* "Behandlung von akuten Sprung-gelenksdisotrionen: Doppelblindstudie zum Wirksamkeitsnachweis eines Homöopathischen Salbenpraparats," *Fortschr. Medicine,* 1988, 106:96–100. **24.** W. Thiel and B. Borho, "Die Therapie von Frischen, Traumatischen Blutergussen der Kniegelnke (Hamartros) mit Traumeel N Injectionslogung," *Biol. Medizin,* 20:506. **25.** E. Ernst, T. Saradeth, and K. L. Resch, "Complementary Treatment of Varicose Veins: A Randomised, Placebo-controlled, Double-blind Trial," *Phlebology,* 1990; 157–163. **26.** A. V. Williamson, W. L. Mackie, W. J. Crawford, *et al.,* "A Study Using Sepia 200c Given Prophylactically Postpartum to Prevent Anoestrus Problems in the Dairy Cow," *British Homoeopathic Journal,* 1991, 80:149. See also by the same researchers: "A Trial of Sepia 200," *British Homoeopathic Journal,* 1995, 84:14–20. **27.** G. Both, "Zur Prophylaxe und Therapie des Metritis-Mastitis-Agalactic: Komplexes des Schweines mit Biologischen Arzneimitteln," *Biologische Tiermedizen,* 1987, 4:39. **28.** M. Labrecque, D. Audet, L. G. Latulippe, *et al.,* "Homeopathic Treatment of Plantar Warts," *Canadian Medical Association Journal,* 1992, 146(10):1749–53. **29.** R. Gupta, O. P. Bhardwaj, and R. K.

Manchanda, "Homoeopathy in the Treatment of Warts," *British Homoeopathic Journal*, April 1991, 80, 2:108–11. **30.** W. E. Boyd, "The Action of Microdoses of Mercuric Chloride on Diastase," *British Homoeopathic Journal*, 1941, 31:1–28: 1942, 32:106–11. **31.** D. Mock, "What's Going on Here, Anyway?—A Review of Boyd's 'Biochemical and Biological Evidence of the Activity of High Potencies,'" *Journal of the American Institute of Homeopathy*, 1969, 62:197. **32.** K. Linde, W. B. Jonas, D. Melchart, *et al.*, "Critical Review and Meta-Analysis of Serial Agitated Dilutions in Experimental Toxicology," *Human and Experimental Toxicology*, 1994, 13:481–92. **33.** A. R. Khuda-Bukhsh, and S. Banik, "Assessment of Cytogenetic Damage in X-irradiated Mice and Its Alteration by Oral Administration of Potentized Homeopathic Drug, Ginseng D200," *Berlin Journal of Research in Homeopathy*, 1991, 1, 4/5:254. Also, A. R. Khuda-Bukhsh and S. Maity, "Alteration of Cytogenetic Effects by Oral Administration of Potentized Homeopathic Drug, Ruta graveolens, in Mice Exposed to Sub-lethal X-radiation," *Berlin Journal of Research in Homeopathy*, 1991, 1, 4/5:264. **34.** J. Bildet, M. Guyot, F. Bonini, *et al.*, "Demonstrating the Effects of Apis mellifica and Apim virus Dilutions on Erythema Induced by U.V. Radiation on Guinea Pigs," *Berlin Journal of Research in Homeopathy*, 1990, 1:28. **35.** P. C. Endler, W. Pongratz, G. Kastberg, *et al.*, "The Effect of Highly Diluted Agitated Thyroxine on the Climbing Activity of Frogs," *Veterinary and Human Toxicology*, 1994, 36:56. Also, P. C. Endler, W. Pongratz, R. van Wijk, *et al.*, "Transmission of Hormone Information by Non-molecular Means," *FASEB Journal*, 1994, 8, Abs.2313. **36.** J. L. Demangeat, *et al.*, "Modifications des Temps de Relaxation RMN a 4 z des Protons du Solvant dans les Tres Hautes Dilutions Salines de Silice/lactose," *Journal of Med. Nucl. Biophy*, 1992, 16:35–45. **37.** J. Benveniste, "Further Biological Effects Induced by Ultra High Dilutions: Inhibition by a Magnetic Field," in P. C. Endler and J. Schulte, (eds.), *Ultra High Dilution*. Dordrecht: Kluwer Academic, 1994, 35. Also, J. Benveniste, B. Arnoux, and L. Hadji, "Highly Dilute Antigen Increases Coronary Flow of Isolated Heart from Immunized Guinea-pigs," *FASEB Journal*, 1992, 6, Abs.1610. **38.** C. Doutremepuch, O. de Seze, D. Le Roy, *et al.*, "Aspirin at Very Ultra Low Dosage in Healthy Volunteers: Effects on Bleeding Time, Platelet Aggregation and Coagulation," *Haemostasis*, 1990, 20:99. **39.** Roeland van Wijk and Fred A. C. Wiegant, *Cultured Mammalian Cells in Homeopathy Research: The Similia Principle in Self-Recovery*. Utrecht; University of Utrecht, 1994. **40.** E. Davenas, F. Beauvais, J. Amara, *et al.*, "Human Basophil Degranulation Triggered by Very Dilute Antiserum Against IgE," *Nature*, June 30, 1988, 333:816–18. **41.** J. Maddox, "When to Believe the Unbelievable," *Nature*, June 30, 1988, 333:787. **42.** J. Maddox, J. Randi, and W. Stewart, "'High-dilution' Experiments a Delusion," *Nature*, July 28, 1988, 334:443–47. **43.** J. Benveniste, E. Davenas, B. Ducot, *et al.*, "L'agitation de Solutions Hautement Diluées n'induit pas d'activité Biologique Specifique," *C. R. Acad. Sci. Paris*, 1991, 312:461. **44.** Reilly *et al.*, 1994. See note 6. **45.** Paolo Bellavite and Andrea Signorini, *Homeopathy: A Frontier in Medical Science*. Berkeley: North Atlantic, 1995.

5. WHAT SKEPTICS SAY AND HOW TO RESPOND TO THEM

1. Abraham Maslow, *Towards a Psychology of Science*. Princeton: Van Nostrand, 1968. **2.** Thomas Kuhn, *The Structure of Scientific Revolutions*. Chicago: University of Chicago, 1962. **3.** In James Gorman, "Take a Little Deadly Nightshade and You'll Feel Better," *New York Times Sunday Magazine*, August 30, 1992. While *Consumer Reports* is usually an excellent resource for impartial information about products, they have had a longtime bias against homeopathy. Surprisingly, rather than test as they do in the case of virtually every other subject upon which they write, *Consumer Reports* has published articles critical of homeopathy without any testing whatsoever of homeopathic medicines. **4.** *L'Homéopathie en 1993*. Lyons: Syndicat National de la Pharmacie Homéopathique, 1993 (Quoting COFREMCA and IFOP public opinion surveys). **5.** Lynn Payer, *Medicine and Culture*. New York: Holt, 1988. **6.** Peter Fisher and Adam Ward, "Complementary Medicine in Europe," *British Med-*

ical Journal, July 9, 1994, 309:107–10. **7.** Richard Wharton and George Lewith, "Complementary Medicine and the General Practitioner," British Medical Journal, June 7, 1986, 292:1498–1500. Also, E. Anderson and P. Anderson, "General Practitioners and Complementary Medicine," Journal of the Royal Academy of General Practitioners, 1988, 38:511–14. **8.** J. Kleijnen, P. Knipschild, and G. ter Riet, "Clinical Trials of Homoeopathy," British Medical Journal, February 9, 1991, 302:316–23. **9.** David Reilly, Morag Taylor, C. McSharry, et al., "Is Homoeopathy a Placebo Response? Controlled Trial of Homoeopathic Potency, with Pollen in Hayfever as Model," Lancet, October 18, 1986, 881–86. **10.** Petr Skrabanek, Lancet, November 8, 1986, 1107. **11.** Health Physics, May 1987. **12.** Deborah Daly, "Alternative Medicine Courses Taught at U.S. Medical Schools: An Ongoing Listing," Journal of Alternative and Complementary Medicine, 1995, 1, 1:111–13. **13.** Lynn Payer, Disease-Mongers. New York: John Wiley, 1992. **14.** R. L. Avina and L. J. Schneiderman, "Why Patients Choose Homeopathy," Western Journal of Medicine, April 1978, 128:366–69. **15.** Martin Walker, Dirty Medicine. London: Slingshot, 1994. **16.** Office of Technology Assessment, Assessing the Safety and Efficacy of Medical Technology. Washington, D.C.: U.S. Government Printing Office, 1978. **17.** D. T. Reilly and M. Taylor, Developing Integrated Medicine: Report of the Research Council for Complementary Medicine (RCCM) Research Fellowship in Complementary Medicine 1987-90. Glasgow: University of Glasgow, 1990.

6. THE INTERFACE BETWEEN HOMEOPATHY AND CONVENTIONAL MEDICINE

1. K. J. Thomas, et al., "Use of Non-orthodox and Conventional Health Care in Great Britain," British Medical Journal, January 26, 1991, 302, 6770, 207–10. **2.** Jennifer Jacobs, L. Jimenez, L. Margarita, and Stephen S. Gloyd, "Treatment of Acute Childhood Diarrhea with Homeopathic Medicine: A Randomized Clinical Trial in Nicaragua," Pediatrics, May 1994, 93, 5:719–25. **3.** A. R. Khuda-Bukhsh and S. Banik, "Assessment of Cytogenetic Damage in X-irradiated Mice and Its Alteration by Oral Administration of Potentized Homeopathic Drug, Ginseng D200," Berlin Journal of Research in Homeopathy, 1991, 1, 4/5:254. Also, A. R. Khuda-Bukhsh and S. Maity, "Alteration of Cytogenetic Effects by Oral Administration of Potentized Homeopathic Drug, Ruta graveolens in Mice Exposed to Sub-lethal X-radiation," Berlin Journal of Research in Homeopathy, 1991, 1, 4/5:264. **4.** David Reilly, Morag Taylor, Neil Beattie, et al., "Is Evidence for Homoeopathy Reproducible?" Lancet, December 10, 1994, 344:1601–6. **5.** British Medical Association, Complementary Medicine: New Approaches to Good Practice. Oxford: Oxford University, 1993, 9. **6.** Universal News Services, June 16, 1994. **7.** David M. Eisenberg, Ronald C. Kessler, Cindy Foster, et al., "Unconventional Medicine in the United States," New England Journal of Medicine, January 28, 1993, 328, 4:246–52. **8.** Complementary Medicine, 36. **9.** Social Security Statistics, CNAM 61, French Government Report, January 1991. **10.** British Homoeopathy Research Group, Communication 23, April 1994, 18.

Part II.   Common Concerns of Consumers

8. SEEKING PROFESSIONAL HOMEOPATHIC CARE

1. Jennifer Jacobs, Presentation at Annual Conference of the National Center for Homeopathy, 1993, Alexandria, Virginia (paper updated and recently submitted to a professional public health journal). **2.** David M. Eisenberg, Ronald C. Kessler, Cindy Foster, et al., "Unconventional Medicine in the United States," New England Journal of Medicine, January 28, 1993, 328, 4:246–52. **3.** Rima Handley, A Homeopathic Love Story. Berkeley: North Atlantic, 1990. **4.** Jacobs, *op. cit.* **5.** *Statistical Studies,* CNAM (France's Health Care Insurance Agency), January 1991.

10. COMBINATION HOMEOPATHIC MEDICINES

1. David Reilly, Morag Taylor, C. McSharry, *et al.,* "Is Homoeopathy a Placebo Response? Controlled Trial of Homoeopathic Potency, with Pollen in Hayfever as Model," *Lancet,* October 18, 1986, 881–86. **2.** J. Zell, W. D. Connert, J. Mau, *et al.,* "Behandlung von akuten Sprung-gelenksdisotrionen: Doppelblindstudie zum Wirksamkeitsnachweis eines Homöopathischen Salbenpraparats," *Fortschr. Medicine,* 1988, 106:96–100. **3.** P. Dorfman, M. N. Lasserre, and M. Tetau, "Preparation a l'accouchement par Homéopathie: Experimentation en double-insu versus Placebo," *Cahiers de Biotherapie,* April 1987, 94:77–81. **4.** G. Aulagnier, "Action d'un Traitement Homéopathique sur la Reprise du Transit Post Operatoire," *Homéopathie,* 1985, 6:42–45. **5.** E. Ernst, T. Saradeth, and K. L. Resch, "Complementary Treatment of Varicose Veins: A Randomised, Placebo-controlled, Double-blind Trial," *Phlebology,* 1990, 157–63. **6.** Rima Handley, *A Homeopathic Love Story.* Berkeley: North Atlantic, 1990.

12. PRACTICAL ISSUES IN USING HOMEOPATHIC MEDICINES

1. W. Pongratz and M. Haidvogl, "Effect of Microwaves on Potencies," *Homöopathie in Osterrich,* 1994, 5:14–15.

Part III.   Can Homeopathy Help Me?

CONDITIONS OF INFANTS

1. Joe Graedon, *The People's Pharmacy.* New York: St. Martin's, 1985, 372.

CHILDREN'S CONDITIONS

1. Jennifer Jacobs, L. Margarita Jimenez, and Stephen S. Gloyd, "Treatment of Acute Childhood Diarrhea with Homeopathic Medicine: A Randomized Clinical Trial in Nicaragua," *Pediatrics,* May 1994, 93, 5:719–25. **2.** Robert L. Williams, *JAMA,* September 15, 1993. **3.** Adrienne Brooks, "Middle Ear Infections in Children," *Science News,* November 19, 1994, 146:332–33. **4.** U.S. Department of Health and Human Services, *Child Health USA '93.* Washington, D.C.: U.S. Government Printing Office (ISBN: 0-16-043116-6), 26. **5.** *FDA Drug Review: Postapproval Risks 1976–85,* GAO/PEMD-90-15. Gaithersburg, MD. **6.** "Highlights of Drug Utilization in Office Practice; National Ambulatory Medical Care Survery, 1985," *NCHS Advance Data,* May 19, 1987, 134.

WOMEN'S CONDITIONS

1. Harris L. Coulter, *Divided Legacy: The Conflict Between Homoeopathy and the American Medical Association.* Berkeley: North Atlantic, 1975, 116. **2.** Maria Luisa Queralt Gimeno, "Research and Practical Application of the Treatment of Forty Women with Ovarian Cysts," 45th Congress of the International League for Homeopathic Medicine, Barcelona, Spain, May 1990. **3.** Chellis Glendenning, *When Technology Wounds.* New York: Morrow, 1990.

PREGNANT AND LABORING WOMEN

1. Yvonne Brackbill, *et.al., Medication in Maternity.* Ann Arbor: University of Michigan, 1985, 51–55. **2.** From the foreword to Richard Moskowitz, M.D., *Homeopathic Medicines for Pregnancy and Childbirth.* Berkeley: North Atlantic, 1992. **3.** P. Dorfman, M. N. Lasserre, and M. Tetau, "Preparation a l'accouchement par Homéopathie: Experimentation en double-insu versus Placebo," *Cahiers de Biotherapie,* April 1987, 94:77–81. Note: Copies of this study translated into English are available for $2 from Homeopathic Educational Services (page 366). **4.** P. Eid, E. Feliisi, and M. Sideri, "Applicability of Homeopathic Caulophyllum thalictroides During Labour," *British Homoeopathic Journal,* 82:245. See also P. Eid, E. Felisi, and M. Sideri, "Super-placebo ou Action Pharmacologique? Une Etude en Double Aveugle, Randomisée avec un Remède Homéopathique (Caulophyllum thalictroides) dans le Travail de l'accouchement. *Proceedings of the 5th Congress of the O.M.H.I.* Paris, October 20–23, 1994. **5.** World Health Organization, "Appropriate Technology for Birth," *Lancet,* August 24, 1985, 8452:436.

MEN'S AILMENTS

1. A. F. Vozianov and N. K. Simeonova, "Homoeopathic Treatment of Patients with Adenomas of the Prostate," *British Homoeopathic Journal,* July 1990; 79:148–51. **2.** T. Adler, "Just Say No to Prostate Cancer Screening," *Science News,* September 17, 1994, 146:180.

CONDITIONS OF THE ELDERLY

1. *Toronto Globe and Mail,* June 4, 1994. **2.** S. M. Willcox, D. V. Himmelstein, and S. Woolhandler, "Inappropriate Drug Prescribing for the Community-dwelling Elderly," *JAMA,* July 27, 1994, 272:292. **3.** *Canadian Medical Association Journal,* June 4, 1994. **4.** M. E. Ferry, *et al.,* "Physicians' Knowledge of Prescribing for the Elderly," *Journal of the American Geriatric Society* 1985, 33:616. **5.** Gina Kolata, "Study Faults Prescriptions for Elderly," *New York Times,* July 26, 1994. **6.** Arthur A. Levin, "New Report on Drugs and the Elderly," *Healthfacts,* May 1989. **7.** Jonathan King, "The Problem with Pills," *View,* Group Health Cooperative, Seattle, May–June 1983, 48. **8.** Andrew Lockie, "A Comparison of Alumina—The Drug Picture—and Alzheimer's Disease—The Disease Picture," *British Homoeopathic Journal,* April 1984, 73:92–94.

COMMON INFECTIONS

1. Thomas L. Bradford, *The Logic of Figures, or the Comparative Results of Homoeopathic and Other Treatments.* Philadelphia: Boericke and Tafel, 1900. See also Harris L. Coulter, *Divided Legacy: The Conflict Between Homoeopathy and the American Medical Association.* Berkeley: North Atlantic, 1975. **2.** "Those Overworked Miracle Drugs," *Time,* August 17, 1981, 63. **3.** Sharon Begley, "The End of Antibiotics," *Newsweek,* March 28, 1994, 49. **4.** "Antimicrobials for Treating Ulcers," *American Druggist,* May 1994, 35. **5.** E. de Lange de Klerk, J. Blommers, D. J. Kuik, *et al.,* "Effect of Homoeopathic Medicines on Daily Burden of Symptoms in Children with Recurrent Upper Respiratory Tract Infections," *British Medical Journal,* November 19, 1994, 309:1329–32. **6.** C. A. Gassinger, G. Wunstel, and P. Netter, "Klinische Prüfung zum Nachweis der therapeutischen Wirksamkeit des homöopathischen Arzneimittels Eupatorium perforiatum D2 (Wasserhanf composite) bei der Diagnose 'Grippaler Infekt,'" *Arzneimittelforschung,* 1981, 31:732–36. **7.** L. R. Bordes and P. Dorfman, "Evaluation de l'activité Antitussive du Sirop Drosetux: Etude en Double Aveugle versus Placebo," *Cahiers d'Otorhinolaryngologie,* 1986, 21:731–34. **8.** J. P. Ferley, D. Zmirou, D. D'Admehar, *et al.,* "A Controlled Evaluation of a Homoeopathic Preparation in the Treatment of Influenza-like Syndrome," *British Journal of Clinical Pharmacology*, March 1989, 27:329–35. **9.** A. George Veasy, *et al.*, "Resurgence of Acute Rheumatic Fever in the Intermountain Area of the United States," *New England Journal of Medicine*, February 19, 1987; 316:421–26.

HEADACHES

1. Dorothy J. Cooper, "Migraine: A Homoeopathic Approach," *British Homoeopathic Journal*, January 1984, 73, 1:1–9. **2.** Bruno Brigo, "Le Traitement Homéopathique de la Migraine: Une Etude de 60 cas, controllée en Double-aveugle," *Journal of LMHI*, 1987.

DIGESTIVE DISORDERS

1. Jennifer Jacobs, L. Margarita Jimenez, and Stephen S. Gloyd, "Treatment of Acute Childhood Diarrhea with Homeopathic Medicine: A Randomized Clinical Trial in Nicaragua," *Pediatrics*, May 1994, 93, 5:719–25. **2.** V. W. Rahlfs and P. Mossinger, "Asafoetida bei Colon Irritabile," *Deutsche Medizinische Wochenschrift*, 1978, 104:140–43.

SKIN CONDITIONS

1. D. S. Spence, "Homoeopathic Treatment of Eczema: A Retrospective Survey of 130 Cases," *British Homoeopathic Journal*, April 1991, 80, 2:74–81. Homeopathic treatment was individualized according to constitutional characteristics, miasmatic tendencies (see Chapter 2 for a discussion on miasms), causative factors, and local symptoms. The most common medicines prescribed were *Sulphur, Kali sulphuricum,* and *Pulsatilla.* The researcher treated forty adult patients with an average duration of eczema of 18.27 years. Over 85 percent of these patients were better or much better after an average 1.8 years of treatment. *Sulphur* and *House dust mite* in potency were the most commonly prescribed homeopathic medicines for adults, with *Cat fur* and *Dog fur* in potency being a close third and fourth. *Sulphur, Arsenicum,* and *Natrum mur* were the most common constitutional remedies. The 6c, 12c, and 30c were by far the most common potencies used, except when the practitioner was prescribing a constitutional medicine or a miasmatic remedy and was confident in its correct prescription. **2.** M. Labrecque, D. Audet, L. G. Latulippe, *et al.*, "Homeopathic Treatment of Plantar Warts," *Canadian Medical Association Journal*, 1992, 146(10):1749–53. **3.** R. Gupta, O. P. Bhardwaj, and R. K. Manchanda, "Homoeopathy in the Treatment of Warts," *British Homoeopathic Journal*, April 1991, 80, 2:108–11. This study, as noted in Chapter 4, was a review of 66 patients with varying types of warts (33 common warts, 20 plantar warts, 13 flat warts). Not counting the 14 patients who dropped out of the study, 90 percent of patients had their warts disappear after an average of four months, including 21 of 22 people with common warts (9 with *Thuja*, 3 with *Nitric acid*, 2 with *Calcarea carb*, 2 with *Natrum mur*, 2 with *Ruta*, 1 each with *Causticum, Antimonium crud,* and *Opium*). Eighteen of the 19 people with plantar warts (12 with *Ruta*, 3 with *Thuja*, 2 with *Antimonium crud* and 1 with *Calcarea carb*) had their warts disappear. Although *Thuja* is the most important remedy for warts, it was prescribed in only 3 of the 19 patients with plantar warts and was successful in each. *Ruta* was the most common remedy for plantar warts. It is indicated for treating sore warts with a smooth surface, though it was successfully given for plantar warts irrespective of any specific indications. Nine of the 12 people with flat warts experienced successful treatment (6 with *Ruta*, 2 with *Thuja*, and 1 with *Antimonium crud*). The remedies were prescribed in varying potencies. When prescribed in the 30th potency, they were given three times daily. When prescribed in the 200th potency, they were given twice daily. Higher potencies were prescribed once a day until improvement started. These dosages were used by professional homeopaths; it is generally recommended that nonprofessionals use lower potencies such as the 6, 12, or 30th.

ALLERGIES

1. C. H. Blackley, "Experimental Researches on the Nature and Causes of Catarrhus aestivus," *British Journal of Homoeopathy,* 1871, 29:238–86, 477–501, 713–36. **2.** Sheldon G. Cohen, "The American Academy of Allergy: An Historical Review," *Journal of Allergy and Clinical Immunology,* 1979, 64, 5:332–466. **3.** David Taylor-Reilly, Morag Taylor, C. McSharry, *et al.,* "Is Homoeopathy a Placebo Response? Controlled Trial of Homoeopathic Potency, with Pollen in Hayfever as Model," *Lancet,* October 18, 1986, 881–86. **4.** David Reilly, Morag Taylor, Neil Beattie, et al., "Is Evidence for Homoeopathy Reproducible?" *Lancet,* December 10, 1994, 344:1601–6.

ARTHRITIS

1. R. G. Gibson, S. Gibson, A. D. MacNeill, *et al.,* "Homeopathic Therapy in Rheumatoid Arthritis: Evaluation by Double-blind Clinical Therapeutic Trial," *British Journal of Clinical Pharmacology,* 1980, 9:453–59. **2.** M. Shipley, H. Berry, G. Brosler, *et al.,* "Controlled Trial of Homoeopathic Treatment of Osteoarthritis," *Lancet,* January 15, 1983, 97–98.

AIDS

1. P. A. Volberding, S. W. Lagakos, J. M. Grimes, *et al.,* "A Comparison of Immediate with Deferred Zidovudine Therapy for Asymptomatic HIV-Infected Adults with CD4 Cell Counts of 500 or More per Cubic Millimeter," *New England Journal of Medicine,* August 17, 1995, 333, 7:401–407. (One important benefit of AZT is that it seems to prevent the transfer of HIV to infants of infected mothers.) **2.** René Dubos, *The Mirage of Health.* San Francisco: Harper and Row, 1959, 93–94. **3.** Claude Bernard, *Principles de Médecine Experimentale.* Paris: Presses Universitaires de France, 1947, 160–61. **4.** I. Wolffers and S. de Moree, "Use of Alternative Treatments by HIV+ and AIDS Patients in the Netherlands, *Ned Tijdschr Geneeskd.,* February 5, 1994, 138(6):307–10. **5.** D. P. Rastogi, V. P. Singh, V. Singh, *et al.,* "Evaluation of Homoeopathic Treatment in 129 Asymptomatic HIV Carriers," *British Homoeopathic Journal,* January 1993, 82:4–8. The diagnoses of all patients in this study were initially confirmed by the two accepted laboratory analyses, ELIZA and the Western Blot, which were performed by a World Health Organization–recognized center in India. After homeopathic treatment, twelve patients who initially tested HIV+ on the ELIZA test were found to be HIV- later. The initial report on this study showed that only two of these twelve patients were tested again through the Western Blot, which opened the study up to criticism because the ELIZA test is known to have errors and requires a confirmatory test with the Western Blot. Because of the extremely atypical result of this study, the editor of the homeopathic journal in which it was published was so startled that he wrote an editorial questioning its authenticity. (P. Fisher, "When to Believe the Unbelievable," *British Homoeopathic Journal,* January 1993, 82:2–3.) However, since this editorial, the authors have confirmed that an additional nine of the original twelve patients tested negative according to the Western Blot, plus an additional two people changed from HIV+ to HIV-. (D. P. Rastogi, "Asymptomatic HIV Carriers," *British Homoeopathic Journal,* January 1994, 83:54.) **6.** D. P. Rastogi, V. Singh, S. K. Dey, *et al.,* "Research Studies in HIV Infection with Homoeopathic Treatment," *CCRH* (the Indian government's Central Council for Research in Homoeopathy) *Quarterly Bulletin,* 1993, 15, 3/4:1–6. **7.** V. Singh, D. P. Rastogi, S. K. Dey, *et al.,* "Homoeopathic Drugs as Immunomodulators: A Study of 34 HIV Subjects," International Conference on AIDS, August 7–12, 1994:10(1):218. (abstract PB0301). **8.** Laurence Badgley, *Journal of the American Institute of Homeopathy,* March 1987, 80:8–14. **9.** L. M. Singh and G. Gupta, "Antiviral Efficacy of Homoeopathic Drugs Against Animal Viruses," *British Homoeopathic Journal,* July 1985, 74:168–74. **10.** *Ibid.* **11.** E. Davenas, B. Poitevin, and J. Benveniste, "Effect on Mouse Peritoneal Macrophages of Orally Administered Very High

Dilutions of Silica," *European Journal of Pharmacology*, 1987, 135:313–19. **12.** R. G. Gibson, S. Gibson, A. D. MacNeill, *et al.*, "Homoeopathic Therapy in Rheumatoid Arthritis: Evaluation by Double-Blind Clinical Therapeutic Trial," *British Journal of Clinical Pharmacology*, 1980, 9:453–59. **13.** M. Bastide, V. Daurat, M. Doucet-Jabeuf, *et al.*, "Immunomodulatory Activity of Very Low Doses of Thymulin in Mice," *International Journal of Immunotherapy*, 1987, 3:191–200. See also V. Daurat, P. Dorfman, and M. Bastide, "Immunomodulatory Activity of Low Doses of Interferon in Mice," *Biomedicine and Pharmacotherapeutics*, 1988, 43:197–206.

HEART DISEASE

1. M. Bignamini, *et.al.*, "Controlled Double-blind Trial with Baryta carbonica 15CH versus Placebo in a Group of Hypertensive Subjects Confined to Bed in Two Old People's Homes," *British Homoeopathic Journal*, July 1987, 76, 3:114–19. **2.** V. Baumans, *et al.*, "Does Chelidonium 3x Lower Serum Cholesterol?" *British Homoeopathic Journal*, January 1987, 76, 1:14–15. **3.** Michael Murray, *Natural Alternatives to Over-the-Counter and Prescription Drugs*. New York: Morrow, 1994, 53–54. **4.** N. I. Foster and N. D. Heindel, "The Discovery of Nitroglycerine: Its Preparation and Therapeutic Utility," *Journal of Chemical Education*, April 1981, 58, 4:364–65.

CANCER

1. J. Cairns, "The Treatment of Diseases and the War Against Cancer," *Scientific American*, 1985, 253:59. See also J. C. Bailar and E. M. Smith, "Progress Against Cancer?" *New England Journal of Medicine*, May 8, 1986, 314:1231. **2.** Tim Beardsley, "A War Not Won," *Scientific American*, January 1994, 130–38. **3.** A. H. Grimmer, "Some Cancer Remedies and Their Indications," *Homoeopathic Recorder*, 4-1937, 52(4). **4.** J. De Gerlach and M. Lans, "Modulation of Experimental Rat Liver Carcinogenesis by Ultra Low Doses of the Carcinogens," in M. Doutremepuich, *Ultra-Low Doses*. Washington, D.C./London: Taylor and Francis, 1991. **5.** J. T. Safrit and B. Bonavida, "Sensitivity of Resistant Human Tumor Cell Lines to TNF and Adriamycin Used in Combination," *Cancer Research*, 1992, 52: 6630–37. **6.** A. R. Khuda-Bukhsh and S. Banik, "Assessment of Cytogenetic Damage in X-irradiated Mice and Its Alteration by Oral Administration of Potentized Homeopathic Drug, Ginseng D200," *Berlin Journal of Research in Homeopathy*, 1991, 1, 4/5:254. Also, A. R. Khuda-Bukhsh and S. Maity, "Alterations of Cytogenetic Effects by Oral Administration of a Homeopathic Drug, Ruta graveolens, in Mice Exposed to Sub-lethal X-radiation, *Berlin Journal of Research in Homeopathy*, 1991, 1, 4/5:264. Researchers from the Department of Zoology at the University of Kalyani, India, tested homeopathic medicines for potential protective effects from radiation-induced damage. Mice treated with sublethal doses of radiation were found to have experienced significantly less damage when given either *Ruta 30x* or *200x* or *Ginseng 6x, 30x, or 200x*, as compared with mice given potentized doses of ethanol (the placebo group). The mice were given one of these remedies in a single potency before and after radiation exposure. **7.** G. W. Bradley and A. Clover, "Apparent Response of Small Cell Lung Cancer to an Extract of Mistletoe and Homoeopathic Treatment," *Thorax*, 1989, 44:1047–48. **8.** S. Gabius, S. Joshi, S. S. Kayser, *et al.*, "The Galactoside-specific Lectin from Mistletoe as Biological Response Modifer," *International Journal of Oncology*, 1992, 1, 6:705. Also L. A. Anderson and J. D. Phillipson, "Mistletoe: The Magical Herb," *Pharmaceutical Journal*, 1982, 229:437. G. Koopman, *et al.*, "In vitro Effects of Viscum Album Preparations on Human Fibroblasts and Tumour Cell Lines," *British Homoeopathic Journal*, 1990, 79:12–18.

PSYCHOLOGICAL CONDITIONS

1. Charles Frederick Menninger, "Some Reflections Relative to the Symptomatology and Materia Medica of Typhoid Fever," *Transactions of the American Institute of Homoeopathy,* 1897, 430. **2.** Edward C. Whitmont, *The Alchemy of Healing.* Berkeley: North Atlantic, 1993, 37–38. **3.** "High Anxiety," *Consumer Reports,* January 1993, 19–24. **4.** Seldon H. Talcott, "The Curability of Mental and Nervous Diseases Under Homoeopathic Medication," *Transactions of the American Institute of Homoeopathy,* 1891, 875–86. **5.** P. Benzecri, "Comparaison entre quatre méthodes de sevrage après une thérapeutique anxiolytique, *Les Cahiers de l'Analyse des Connées,* 1991, 16, 4:389–402. **6.** S. Lipper and D. S. Werman, "Schizophrenia and Intercurrent Physical Illness: A Critical Review of the Literature," *Comprehensive Psychiatry,* January–February 1977, 18:1:11–22. There is a similar observation of reduction in physical illness in people suffering from Alzheimer's disease. See G. P. Wolf-Klein, *et al., Journal of the American Geriatrics Society,* March 1988, 36:2219.

DRUG, ALCOHOL, AND NICOTINE ADDICTION

1. J.P.S. Bakshi, "Homoeopathy: A New Approach to Detoxification," Indian Foundation for Medical Research and Education and the Delhi Police Foundation for Correction, Deaddiction and Rehabilitation, National Congress on Homoeopathy and Drug Abuse, March 16–18, 1990, New Delhi. Also published in *Journal of the OMHI* (International Homeopathic Medicine Organization), 1993, 6(2):24–32.

CONDITIONS OF TRAVEL AND RECREATION

1. C. F. Claussen, *et al.,* "Homöopathische Kombination bei Vertigo and Nausea," *Arzneim.-Forsch/Drug Res.,* 1984, 34:1791–98. **2.** V. R. Subramanyam, *et al.,* "Homoeopathic Treatment of Filariasis," *British Homoeopathic Journal,* July 1990, 79:157–60. This study investigated the treatment of human lymphatic filariasis, which is caused by a type of roundworm and affects approximately 90 million people in endemic areas. This single-blind study of 165 people showed a statistically significant difference in those given an individualized homeopathic medicine, as compared with those given a placebo. Compared to people given a placebo, over twice as many people who were given homeopathic medicines experienced a significant decrease in the frequency, duration, and intensity of their symptoms.

INJURIES

1. Robert Becker, *Cross Currents.* Los Angeles: Tarcher, 1990.

PRE- AND POSTSURGICAL TREATMENT

1. J. P. Alibeau and J. Jobert, "Aconit en Dilution Homéopathique et Agitation Post-Operatoire de l'enfant," *Pediatrie,* 1990, 45 (7–8):465–66. **2.** J. Baillargeon, *et al.,* "The Effects of Arnica Montana on Blood Coagulation: A Randomized Controlled Trial," *Canadian Family Physician,* November 1993, 39:2362–67. **3.** C. Amodeo, *et al.,* "The Role of Arnica in the Prevention of Venous Pathology from Long-term Intravenous Therapy: Evaluation of Platelet Aggregation," Ninth National Conference of the Italian Society for Vascular Pathology, Capanello, June 6–9, 1987. The study included 39 patients, including 21 undergoing intravenous feeding, 9 in infusion protracted beyond seventy-two hours, and 9 in chemotherapeutic treatment.

Watson, Lyall, 304
Webster, Daniel, 33
Weight loss, 160
Westchester County Prison and Jail
    (New York), 319
Whitmont, Dr. Edward C., 303–
    304
Whooping cough, 328
Women's conditions, 189–204
World Health Organization, xiv, 39,
    69, 203

Wound infection, 347
Wrigley, William, 33

X-rays, 57

Yeast infection, 192–194
Yellow fever, 223, 286
Yoga, 88
Young, Eliza Flagg, 189

Zand, Dr. Janet, 314–315

HOMEOPATHIC MEDICINE INDEX

ABOUT THE AUTHOR

Dana Ullman, M.P.H. (master's in public health, University of California at Berkeley), is one of America's leading spokespersons for homeopathic medicine. He has written five books, including *Everybody's Guide to Homeopathic Medicines* (with Stephen Cummings, M.D.), *Homeopathic Medicine for Children and Infants*, *The One-Minute (or So) Healer*, and *Discovering Homeopathy*. He has also had his writing published in the *Western Journal of Medicine*, *Social Policy*, *Utne Reader*, *Futurist*, and *The Reader's Digest Family Guide to Natural Medicine*, and he is regularly quoted in the leading national media.

His company, Homeopathic Educational Services, has published more than thirty homeopathic books, including many leading texts for consumers and professional homeopaths.

Dana Ullman serves on the Advisory Council of the Alternative Medicine Center at Columbia University's College of Physicians and Surgeons and is a consultant to Harvard Medical School's Center to Assess Alternative Therapy for Chronic Illness.

He is a regular speaker at universities, medical schools, pharmacy schools, and hospitals. Among the schools where he has spoken are UCSF School of Medicine, Stanford School of Medicine, Duke Medical School, UC Berkeley, New York University, and the University of Illinois.

Besides serving as an educator, Dana Ullman has developed a line of homeopathic medicines called Medicine From Nature, which are manufactured by Nature's Way, a leader in the natural products industry.

COMPLETE YOUR HOMEOPATHIC MEDICAL LIBRARY
WITH OTHER BOOKS FROM JEREMY P. TARCHER/PUTNAM.

EVERYBODY'S GUIDE TO HOMEOPATHIC MEDICINES: Taking Care of Yourself and Your Family with Safe and Effective Remedies (Revised & Expanded) by Stephen Cummings, M.D., and Dana Ullman, M.P.H.

Written by a physician and the leading homeopathic educator in America, this revised and expanded edition is one of the most popular and authoritative guides to homeopathy available.

$10.95 ($14.95 CAN)   ISBN 0-87477-614-4

THE ONE-MINUTE (OR SO) HEALER
500 Quick and Simple Ways to Heal Yourself Naturally
by Dana Ullman, M.P.H.

This book offers you the most simple, safe, quick, and effective natural remedies for treating and preventing common day-to-day health problems.

$8.95 ($11.75 CAN)   ISBN 0-87477-667-8

HOMEOPATHIC MEDICINES FOR CHILDREN AND INFANTS
by Dana Ullman, M.P.H.

The nation's leading homeopathic educator provides everything parents need to know about treating their children's ailments at home with safe and effective homeopathic medicines.

$11.95 ($15.75 CAN)   ISBN 0-87477-692-9

HOMEOPATHIC MEDICINE AT HOME
Natural Remedies for Everyday Ailments and Minor Injuries
by Maesimund B. Panos, M.D., and Jane Heimlich

A classic! The complete handbook for anyone desiring safe and natural remedies for accidents, emergencies, and minor ailments. Highly recommended by homeopathic doctors around the world as *the* best first book for the lay reader.

$10.95 ($14.95 CAN)   ISBN 0-87477-195-1

To order call 1-800-788-6262 or send your order to:

Jeremy P. Tarcher, Inc.
Mail Order Department
The Putnam Berkley Group, Inc.
P.O. Box 12289
Newark, NJ 07101-5289

Subtotal $	_____
Shipping and handling	_____
Sales tax (CA, NJ, NY)	_____
Canada GST	_____
Total amount due	_____

Payable in U.S. funds (no cash orders accepted). $15.00 minimum for credit card orders.
*Shipping and handling: $2.50 for one book, $0.75 for each additional book, not to exceed $6.25.

Enclosed is my ❑ check ❑ money order
Please charge my ❑ Visa ❑ MasterCard ❑ American Express

Card # _____ Expiration date _____

Signature as on credit card _____

Daytime phone number _____

Name _____

Address _____

City_____ State _____ Zip_____

Please allow six weeks for delivery. Prices subject to change without notice.